RESEARCH:
The Validation of Clinical Practice

Edition 3

RESEARCH:
The Validation of Clinical Practice
Edition 3

OTTO D. PAYTON, Ph.D., P.T., F.A.P.T.A.
Professor of Physical Therapy
School of Allied Health Professions
Medical College of Virginia
Virginia Commonwealth University
Richmond, Virginia

 F. A. Davis Company • Philadelphia

F. A. Davis Company
1915 Arch Street
Philadelphia, PA 19103

Printed in the United States of America

Last digit indicates print number: 10 9 8 7 6 5 4 3 2 1

Acquisitions Editor: Jean-François Vilain
Production Editor: Arofan Gregory
Cover Design By: Donald B. Freggens

As new scientific information becomes available through basic and clinical research, recommended treatments and drug therapies undergo changes. The author(s) and publisher have done everything possible to make this book accurate, up to date, and in accord with accepted standards at the time of publication. The authors, editors, and publisher are not responsible for errors or omissions or for consequences from application of the book, and make no warranty, expressed or implied, in regard to the contents of the book. Any practice described in this book should be applied by the reader in accordance with professional standards of care used in regard to the unique circumstances that may apply in each situation. The reader is advised always to check product information (package inserts) for changes and new information regarding dose and contraindications before administering any drug. Caution is especially urged when using new or infrequently ordered drugs.

Payton, Otto D.
    Research, the validation of clinical experience / Otto D. Payton — Ed. 3.
        p.   cm.
    Includes bibliographical references and index.
    ISBN 0-8036-6799-X
    1. Physical therapy—Research—Evaluation. 2. Occupational therapy—Research—Evaluation. I. Title.
    [DNLM: 1. Occupational Therapy. 2. Physical Therapy.
    3. Research. WB 25 P347r 1993]
    RM708.P38   1993
    615.8'2'072—dc20
    DNLM/DLC
    for Library of Congress   93-26828
                                                                                        CIP

**To My Students:
Past, Present, and Future**

Introduction

The purpose of this book is to provide a basic text that examines and explains the process by which we can test and improve what we do, as health professionals, to and for our clients or patients. The intended audience is entry-level students in the fields of occupational therapy and physical therapy. As future health professionals they should be prepared to defend, with rational and scientific evidence, the appropriateness and effectiveness (i.e., the validity) of their practice and procedures. To more fully understand the scientific basis of practice, the student-clinician must understand the process by which that basis of practice is defined. Understanding the process will also help students to read, or hear, the scientific statements of other professionals; interpret them correctly; incorporate them into their own practice, if appropriate; and question insupportable claims.

What I am talking about, of course, is research, a word much maligned and unreasonably feared by some people who do not understand the process. All the word "research" means is a systematic search for reliable knowledge. Kerlinger[1] has called science a "systematic, controlled extension of common sense." Most of this book will be about reading and interpreting the research of others, which is its primary purpose. However, accurate research reading skills are necessary prerequisites to later performance skills. To some will come the incentive and the opportunity to contribute to that body of knowledge that supports and sustains clinical practice. This text lays the foundations for those contributions.

The following five basic principles form the foundation for this text:

1 Research is important to therapy because it is the major tool available to us for validating our services to people in our role as therapists. Although most of the people we serve are clients (usually called patients in this text), we should also include students and co-workers with whom we interact as therapists as

1

people who expect valid services from us, for example, instruction or supervision.

2   Using research effectively as a tool for understanding is a skill that can be learned. There are two corollaries to this principle: (a) to become skillful in reading or doing research, one needs concepts, principles, and practice, and (b) among these important concepts and principles are some related to measurement and to the scope and limitations of different research designs.

3   Validity and reliability are special characteristics that are important to measurement and research design.

4   A model of therapeutic practice is useful in looking at what we know now and what we need to know in order to substantiate what we do as therapists.

5   Theories and models are better guides to knowledge than trial and error.

Although this third edition incorporates more statistical concepts than were found in the earlier editions, it still emphasizes a nonmathematical approach to understanding the research process. It attempts to give the reader those concepts necessary to read and understand scientific literature, including the *meaning* of statistics and how statistics may be interpreted for practical use. Some of the information in this book will also lay the foundation for selecting statistical tools, but I do not want statistics and mathematics to interfere with the reader's understanding of basic concepts. Most of the students and faculty who have used this textbook over the years have been very supportive of this cognitive, nonmathematical approach to understanding the research process. As Wang and associates[2] have so clearly stated, "Be assured that you can have a good conceptual understanding of statistics without a good mathematical background."

Basic arithmetic will suffice for understanding this text. Basic statistical tools are introduced in the text as they relate to the designs being discussed. The writing of scientific reports will not be dealt with extensively; Appendix A provides an outline for writing a research protocol, and additional writing references are given in Appendix D. The statistical references in Appendix D will provide formulas and calculations for most statistical tests. Appendix F contains a summary of all the statistics presented in the text.

About half of the text has been rewritten. Most of the examples and illustrations have been updated, and more examples from the literature have been incorporated into the text. More statistical concepts and examples have been incorporated into the relevant chapters, and there is a fuller discussion of the use of computers in statistical analysis and literature searches. The material on writing grant proposals and on ethics has been expanded. Two glossaries have been added; one for general concepts and one for statistical terms and formulas.

The concepts and principles presented in the text are illustrated with teaching examples from the literature of occupational therapy, physical therapy, and related fields. The reader is asked to be ecumenical in approaching the examples, as it was not always possible to find ones that would appeal immediately to both physical and occupational therapists. As in the earlier editions, goniometry was chosen because both disciplines use it.

In addition, the reprints in Appendix C are used throughout the text to examine, analyze, and exemplify the concepts being developed. These reprints give students an opportunity to check their understanding of the textual material. Only articles that can be presented in positive and complementary ways are used. In some instances, only part of an article is used to make a point.

The question may be posed by beginning students as to whether students and practitioners in the allied health professions need the kind of knowledge and skills dealt with in this text. The *Standards of Practice for Physical Therapy* adopted by the House of Delegates of the American Physical Therapy Association in 1990 state in Article 16 that the physical therapist is expected to use research findings in practice and promote and encourage or participate in research activity.[3] The *Quality Assurance Manual* is a guide to the daily use of the research process and a method of assessing quality of patient care.[4] Quality assurance activities are the norm expected of all practitioners.

Both occupational and physical therapy include the teaching of basic research skills in the standards for accreditation of entry-level educational programs. Among other reasons, the professions cite the expectations in quality assurance and the expectations of the federal government for the most effective care as expressed through legislation pertaining to diagnostic-related groups (DRGs). The accreditation standards in physical therapy state that the new graduate will "practice in an ethical, legal, safe, caring, and effective manner which is demonstrated by practicing with a knowledge of ... the scientific basis and effectiveness of physical therapy evaluation, prevention, and treatment procedures" and will "apply basic principles of the scientific method to read and interpret professional literature, to participate in clinical research activities, and to critically analyze new concepts and findings provided."[5]

It seems clear, then, that practitioners and physical therapy students need certain fundamental skills in understanding research and interpreting research studies. They are also strongly encouraged, wherever possible and especially in quality assurance programs, to participate in research activities.

A similar story may be told for the discipline of occupational therapy. The *Essentials and Guidelines of an Accredited Educational Program for the Occupational Therapist* state that upon completion of the course of study the student shall be able to recognize the necessity for and value research for both clinical practice and professional development, know the essential components of a research protocol, interpret studies related to occupational therapy, and apply research results to occupational therapy services.[6] The *Standards of Practice for Occupational Therapy* adopted in 1985 state that recent developments in research and theory are to be used in quality assurance programs and that the practicing therapist should facilitate research on the practice of occupational therapy.[7] The American Occupational Therapy Association (AOTA) code of ethics addresses the clinician's responsibility for maintaining the standards of practice of the profession.[8]

In a recent issue of the *American Journal of Occupational Therapy,* Nedra Gillette[9] wrote, "The major challenge facing the profession of occupational therapy today is the critical need for research that validates claims made for the therapist's use of occupations. . . . Credibility . . . is gained only through exemplary practice, and exemplary practice is largely grounded in research that has tested and refined the treatment strategies that emerge in the practice arena." Commenting on the need for research to substantiate the practice of his discipline, Dr. Charles Christiansen[10] wrote, "For progress to occur, the enterprise of research in a practice profession requires educated persons who have the spirit of inquiry necessary to advance knowledge as well as the skills required to plan and conduct useful studies." Christiansen estimated that 14 percent of the articles published in the occupational therapy literature in 1949 were research based, whereas the percentage in 1989 was 60 percent; hence, without a knowledge of research methodology, today's occupational therapist would not be able to understand 60 percent of the professional literature. "These advancements are more accurately explained by the profession's philosophical commitment to research and the structures created within this climate of support."[11] He goes on to discuss the American Occupational Therapy Foundation as one of the structures that supports research in occupational therapy.

In today's competitive environment, survival in the health and human service systems requires excellence in performance. It is proposed here that research is the key and pivotal force for achieving professional excellence because only through scientific inquiry can occupational therapy develop as an academic discipline and an applied science. Research is also the essential ingredient in Association efforts to promote job security, secure reimbursement for services, enhance the profession's public image and influence public policy.[12]

A recent editorial in *Physical Therapy* noted the need for objective data, both positive and negative, which support the outcomes of physical therapy interventions. Declarative statements of effectiveness without scientific support will ultimately do more harm than good.[13] A previous editorial stated: "Entry-level students must develop an appreciation of science and scientific practice, and they must be capable of reading research reports. . . . All practitioners should be scientific, but not all will do research. That is true of all professions, even of those with far more educational resources than we have in physical therapy."[14] Tracy's[15] review of literature in the *Journal of Physical Therapy Education* has suggested that teaching research in an entry-level curriculum can facilitate the learning of critical thinking, which is so important in clinical practice.

Each chapter begins with a list of objectives so that readers can be alert to the main points in studying and working with that chapter. At the end of each chapter, questions are provided so that readers can assess their mastery of subject matter.

In a group setting, such as a classroom or in-service study group, the teacher or leader may wish to assign supplemental reading to give students more practice in identifying key concepts and principles. A useful instructional-learning strategy is to have participants report on current journal articles of interest, emphasizing the question asked, the research design, methods of data treatment, interpretation and results, and the compatibility of the various elements in the research project. This method can also be used by clinicians in their in-service programs to develop skill in critical reading. Independent readers may simply work on their own to develop the same skills as they read.

Rather than use the traditional masculine gender as representing both sexes or the awkward he or she, his or her notations, I have elected to use both masculine and feminine genders indiscriminately in this text. In this way the text may be more reflective of real life and not of a particular bias.

Acknowledgment of intellectual indebtedness is an impossible task. So many people have influenced and informed my thinking that a list will not be attempted. However, special recognition should be made of my students, who, over the years, have listened to the spoken version of this book in class and helped to clarify ideas and methods of presentation. I would also like to acknowledge with gratitude all those therapists, faculty, students, and clinicians who took the time to provide helpful feedback on the first and second editions. Many of their suggestions have strengthened the text, and their help is gratefully acknowledged. The continued support of the staff of F.A. Davis is also appreciated.

References

1. Kerlinger, FN: Foundations of Behavioral Research, ed 2. Holt, Rinehart & Winston, New York, 1973, p 3.
2. Wang, M, Airhihenbuwa, CO, and Okolo, EN: Data analysis and selection of statistical

methods. In Okolo, EN (ed): Health Research Design and Methodology. CRC Press, Ann Arbor, 1990, p 151.

3. American Physical Therapy Association: Standards of Practice for Physical Therapy. Alexandria, VA, 1990.

4. American Physical Therapy Association: Quality Assurance Manual. Alexandria, VA, 1990.

5. Commission of Accreditation. Accreditation Handbook. American Physical Therapy Association. Alexandria, VA, 1990.

6. American Occupational Therapy Association: Essentials and Guidelines of an Accredited Educational Program for the Occupational Therapist. Rockville, MD, 1991.

7. American Occupational Therapy Association: Standards of Practice for Occupational Therapy. Rockville, MD, 1985.

8. American Occupational Therapy Association: Occupational therapy code of ethics. AJOT 42:795, 1988.

9. Gillette, N: The challenge of research in occupational therapy. AJOT 45:660, 1991.

10. Christiansen, C: Research: Looking back and ahead after four decades of progress. AJOT 45:391, 1991.

11. Ibid., p 392.

12. Gilfoyle, EM, and Christiansen, CH: Research: The quest for truth and the key to excellence. AJOT 41:7, 1987.

13. Rothstein, JM: Believe it or not! Phys Ther 72:557, 1992.

14. Rothstein, JM: Living without student research projects. Phys Ther 72:332, 1992.

15. Tracy, JE: Role of research in the entry-level physical therapy curriculum. JPTE 6:28, 1992.

Everything should be made as simple as possible, but not one bit simpler.

ALBERT EINSTEIN

1

Basic Concepts in Research

OBJECTIVES

1 Discuss the role of research in professional development.

2 Discuss four ways of knowing

3 Define and illustrate the following terms: research, fact, data, data set, variable, independent variable, dependent variable, concept, principle, population, sample, parameter, statistic, hypothesis, alternate hypothesis, null hypothesis.

4 Outline the scientific method and state some of its underlying assumptions.

5 Identify the purpose and question in a given research report.

6 State several typical assumptions underlying many clinical research problems, and identify them in the literature.

7 Define primary and secondary sources, and list several common fallacies in citing authorities.

8 Define several research questions based on one goal, and state the null and alternate hypotheses for each question.

7

Role of Research

Research should begin with an intellectual itch that needs scratching. The "itch" is the question, and the "scratching" is the process of finding an answer. You may be driven by purely intellectual curiosity, or you may need an answer in order to solve a clinical or professional problem. Many important questions start with What? How? When? What works? How does it work? Under what circumstances or conditions does it work?

The answer to the question comes in the form of reliable facts, concepts, or principles that may be used either to generate more comprehensive principles or to assist in solving a practical problem. For example, you might need to know why some patients in a given disease category respond well to a treatment procedure while other patients who are apparently comparable do not. You want this information in order to improve the quality of care in your clinic. So the basic role of research is to provide answers to questions. In answering the question, the research may explain observed facts, discover and interpret new facts, try new ideas or techniques, or test theory. Research is used to establish what is and to explore the conditions under which something occurs. It is fun as well as work.

Clinical questions can best be answered by clinicians who have the knowledge and skills to see the important questions, hypothesize reasonable answers, and apply the therapeutic techniques to be tested. Not only must clinicians understand and appreciate the role of research; there must also be a productive interaction between clinical practice and the research process. Lieske[1] observes that,

As the dynamics of health care economics unfold over the next decade, we are assured that a new health care delivery system will emerge. Professional activities and traditions will be altered, with economics as the driving force in this new environment. This will result in competition among physicians, nurses, and other care providers for their respective share of available funds. To compete effectively in this arena, it is imperative that nursing validate the aspects of health care that are predominantly and appropriately the concerns of nurses. Clinical nursing research is an essential element in this validation process.

What Lieske says of nursing obviously applies to the therapies as well.

All professional clinicians should be responsible for making some contribution to the scientific validation of their practice. That means research—the discovery and validation of the concepts and principles on which practice is based. The research mentality (and it is as much a state of mind as a process) should be an everyday working tool of the practitioner. Research is not the esoteric enterprise of people in ivory towers, nor is it the exclusive domain of people in laboratories isolated from everyday life. It is an attitude and a process used by professional people to increase practical knowledge and clinical skills.

Ways of Knowing

How does one "know" something? How does one know that a given fact is so? How does one know that a given procedure tests what it is supposed to test, that it works every time and is dependable? How does one know the causes of certain client reactions to therapeutic interventions? In other words, what are the sources of reliable knowledge? Dickoff and James[2] have defined four major ways in which people arrive at knowledge. These are modified from an original formulation by the philosopher Charles Peirce.[3]

The first way is tenacity, or intuition. This method has been used by humans since the beginning of our existence. Unfortunately, this method may sometimes spill over into clinical practice, and the clinician will say, "I know this is so simply because I know it. Everybody knows it." There is an important place in human knowing for intuition, and it has an important role to play in the scientific method. Intuition is useful in defining the question and providing clues as to where answers may be found, but it is not an appropriate method for validating the answer.

The second way of knowing is the way of authority: "I know that this is so because _____[some authority] said so." In the past, authorities have said that the earth was flat. Some of today's authorities may be making equally erroneous statements. Authority figures who use tenacity, some other authority, or pure reason as the basis for their pronouncements may be just as mistaken as anyone else. On the other hand, authorities in the field are frequently right and can be good sources of information. Where important or highly complex questions are involved, it is best to check out the basis of "authoritative" statements.

The third way of knowing is often called the a priori method, which means the use of reason alone, without experimental evidence. It is the method of the armchair philosopher. Taken to the extreme, it is called rationalism. Reason is an extremely useful tool; it has helped humanity to achieve great things. But reason is only a tool, and how it is used makes a great deal of difference. If one applies the rules of logic to abstract ideas and verbalizations without ever checking them against concrete realities, one can easily fall into error. An excellent example of this, as well as an example of the abuse of authority, is the work of Galen. His dogmatic textbook on medicine became *the* medical textbook of the Middle Ages. Because it was not based on observation, it contained more errors than it should have, even in that age. Unfortunately, it supplanted the writings of Hippocrates, whose work was based on direct observation of the phenomena he discussed.

The fourth way of knowing is that combination of methods and procedures which has come to be known as the "scientific method." This may be called "experience," but it is experience of a special kind. The scientific method combines intuition, authority, and reason. Intuition is a guide to the really important questions and the best place to look for the answer; authority tells us what has already been discovered by valid and reliable means; and reason enables us to abstract concepts and principles from observed data. Reason is essential for interpreting what the facts mean and how they may best be used to solve practical problems. The scientific method adds something else that is equally important: observation. The direct or indirect observation of some aspect of reality and the careful recording of what is observed are important elements in the scientific process that has created our present-day technology. Extreme dependence on observation alone is called empiricism. The scientific method is outlined in more detail later on in this chapter.

Definition of Terms

A number of terms that are commonly used in scientific research need to be discussed and defined.* **Research** is the goal-directed process of looking for a specific answer to a specific question in an organized, objective, and reliable way. The process of inquiry may include experimentation, but it always involves collection, analysis, and interpretation of data for the purpose of generating new knowledge. Research is not just a search for what others have discovered, as in a library search; it is a rigorous search for new knowledge. Research is a tool of science, and the purpose of science is to develop theories that will *explain, predict,* and *control* behavior. Health science research—be it in physical therapy, occupational therapy, or some other discipline—is directed toward the development of an organized body of valid and reliable knowledge about the events of concern to the health scientist. For the clinician, the observable behavior of patients, particularly those behaviors that are influenced through the therapeutic process, are of central importance. The purpose of gathering this scientific body of knowledge is to enable the clinician to determine which conditions produce desirable reactions in clients, to justify treatment selection, to justify reinbursement, and so forth.

Facts are records of events—for example, Mr. Smith's blood pressure at 8 A.M. or the distance George walked in the hallway this morning. **Data** are measurements or records of facts made under specific conditions. If a therapist observes that "depressed patients are quiet," this is not a statement of scientific fact, and thus is not a datum. We cannot tell from the statement whether it is based on direct observation of one person or an opinion gathered from reading. We do not know under what circumstances

---

*See also the glossary of terms in Appendix E.

the observation was made, and there is no indication of the possible exceptions. Are there any depressed patients who are not quiet under certain circumstances? If the same therapist records that when Ms. Smith was observed unobtrusively for 10 minutes while she was in a group of people who were talking to each other, she was quiet throughout the 10-minute period, that is a datum. Broadly, data are all measurements made in the course of a study: age, sex, scores on tests, and so forth.

A **data set** is a group (2 or more) of recorded observations made on a defined sample of subjects. For example, if the same kind of observation is recorded in the same way under the same circumstances for 20 different people who were diagnosed as depressed, we now have a data set—20 recorded observations—upon which to make a generalization. A data set is any set of measurements on the same variables; there can be a data set for the age of the sample, a data set for their scores on an intelligence test, and so forth.

Using our data set of 20 recorded observations, we might now make the generalization that 80 percent of the people who are diagnosed as depressed are quiet, where "quiet" is defined as not taking part in a conversation in a social situation. On the basis of that generalization, we might make a prediction that 80 percent of the next sample of 20 depressed people who are observed will be quiet under similar circumstances. Prediction is the ultimate goal of most scientific inquiry.

A **variable** is an observable and measurable characteristic or event that can assume a range of values on some dimension; for example, weight is a characteristic of many objects and can assume a range of values on a metric scale. Hence, weight is a variable on which we can gather data. A researcher who is interested in the variable "weight of children on their 10th birthday" observes the fact of weight in each of several children on their 10th birthday and records those weights as a data set. If a characteristic or event has only one value, it is called a constant, not a variable. More will be said about the values assigned to variables in the chapter on measurement.

An **independent variable** (IV), also called an *experimental variable*, is the variable being studied; for example, the influence of exercise. The IV is often manipulated by the researcher to see what effect that manipulation will have on the dependent variable. A **dependent variable** (DV), also called the criterion, is the result or measured outcome of the action of the IV; for example, strength. For the beginning student these may be confusing concepts because both the IV and the DV can be measured; so much exercise produces so much change in strength. The differences should become clear as illustrations are provided throughout the text.

A **concept** describes some regularity or relationship within a group of facts and is designated by some sign or symbol, usually verbal. Most nouns symbolize concepts: goniometer, patella, hemiplegia, school, freedom. A concept is an abstract idea generalized from particular instances. One has a concept of a phenomenon when one is familiar enough with its essential features so that new examples of that same phenomenon can be recognized and classified wherever they are seen. The essence of concept formation is the ability to disregard the nonessential differences and pay attention to the essential characteristics of an item in order to classify it. For example, one has a concept of a goniometer if all examples can be properly classified as goniometers and all nonexamples can be classified as not-goniometers. Nonessential aspects such as size, material, angles of 180° or 360°, or universal or specialized status are disregarded and the essential aspects are identified. As the neuron is the basic unit of the nervous system, so the concept is the basic unit of thought.

A **principle** states a relationship between two or more concepts. For example, if one has the concepts "patellar bone," "tendon," and "quadriceps muscle" and a concept of what the word "embedded" means, then one is in a position to understand the principle that the patellar bone is embedded in the tendon of the quadriceps muscle. It would be incorrect to say that the quadriceps muscle is embedded in the tendon of the patellar bone; that is a completely different relationship. This expression of a correct relationship is also called a rule, or a generalization, or sometimes even a law.

The goal of research is to develop concepts and principles that are based on observed facts and to establish these concepts and principles to the point where they are useful for predicting future events. To give a simple example, Newton's first law is a principle that states, in part, that a body at rest will remain at rest unless some force acts to move it. Using this principle we can predict that if you rest a coffee cup carefully on the desk in front of you, it will stay there until something is done to move it. The cup will not unpredictably go wandering across the top of the desk or into your lap. In similar ways we can use concepts and principles to predict the behavior of patients in the clinical setting. This is the ultimate goal of clinical research.

At this point the reader should be able to discern a progression from (1) the collection of data based on controlled observations of the facts in specific situations, to (2) the formation in the mind of concepts and principles, to (3) the prediction of future events based on principles. Research is the process of observing new facts, forming new concepts, establishing new or more comprehensive principles and thus adding to the body of knowledge with which we predict or control our environment or our behavior. All of this process is under the discipline of probability. The clinical scientist makes decisions based on inferences that can never be absolutely certain; they are only probably true. Probability will be discussed at greater length in the next chapter.

When one is tentatively putting concepts into a new, *possible* relationship, that possible relationship is called a **hypothesis**. A hypothesis is a statement of what one might expect to occur if certain concepts and relationships hold true. Hypotheses are often stated in an *if-then format*: for example, *if* high SAT scores are associated with success in college, *then* the students in a given program with high SAT scores will have high GPAs. To test this hypothesis, the researcher would collect data (SAT scores and GPAs of a group of college students), and test the data to see if the hypothesis (the relationship) holds true. If the data support the hypothesis, then a new principle has been established. The if-then hypotheses is restated as a new principle: college students with high SAT scores earn high GPAs.

At this point it might be well to differentiate between goal, purpose, and hypothesis in scientific inquiry. A *goal* is a general, comprehensive statement of intention; a *purpose* is more specific; a *hypothesis* is most specific. For example, one might have as a goal the improvement of the functional abilities of the upper extremities of brain-damaged patients. One of many related purposes might be to test the validity of selected Rood techniques for facilitating control of the upper extremities. One of many hypotheses related to that one purpose might be that if extensor tone is increased through stimulation of the tonic labyrinthine reflex and vibration of extensor musculature, then spastic children with cerebral palsy who fulfill certain criteria should have more functional use of their elbow extensors after vibration of the triceps in the inverted position. (Hypotheses will be further defined later in this chapter.)

Population refers to all the actual data that could potentially be collected on a well-described variable. Examples include the IQ of all 12-year-old children with cerebral palsy in public school systems in the state of Michigan, or the range of motion in all osteoarthritic knee joints, or the GPA of all physical therapy students in the United States, or the score on the Peabody Picture Vocabulary Test of all hemiplegic patients admitted to occupational therapy inpatient services in public general hospitals in Canada. A **sample** consists of all the observations of a variable actually measured. In common practice, "population" and "sample" are often used to refer to the people from whom the data are collected. Usually a sample is a subset of a population, but occasionally sample and population are identical. The process of selecting a sample from a population will be discussed in the next chapter. Examples of a sample include the measured IQ of 50 randomly selected 12-year-old children with cerebral palsy in three public schools in Michigan; the range of motion of all osteoarthritic knee joints seen in one clinic during 1993; the GPA of all physical therapy students in 15 randomly selected schools in the United States; and the scores on the Peabody Test for all hemiplegic patients admitted to the occupational therapy inpatient service in one general hospital in Quebec in 1992.

A **statistic** is a numerical statement about a group of observations. It is a mathematical tool that serves two purposes: it summarizes data, and it makes a mathematic statement of the confidence that can be placed in a particular principle, generalization, or hypothesis—a statement of probability. In other words, statistics are mathematic ways of making large amounts of data more manageable and of stating the chances of a prediction based on the summarized data being right or wrong. This latter purpose often involves estimating some characteristic in a population on the basis of the observed values of that characteristic in a sample. A mathematical statement about observations actually made on a sample is called a *statistic*; an estimation of the value of the same variable in a population is called a **parameter**. Types of statistics and the interpretation of statistical information is dealt with more fully in subsequent chapters.

The Scientific Method

Some writers contend that there is no such thing as the scientific method. Insofar as different scientists put their individual stamp on what they do, and do not follow a rigid set of procedures step by step, this is true. However, it is also true that a generally recognized pattern is inherent in most scientific endeavors, and at certain stages of the process careful discipline and strict controls are essential. The core of the scientific method concerns the problem, the data, and the inference. This section presents a generalized pattern of the chain of reasoning in the scientific approach to problem solving. The differences between scientific problem solving— that is, research as we have defined it—and clinical problem solving with patients is briefly discussed later in this chapter.

ASSUMPTIONS OF THE SCIENTIFIC METHOD

Before we look at the pattern of the scientific process itself, let us look at some of the assumptions underlying the process or method. Most scientists do not give these assumptions a great deal of thought from day to day, and that is why they are called assumptions. Nevertheless, they are the basis of the researchers' daily activities in the same way that a foundation supports a building. The clearest statement of these assumptions that I know of was made by Dressel and Mayhew[4] in a 1954 study sponsored by the American Council on Education:

1 **Principle of Objectivity:** A scientist cultivates the ability to examine facts and suspend judgment with regard to his observations, conclusions, and activities.

2 **Principle of Consistency:** A scientist assumes that the behavior of the universe is not capricious, but is describable in terms of consistent laws,

such that when two sets of conditions are the same, the same consequences may be expected.

3 **Principle of Tentativeness:** A scientist does not regard his generalizations as final, but is willing to modify them if they are contraindicated
by new evidence.

4 **Principle of Causality:** A scientist believes that every phenomenon
results from a discoverable cause.

5 **Principle of Uniformity:** A scientist believes that the forces which are
now operating in the world are those which have always operated, and
that the world and the universe which we see are the result of their
continuous operation.

6 **Principle of Simplicity:** A scientist prefers simple and widely applicable
explanations of phenomena. He attempts to reduce his view of the world
to as simple terms as possible. This principle is related to Occam's Razor
or the Law of Parsimony: the simplest answer which accounts for the
most known facts is the best answer.

7 **Principle of Materiality:** A scientist prefers material and mechanical
explanations of phenomena, rather than those which depend on non-
material forces. [Many social scientists would probably want to modify
this assumption, which was not necessarily written with their interests
in mind.]

8 **Principle of Dynamism:** A scientist expects nature to be dynamic rather
than static, and to show variation and change.

9 **Principle of Relativeness:** A scientist thinks of the world, and of things
in it, as sets of relationships rather than as absolutes.

10 **Principle of Intergradation:** A scientist thinks in terms of continua; he
distrusts sharp boundary lines, and expects to find related classes of
natural phenomena grading imperceptibly into one another.

11 **Principle of Practicality:** A scientist expects that in any situation involving competition among units of varying potentialities, those which work
best under existing circumstances will tend to survive and perpetuate
themselves.

12 **Principle of Continuous Discovery:** A scientist hopes that it will be
possible to go on learning more and more about the material world and
the material universe of which it is a part, until eventually all may be
understood.

13 **Principle of Complementarity:** A scientist attempts to incorporate all
phenomena into a single, consistent, natural scheme, but he recognizes
that contradictory generalizations may be necessary to describe different
aspects of certain things as they appear to us.

14 **Principle of Social Limitation:** The social framework within which a
scientist operates may determine and limit the kinds of problems on

which he works, and the data which he collects, and may also influence his conclusions.

THE RESEARCH PROCESS

The reader should begin to become familiar with the outline of a research protocol to be found in Appendix A. We will refer to this schema frequently throughout the text, and the student will use it in analyzing reports of research and in written exercises. The outline in Appendix A lists all of the topics that one should consider in planning a research project; it is a guide for thinking and planning. Many of the topics in Appendix A form headings and subheadings for a thesis proposal.

What follows is a more general outline of a research proposal. At a later date the reader may return to this section and find that it may serve as a *general* guide to writing a grant proposal. Of course, each granting agency has its own forms, which require that the material be presented in slightly different formats, but the general content is the same for most proposals. For another discussion of grant writing, see Chapter 1 in Okolo.[5]

Step 1: Formulate the Question

The first step in the scientific process is to identify the issues that are vital to your overall goal. What are the critical questions that need to be answered to solve the problem or relieve the concerns that are important to you? There are thousands of unanswered questions in your discipline. Many of them are not worth the time, effort, and money it would take to answer them; they are trivial. Other questions are unanswerable, at least in the immediate future, because they are too complex, because the technology for measuring the important variables is not available, or because the researcher does not have the technical expertise to perform some aspect of the study. Sometimes a study cannot be executed at a particular time or place for very practical reasons such as the absence of a suitable sample of sufficient size. The effective researcher has the basic skills of critical thinking, including the ability to identify the central issues in a topic and the underlying assumptions. Researchable questions address relevant questions that are answerable, all things considered.

Where do good questions come from, other than that intellectual itch mentioned at the beginning of this chapter? They come from experience: your own or someone else's. They come from thoughtful reflection on your daily clinical experience: What produced that reaction in Mr. Jones? How many patients like him would respond the same way? What's different about Mr. Smythers that caused him to respond differently? Is there a demonstrable relationship between your treatment goals and objectives and your treatment plan? What would happen if I changed this or that?

Good questions also come from the experience of others as reported in our professional literature. In particular, theoretical statements of how some aspect of practice works can be a source of important questions; questions generated by theory often make the more significant contributions to our knowledge. Does your question make sense in terms of what is known, or does it challenge what is reported in the literature? Both are potentially fruitful avenues of research. Other sources of important questions are official statements of research priorities such as the one promulgated by the American Physical Therapy Association.[6]

To be researchable, your question needs to meet several practical criteria; the question needs to be important, relevant, measurable, and ethical. Practical research methods, as well as material and financial resources, time, and subjects, need to be available.

Intuition plays a vital role in defining the question, especially if it is intuition based on experience. Insight comes to the prepared mind. Many scientists had seen mold on their petri dishes, but it took Sir Alexander Fleming's intuition to ask the critical questions that led to the discovery of penicillin.

Once a question has been formulated it often needs to be subdivided into a number of smaller, more manageable questions. Do the methods of stimulation and inhibition proposed by Margaret Rood really work? This is an interesting question, but it is too broad, too vague. Does 2 minutes of rapid brushing followed by 30 seconds of slow icing on the triceps of a spastic child with cerebral palsy placed in the inverted position facilitate motion in elbow extension as measured by active range of motion? This is the kind of question that you can begin to answer, and even that question must be narrowed down and provided with a definition of terms before it becomes a workable research question. The final question should be precise and grammatically correct and should state exactly what you expect to learn as a result of the study. Frequently, but not always, the research question will need to be stated as a hypothesis. Stating the hypothesis is discussed in detail shortly.

Frequently a researcher will want to ask one or more subquestions. These subquestions may seek information that is an essential prerequisite to the main question. For example, your main question may be, Is there a correlation between age and the number of professional journals reviewed by practicing therapists? Before you can answer that question, you may need to ask a subquestion: How old is each therapist in my sample? On the other hand, subquestions may extend your main question in some way. For example, the main question may be extended by asking, How many of the journals reviewed are subscribed to by the therapists, and how many do they review in the library?

In writing research questions for grant proposals, one should read very carefully the stated purposes of the grant source or agency. If the agency is interested only in children, can your question be answered with subjects that are children? If the granting source is interested in vocational rehabilitation, can you phrase your question so that it addresses both your interests and those of the funding source? Are there key words in the stated purpose of the funding source that can be incorporated into your question? Do not mimic the wording of the grant guide, but use some of their key words and phrases in your discussion of the question. It may be helpful if key concepts of interest to the funding agency are reflected in the title of your proposal. Also be sure that the key interests of the funding source are prominent in the abstract and summary of the proposal.

Step 2: Review the Literature

The second step is to find out whether or not someone else has already answered your question convincingly; there is no point in reinventing the wheel. (You can, however, test to see if someone else's wheel is really round or if it will support a wheelbarrow.) Replication of a study is theoretically important but sometimes hard to get published; replication of another work with some extension is more commonly the way knowledge is built up. There may also be a lot of information in the literature that is related to your topic and will help you formulate your question better and understand its implications, even though a direct answer to your specific question is not provided.

This step usually involves a systematic review of the literature. In developing fields of study, however, do not discount the knowledge of experts from nonwritten sources. These individuals may have very useful ideas, insights, and experiences that could facilitate your own search for understanding. Is what is known in your area of interest stated in any kind of a theoretical format? If so, theory may help you clarify your question and state it in a more useful form. Before you accept the conclusion of other researchers, however, be sure to check the basis on which they make their statements or conclusions. Is it their considered opinion, or is it a statement based on the interpretation of data gathered in a scientific way? Are the author's statements based on generalized experiences, or are they based on carefully controlled observation? The careful researcher should be able to distinguish these various types of conclusions in the literature. The ability to make such distinctions is one of the major goals of this text.

The review of literature may also help you with methodological issues. Have others tried to answer your question and arrived at no specific conclusion? Perhaps their work will help you find better methods for collecting data relevant to your question. This systematic review of what is known about your topic generally takes place in the library. Doing library research is discussed in more detail in Chapter 10.

Many granting agencies limit the number of allowable citations to the literature. Hence, it is important to select those references that (1) provide most support for your statement, (2) demonstrate the effectiveness of the methodology you have chosen for answering similar questions, and (3) demonstrate your track record in research (if this can be done within the frame of the question addressed; otherwise leave your publications in your curriculum vitae).

Step 3: Develop and Execute a Plan

The third step in the scientific method is to develop a plan (including a research design) for gathering reliable data from a set of controlled observations that answer the research question. This plan includes some form of measurement. The observations usually involve measuring some phenomena and recording the observations as numerical data. Much more is said about the construction of the plan in subsequent chapters. At this point it is important to realize that researchers do not simply go out and gather facts; they make and record observations according to a precise plan and in controlled ways that usually involve measurement. The plan defines in advance important questions. For example, what will the data look like: answers to a questionnaire, shoulder ranges of motion, scores on a pain scale? How are the data related to the question? How will the data be analyzed? Because physical and occupational therapy are practical disciplines rather than basic sciences, the data collection methods may be diverse, using methods developed in the biological and social sciences, medicine, and nursing. The research plan also needs to specify the population and sample of the study and how the sample will be defined and chosen. This is discussed more fully in Chapter 2. How will the sample be recruited? How will the rights of subjects be safeguarded? What controls will be imposed on the sample and the research design? Will part or all of the plan be pretested before the definitive study is started?

In a grant proposal the research plan may be developed through several subsections of the narrative. An introduction gives the grant reader an overview of the topic area—for example, stroke rehabilitation—and a specific statement of the problem to be addressed if the grant is funded— for example, do integrated PT and OT interventions improve functional outcomes in hemiplegic patients? Specific objectives of the proposal are stated in terms of measurable outcomes. The grant writer needs to convince the grant reviewer that these objectives are important, that they solve, or contribute to the solution of, the central problem, and that they are related to the stated interests of the grant agency.

A methodology section details a step-by-step sequence of activities that the researcher will perform in the process of executing the proposal. Specific methods must be stated for meeting each objective and for solving the problem. The writer may be expected to suggest what the outcomes will look like: for example, higher scores on the Barthel index. The narrative also states how the researcher plans to disseminate the results of the study: for example, by publication in a referred journal or presentation at an appropriate professional conference.

Personnel, equipment, and other needed resources are usually specified in the budget section of grant applications. Each item in the budget requires a statement justifying its need and relating the personnel and equipment to the objectives and problem in the narrative part of the proposal. If money is not requested for space, the application needs to indicate that space is available. It is often helpful (or even required by some grant sources) to indicate that some space, resources, and equipment will be provided by the researcher. Grants are almost always given for a specific time. The proposal needs to demonstrate that the objectives of the proposal can be met within the specified time frame.

Step 4: Interpret Your Data

After the research plan has been carried out, the data must be examined with an unbiased and critical eye. What do the data mean? Critical thinking skills needed at this point include the ability to evaluate the evidence so as to distinguish essential, relevant, verifiable data from biased, incidental, irrelevant, and unverifiable data. Data must be interpreted in light of the question you set out to answer. Is the answer one you had expected or is it different? What are all of the possible ways in which your research question could be answered on the basis of the data you have gathered? Of the possible conclusions, which one is most likely to be correct when all aspects of your experiment have been considered? What are your chances of being right if you answer your question in a certain way on the basis of your data? One uses every tool available in working with the data to arrive at their most probable meaning. Conclusions should relate factual data to generalizations made and demonstrate the adequacy and consistency of the data for warranting your conclusions. Again, the intuition of the prepared mind is important. The light shed by the work of other people and the rules of logic are important tools. All of the ways of knowing contribute to the final interpretation and conclusion.

Step 5: Share Your Results

An important step in the validation of clinical practice is to share what you have learned with your colleagues. There are many ways of sharing: in-service educational programs in your department; state, regional, and national meetings of your professional association, including poster and platform presentations; newsletters and bulletins of the special-interest groups within your profession; and professional journals. Crucial to all of these forms is the correct use of language. There are many good reference books on clear communication; some of them are included in the additional reading list at the end of this chapter and in Appendix D. The ability to express your results understandably is attained through thoughtful practice—the same process that will refine your clinical skills.

Step 6: Institute Change

What difference has your research made and for whom? On the basis of what you have learned, what changes are you justified in making in your clinical practice? Do not expect the answer to these questions to be momentous. Few of us are Nobel Prize winners whose discoveries reshape the ways people live. On the other hand, if your question was important and relevant to some aspect of practice, then the answer should have some effect on that practice. Sometimes we act with more confidence because our research has confirmed what we previously only hypothesized was happening. Sometimes our research alters slightly the types of patients who receive specific treatments or changes timing, dosage, or frequency of treatment. The possibilities are endless. The point is that answers to important questions change something.

Ottenbacher[7] has stated that, in occupational therapy "research that establishes a scientific basis for therapy must be produced, and this research must be integrated with clinical practice." He noted that we still do not know a great deal about how to do this, and work needs to be done on how best to produce a smooth, consistent integration of research findings into clinical decision making.

CLINICAL PROBLEM SOLVING

Clinicians need skills in both the clinical problem-solving process and the research process. These processes are related but are not identical. The purpose of the former is to identify and deal with an individual patient's concerns, deficiencies, or problems. A good guide to this process may be found in Rothstein and Echternach.[8] The purpose of the research procedure is to add to the knowledge base of one's discipline. Both methods form questions and hypotheses; both make controlled observations and collect data; both interpret the data in terms of the hypothesis, reach conclusions, and take action.

The most important difference between the two activities is a procedural one. The researcher is expected to suspend all judgment on the meaning of the data until all the data are in. Only then can interpretation occur. This objectivity is considered important to avoid the introduction of bias into data collection and to maintain consistency of methodology. Barrows and Tamblyn[9] and Elstein and associates[10] have demonstrated that physicians had to "unlearn" this system of suspended judgment to become skillful clinical problem solvers. Physicians who were recognized by their peers as skilled clinicians formed tentative hypotheses about the patient's problems very early during patient evaluation, modified those hypotheses as they gathered data, and generated tentative treatment plans as they went along. Payton[11] has demonstrated that physical therapists solve clinical problems in exactly the same way. There is no suspended judgment; the clinician interacts with the data throughout the process. Mitcham[12] has presented a table comparing the research process with the occupational therapy process.

Because of this ongoing interaction between data collection and hypothesis refinement, the clinician has less control over some of the variables than does the researcher. In the chapter on single-case designs, one design is briefly reviewed that allows the researcher to have the same flexibility, but most research designs are applied quite rigidly once the experiment or study is under way.

Practice

Turn now to Appendix C and read the article by Giannini. Read it fairly quickly once to become generally familiar with its content and organization. Read it a second time and identify the major sections of the text: the justification (i.e., purpose), review of the literature, methods of data collection, interpretation of data, and clinical implications. Does it fulfill step 5? Is it clearly written?

We will return to the second, third, and fourth steps in later chapters. Go back now and concentrate on the research question(s) in Giannini. See if you can define the question that these researchers were asking. (*Hint*: It is often expressed as the "purpose of the study.") Is the question clear to you from the way that it is reported in the article? If there are any unusual terms in the statement of the question, are they defined in the text so that you know precisely what the investigators mean by them? What is the overall goal of the specific question being asked? What do you think the clinical significance of the question might be? Do you think that an answer to the question would contribute to the basic knowledge of the profession and thus to the welfare of patients? Remember that most contributions will be quite modest. Highly significant breakthroughs in knowledge may occur only several times in a century, but these breakthroughs usually come because many people have answered many small questions along the way that lead up to the big insight. Do not expect the authors of the article to answer more than the question they specified, but the reader should try to see how this bit of knowledge fits into the big picture. Write a long-term goal for the Giannini article. What do you think their contribution to the big picture is?

You will find that the article by Giannini, like most, will not clearly answer all the questions raised by this text. There are several reasons for this, some of which are practical. One important practical reason is the space limitation imposed on authors by editors. This limitation has become increasingly stringent in recent years with the rapidly rising costs of printing. The next time you are in the library stacks, find a journal that has been in print for 60 years or so and compare it with a current one in terms of length and conciseness of expression; the limitations imposed on the more recent article will be obvious. On the other hand, this need to be concise has often made it easier to find the essential information that the author has to convey. Editors and reviewers provide an important level of quality control. If you want to see a research report with *all* the details stated explicitly, look at a master's thesis or a doctoral dissertation.

Another reason for the missing information is that most authors (and editors) assume that anyone interested enough in the topic to read the article will be familiar with standard terminology in the area of study. They also assume that their readers are sufficiently sophisticated in research methodology to understand some procedures implicitly. Both of these assumptions are often in error, making research especially difficult for the neophyte. For this reason you should have on hand a good collegiate dictionary, a good medical dictionary, and a good book on research methodology when you are studying the literature.

Since it is designed for students, this textbook will raise as many questions as possible. They will not all be applicable to every article. Over the years I have found this point to be worrisome to many students. If you are trying to find all the items in Appendix A in an article, and some are not there, there are at least two possibilities. First, for reasons already stated, the point may be implicit rather than explicit. Second, it may not be appropriate or necessary for that particular study. Examples of this point will be given as we study various research designs. The purpose of raising so many issues in this text is to alert you to possible areas of concern and points of interest as you learn to read professional literature. You will sometimes need to "read between the lines" to find answers. This is not necessarily a criticism of the article; it can be, rather, an instructive experience in logical thinking for you. On the other hand, some writers omit information for less noble reasons. Let us pass over them with the comment that, in literature as in commerce, let the consumer beware.

Assumptions

Every act that we perform rests on assumptions, which are accepted at face value without questioning. These assumptions underlie our behavior, yet we seldom give them a second thought. To give an example, I drive rapidly down the highway on the assumption that the car is going to continue to function in a safe manner. Many thousands of people have died when that assumption proved false; yet we do not give the car a thorough safety check each time before we drive. In the nature of things we cannot be expected to check out every assumption on which we act.

As noted earlier in this chapter, the scientific method also makes some very important assumptions that are seldom checked out. They are "given" background for any scientific endeavor. In addition, some assumptions are particular to each project. The careful researcher takes pains to identify the most important assumptions on which each individual study is based. For example, if we were doing a study of the attitudes of hospitalized patients toward the therapy services in a hospital, one of the things that we would have to assume is that patients answered honestly the questions that were put to them about the services. To be sure, the investigator should attempt to increase the probability that patients will answer honestly. He might distribute an anonymous questionnaire—unsigned and unmarked—to be returned through the hospital mail system, the reasoning being that anonymity will increase the honesty of the responses. However, since we cannot get inside the patients' heads to examine their true feelings, after all precautions have been taken, we must assume that patients have responded honestly.

It is important for the researcher to identify such assumptions; they contribute to the accuracy of the conclusions. It should be remembered, too, that whenever we deal with human subjects, we encounter a multitude of variables that simply cannot be controlled. Assumptions can then be made about the regularity or distribution of those uncontrollable variables. This point is dealt with more extensively in Chapter 2, in the section on sampling.

When we use electronic instruments, we assume that after calibration they are functioning correctly and will record accurately. If we make two measurements on a patient using the same machine, we assume the two measurements are comparable and that any changes recorded are because of changes in the characteristic we are measuring, not in the measuring device.

Carefully identifying our assumptions often gives us clues to controls that we can apply to make our study more valid. For example, by identifying the assumption that an electronic instrument is functioning correctly, we are reminded to check the reliability of the instrument's calibration. Thus, the more assumptions we can identify in a given study, the more information we have to evaluate the results of the study.

In formal research reports, such as theses and dissertations, the assumptions underlying the study are usually stated quite clearly. However, in journal articles, where there is a premium on space, the assumptions are usually unstated. In evaluating a report and making decisions about what actions you are going to take on the basis of the information contained therein, it is important to identify the unstated assumptions and decide whether or not the assumptions are valid.

Return now to the article by Giannini. Are any assumptions identified in the text? Can you identify some of the unstated assumptions on which the work was based? On the basis of what you know now, how would you evaluate these stated and unstated assumptions?

Authoritative Sources

As stated earlier, it is important to review the available information that is relevant to your problem. How is one, however, to distinguish reliable from unreliable sources of information? An important distinction to be made here is that of primary versus secondary sources. If I say that I saw George hit Bill, I am a primary source of information about the incident. However, if I say that Betty told me that she saw George hit Bill, I am a secondary source of information; Betty would be the primary source. In terms of scientific literature, primary sources are those reports written by people who made the original observations on which the conclusions were based. By and large, primary sources in the scientific community are the reports of original investigative studies. Secondary sources encompass the review of literature in a research article. The investigator reviews, in her report, what others have said that is relevant to her question. Another type of secondary source is a textbook, which organizes and summarizes primary sources and interprets them according to the understanding of the textbook author.

Ideally, an investigator should never accept a secondary source if primary sources are available. Secondary sources contain all of the errors, misinterpretations, or biases of the author of the primary source, as well as any misinterpretations or biases by the author of the secondary source. In addition, a secondary source may leave out essential information, which will cause the reader to misinterpret what the original data and conclusions were. Secondary sources rarely give the original data from which conclusions were drawn, so the reader is not able to judge the adequacy of the data for the conclusion or to evaluate the relevance of the data to the question.

Look again at the article by Giannini. Can you tell from reading the review of literature whether the authorities they quoted and the sources they used were primary or secondary? If you wanted to use this article as a foundation for your own study, what parts of this article would be primary information for you and what parts would be secondary? If you wanted to make important decisions based on information supplied by this article as a secondary source, what could you do to strengthen the probability that you were making a good decision? If you use this article as a primary source for making a decision, what kinds of questions should you ask yourself about the information contained in this article before you decide to use it as the basis for a decision?

Hypotheses

More specific characteristics of hypotheses are discussed and illustrated in subsequent chapters. At this time, let us identify only some of the more general features. Blakiston's[13] dictionary defines hypothesis as a "supposition or conjecture put forth to account for known facts." That definition would include clinical hypotheses, discussed earlier, as well as research hypotheses. *Taber's Cyclopedic Medical Dictionary*[14] states that a hypothesis is "1. An assumption not proved by experiment or observation. It is assumed for the sake of testing its soundness or to facilitate investigation of a class of phenomena. 2. A conclusion drawn before all the facts are established and tentatively accepted as a basis for further investigation." In a general sense the research hypothesis is the research question to be answered. However, many purists would insist that the word "hypothesis" applies only to experimental research. The approach in this text is that the research hypothesis is the question to be answered by the research project, regardless of what type of research is being undertaken. (See Chapter 2 for definitions of research types.)

In experimental research the hypothesis takes on two specialized forms that refine the question. One form is called the alternate, or research, hypothesis; the other is called the null hypothesis.

The **alternate hypothesis** in an experimental study can be expressed in the if-then form: If I do this to the patient, then the patient will respond in this way. In practice it usually takes the form of a declarative statement: Active exercise increases measured range of motion in the knee joint more than passive exercise does; clients with a high internal locus of control as measured by the Rotter I-E scale will prefer self-directed individual activities in OT rather than projects done in a group or class. Thus, the alternate hypothesis is an intelligent guess as to the nature of the answer to your basic question; it predicts the outcome of your study.

The **null hypothesis** is crucial to only one specific step in the research procedure, the statistical analysis in a predictive study. The null hypothesis is called "null" because it makes a statement that there is no difference; it predicts that there will be no difference between two or more sets of data—for example, between the experimental and control groups or between two or more treatments. The null hypothesis is important for only one reason: it is the only form of the question to which a statistical test can be applied. It can be understood as the question, *Is there a difference?* If the answer is no, then the null hypothesis is supported and the alternate is rejected. If the answer is yes, then the null hypothesis is rejected and the alternate hypothesis is supported.

The following example illustrates the difference between the two types of hypothesis and other terms that have been introduced in this chapter. Refer to Appendix A to see where these term fit into the research protocol.

1 **Long-range goal:** To improve the functional abilities of hemiplegic patients.

2 **Immediate purpose:** To find a better way to relieve tension in spastic muscles in hemiplegic patients so that the antagonists can be more effectively exercised.

3 **Specific question to be answered by this study:** Will brief ice applications relieve spasticity to the point of increasing the function in the antagonists?

4 **Alternate hypothesis (H_A):** *If* an ice pack ($20°F$) is placed to cover 90 percent of the body of spastic biceps brachii muscle in hemiplegic patients for 5 minutes, *then* active elbow extension with subject in a supine position with the humerus flexed to $90°$ will increase more than in a control group.

5 **Null hypothesis (H_0):** There will be *no statistically significant difference* in active elbow extension between hemiplegic subjects that have had 5 minutes of ice pack applied to the biceps brachii and those who have not received ice treatment. (Position, application, and temperature are assumed to be the same as in the research hypothesis.)

Now look at the article by Giannini. Can you identify null or alternate hypotheses? If these forms are missing, can you supply them?

Let us look at one more set of hypothetical examples. Let us suppose that two clinicians, one a staff physical therapist and the other a staff occupational therapist in a free-standing outpatient clinic administratively associated with St. Hopeless Hospital, are interested in improving joint mobility in clients with physical disabilities.* They decide to conduct a series of experiments to evaluate (1) the accuracy of various tools for measuring joint mobility and (2) several therapeutic procedures for increasing joint mobility. Out of these purposes they develop a series of research questions.

---

*For purposes of illustration in this text, a topic was chosen to which both disciplines can contribute, and a rather traditional service setting was chosen for convenience and simplicity. Readers are encouraged to develop their own list of interesting questions to illustrate the elements of research as they proceed through the text.

1   What measurement tools and therapeutic methods are currently being used by therapists in hospitals and clinics across the country?

2   What is the reliability of standard manual goniometry as used by the therapists in their clinic?

3   Are measurements with the manual goniometer comparable to those obtained with an electrogoniometer (elgon)?

4   Do the medical records of their clinic demonstrate the expected level of use of quantitative goniometry?

5   What is the most accurate measurement tool available for practical daily use?

6   Do goniometric measures of joint mobility predict the client's level of functional ability?

7   Does heat applied prior to active exercise increase joint mobility more than active exercise alone?

8   Which is better for maintaining joint mobility in patients with rheumatoid arthritis: heat and active exercise twice daily, heat and passive exercises twice daily, or a functional activity program twice daily?

9   Does goniometric biofeedback training increase functional ability?

Can you convert questions 2, 6, 7, 8, and 9 into if-then statements? Here are 3, 4, and 5 for examples.

3   If the manual goniometer and the elgon are comparable, then they will produce the same measurements when applied to the same joints. (And if they produce the same measurements, then there will be no statistically significant differences between them.)

4   If the medical records of the clinic demonstrate the minimal expected level of usage for client evaluation, then the therapists' records will contain quantitative goniometric measurements at the intake and terminal client visits (a retrospective study).

5   If one instrument is more accurate than all others tested, then that accuracy will be demonstrated when tested against a known range.

For question 1 there is no null hypothesis. The null hypotheses for 2, 3, and 4 follow.

2   There will be no statistically significant difference between two therapists at St. Hopeless outpatient clinic in the independent measures of several joint ranges of motion using manual goni-

ometers according to the techniques described by Hurt.[15] (In other words, their measures will be about the same.)

3 There will be no statistically significant difference between measurements taken with a standard manual goniometer and with an elgon.

4 There will be no statistically significant difference between the expected and the actual use of quantitative goniometry by occupational and physical therapists at the clinic as demonstrated in the clinic's medical records.

Now try writing null hypotheses for questions 5, 6, 7, 8, and 9. When we reconsider each of these questions in more detail in later chapters, we may polish and refine them considerably. That is how researchers normally work—identifying auxiliary problems, defining terms, and redefining hypotheses until they have a clear, answerable question.

Review Questions

1 An intern says to you that he is surprised that people in your department are involved in research. He asks you the purpose of research in your discipline and who should do it. How would you answer?

2 Define and illustrate four ways of knowing. How does each contribute to the search for knowledge?

3 Define the following terms: research, fact, data, data set, variable, concept, principle, population, sample, parameter, statistic, hypothesis, alternate hypothesis, null hypothesis.

4 Differentiate between goal, purpose, and hypothesis.

5 Outline the scientific method. Using the article by McClain in Appendix C, illustrate the general method of scientific inquiry.

6 What is the purpose of McClain's study? What are the research questions?

7 What assumptions are explicit in McClain's study? What assumptions are implicit?

8 Differentiate between primary and secondary sources. What are the major *potential* sources of error in primary sources? What are the major *potential* sources of error in secondary sources?

9 Look at the article by Light in Appendix C. Identify the alternate hypotheses. What are the null hypotheses in this study? Are they stated?

Additional Readings

Barrass, R: Scientists Must Write. Chapman & Hall, London, 1978.

Brink, PT, and Wood, MJ: Basic Steps in Planning Nursing Research: From Question to Proposal, ed 2. Wadsworth, Monterey, CA, 1983.

Day, RA: How to Write and Publish a Scientific Paper. ISI Press, Philadelphia, 1983.

Dempsey, PA, and Dempsey, AD: The Research Process in Nursing, Parts 1 and 2. Jones & Bartlett, Boston, 1986.

Drew, CJ, and Hardman, ML: Designing and Conducting Behavioral Research, Chapters 1 to 4. Pergamon, New York, 1985.

Huth, EJ: How to Write and Publish Papers in the Medical Sciences. ISI Press, Philadelphia, 1982.

Leedy, PD: Practical Research: Planning and Design, ed 2, Chapters 1 to 7, 12, 13. Macmillan, New York, 1980.

Lieske, AM: Clinical Nursing Research. Aspen, Rockville, MD, 1986.

Lynch, BS, and Chapman, CF: Writing for Communication in Science and Medicine. Van Nostrand Reinhold, New York, 1980.

Zinsser, W: On Writing Well, ed 2. Harper & Row, New York, 1980.

References

1. Lieske, AM: Clinical Nursing Research. Aspen, Rockville, MD, 1986, p 13.
2. Dickoff, JW, and James, PA: Think Island. Paper presented at Physical Therapy Graduate Education Conference, Airlie, VA, 1972.
3. See also Kerlinger, FN: Foundations of Behavioral Research, ed 2. Holt, Rinehart & Winston, New York, 1973.
4. Dressel, PL, and Mayhew, LB: General Education: Explorations in Evaluation. American Council on Education, Washington, DC, 1954, pp 112–113.
5. Okolo, EN (ed): Health Research Design and Methodology. CRC Press, Boca Raton, 1990.
6. American Physical Therapy Association: Plan to Foster Clinical Research in Physical Therapy. Alexandria, VA, 1984.
7. Ottenbacher, KJ, Barris, R, and Van Deusen, J: Some issues related to research utilization in occupational therapy. AJOT 40:111, 1986.
8. Rothstein, JM, and Echternach, JL: Hypothesis-oriented algorithm for clinicians: A method for evaluation and treatment planning. Phys Ther 66:1388, 1986.
9. Barrows, HS, and Tamblyn, RM: Problem-Based Learning: An Approach to Medical Education. Springer, New York, 1980.
10. Elstein, AS, et al: Medical Problem Solving: An Analysis of Clinical Reasoning. Harvard University Press, Cambridge, MA, 1978.
11. Payton, OD: Clinical reasoning process in physical therapy. Phys Ther 65:924, 1985.
12. Mitcham, MD: Integrating research competencies into basic professional education. AJOT 40:787, 1986.
13. Blakiston's New Gould Medical Dictionary, ed 2. McGraw-Hill, New York, 1956.
14. Thomas, CL (ed): Taber's Cyclopedic Medical Dictionary, ed 17. FA Davis, Philadelphia, 1993.
15. Hurt, SP: Joint measurement. AJOT 1:209, 1:281, 2:13, 1948.

*The greatest happiness
of the thinking man is
to have fathomed what
can be fathomed, and
quietly to reverence
what is unfathomable.*

GOETHE

2

Introduction to Research Design

OBJECTIVES

1 Define research design, operational definition, and treatment groups.
2 Define and discuss the general concepts of control and sampling.
3 List the essential characteristics of descriptive research, correlational research, and predictive research.
4 Distinguish between basic and applied research.
5 Discuss the ethics of research on human subjects.

Research Design

You will recall that in Chapter 1 research was defined as a process for finding specific answers to specific questions in an organized, objective, and reliable way. **Research design** refers to those concepts and techniques that make research organized, objective, and reliable. Several specific designs are discussed in Chapters 5 to 9. For now, research design may be perceived as the mechanics by which the project is organized. In this context "organized" means that the relationships between the various components of the project are stated clearly; "objective" and "reliable" mean stating what you did so clearly and in such concrete terms that you or other people could repeat the same study and get the same results. Therefore, the two key elements in research design are defining terms and defining relationships. These definitions must be in operational terms. An **operational definition** refers to phenomena that are concrete, observable, and measurable at some level. (This is dealt with more extensively in Chapter 3 on measurement.) Some variables may be operationally defined only by naming them; that is the lowest level of measurement, but it is measurement.

Let us look at an example of an operational definition. The dictionary defines intelligence as the capacity to apprehend facts and propositions and their relationships. This is fine as far as it goes, but how do you know it when you see it, and how do you measure it? It does not refer to concrete phenomena and therefore is not operationally defined. A much more concrete, specific, technical, and operational definition might be the following: "For this study, intelligence is defined as the total score on the Stanford-Binet Test of Intelligence when administered in the standard, prescribed way." That definition points to a measurable score that can be recognized and compared. It would permit replication of the study. One can see how it would be possible to generate 10 or 15 different operational definitions of intelligence. Accordingly, when reading research materials it is often important to see what definition the author has used so that you will know whether or not it is relevant to your area of interest. For example, if I were looking for articles on motor intelligence and I found a study that used the aforementioned definition, I probably would not pursue the article further. An important principle is contained here: "One achieves more by being able to discuss limited phenomena with precision than by indulging in exchanges of vague generalities."[1]

Glance again at the article by Giannini in Appendix C. Notice all the terms used in paragraph 3. Each of these terms requires a precise definition to be useful in the research, but Giannini and Protas do not define these terms. They assume that any reader interested in their research already knows the accepted definitions of these terms.

Control

One of the most important concepts in research design is control. **Control** is particularly crucial to predictive research, but also has a part to play in correlational and descriptive research. The basic principle is that you should attempt to control all aspects of the research project *except* the one you are studying; this is often referred to as the control of **confounding variables,** that is, variables that will confound or confuse the interpretation of your data if they are not controlled. For example, if you have designed a project to compare treatment A with treatment B, you will collect data on the effects of the two treatments and expect to interpret your data in such a way that you can answer the question, "Which is better, treatment A or treatment B?" You will not be able to make this clear-cut interpretation unless you have controlled your observations—your data collection—so that differences in the data can *only* be attributed to one of the two treatments and not to some other influence that you have failed to eliminate or control.

Consider the example that was used in the hypotheses section of Chapter 1: the effects on active elbow extension of 5 minutes of ice pack applied to the spastic biceps of a hemiplegic patient. Here, treatment A was the ice pack and exercise, while treatment B was the elbow extension exercise without the ice. Suppose that you collected data from a group of hemiplegic patients using this design and it appeared from looking at your data that the patients who received the ice did, indeed, extend their elbows actively to a greater extent than the patients who did not receive the ice. Can you conclude from the data that 5 minutes of ice pack inhibits spasticity and thus facilitates active excursion by the antagonistic muscle? Suppose on closer investigation you discover that most of the patients who got the ice pack had a mild spasticity with good active contraction of the triceps, whereas most of the patients who received no ice were severe spastics with only trace active motion in their triceps. Would you still be able to interpret your data in the same way? Obviously in such a study one important control would be participants who demonstrate approximately the same degree of spasticity in both groups. Suppose one group was composed primarily of young, alert individuals with traumatic hemiplegia, while the other group was composed primarily of elderly individuals with both hemiplegia and a history of cardiovascular problems. Would that influence your interpretation?

The two examples should help to clarify the point. In a good research study as many variables as possible are controlled—except for the variables under study—so that any differences in measured range resulting from the treatment can be attributed to that treatment and not to some uncontrolled variable operating on the subjects.

In health sciences research a number of variables that are frequently important to control come readily to mind: age, sex, severity and length of time since onset of illness, type and dosages of medications, psychological and socioeconomic factors, inpatient or outpatient status, the presence or absence of other diseases or disabilities, and numerous other factors revealed in a good history and physical examination. However, effective control can never be applied in a routine and mechanical way. Every research project, question, and research design needs to be evaluated carefully to define exactly what variables are to be studied and what other variables must be controlled so that they do not contaminate the data.

Sometimes researchers want to control for bias, that is, an unconscious tendency to see what you expect to see or to favor one treatment over another. To deal with this problem, either the experimenter or the patient or both may be blinded to who is in the experimental group and who is in the control group. A **double-blind study** is one in which neither the experimenter nor the patient knows who is getting which treatment. This is easier to do in drug studies than in physical or occupational therapy. Therapists can often do a **single-blind study,** in which the one who does the data collection is "blind" as to which group a patient is assigned. In the earlier example, where treatment A was the ice pack and exercise while treatment B was the elbow extension exercise without the ice, the therapist who did the goniometry could be blind to which treatment a patient was receiving.

This emphasis on control appears again and again throughout this text as we discuss specific research designs and threats to internal and external validity in Chapter 4. Sometimes the researcher must make a trade-off between control and generalizability of conclusions—a little less control to have more generalizability. Look at paragraph 11 in the Beattie case study in Appendix C. How could you use the findings as controls in a study designed to expand Beattie's study to a group of patients? What use could you make of the exclusion criteria listed in the appendix to Beattie's article? What controls do you find in paragraph 5 in the Giannini article? What control is exemplified in the last sentence of paragraph 16?

Sampling

A second concept that is crucial to all research designs is the concept of sampling. A *population* refers to the members of a clearly defined set or class of people, objects, or events that are the focus of an investigation. A **sample** is composed of those subjects selected from a population for research study. To collect data on a group of people, objects, or events and be interested in the interpretation of the data only as it applies to those individuals who were studied is possible but unusual; in such a case the population and sample would be identical. Almost always, however, one hopes that the interpretation can be extrapolated to the larger group of people, objects, or events from which the sample was taken. To make this inference from the sample to the population, it is important that the sample be appropriate to the research question and representative of the population. The researcher usually defines the population first, then looks for ways to select a representative sample.

In reading the literature, defining the appropriate population for a given study is not always as easy as it may seem. For example, the therapists at St. Hopeless Hospital may decide to do a study and draw their sample from those hemiplegic patients who were admitted as inpatients to the hospital during a given calendar year, and their final report may interpret the results as if the population were all the hemiplegic patients in the world. However, is that really so? *Theoretically,* each individual in the population should have an equal opportunity to be in the sample drawn for study, but in this hypothetical example, even individuals with hemiplegia who are admitted to the hospital across the street did not have the opportunity to be in the study, let alone hemiplegic individuals across the country or halfway around the world. Therefore, a strict definition of the population of this study is the hemiplegic patients admitted to St. Hopeless outpatient clinic. We need not be so rigid as to further limit the population to those patients admitted during the specified calendar year of the study. On the other extreme, however, we might not want to include in the population all hemiplegic patients ever admitted to St. Hopeless, which was founded in 1892. Too many factors, both medical and sociological, have changed over such a long period. The population should be similar to the sample in all relevant respects.

This example illustrates some of the difficulties involved in defining the population of a study. Some researchers are more restrictive than others in this regard. Since in most things virtue stands between the two extremes, the approach of this text will be that the population is that group of objects, individuals, or events that resemble the sample in all or most important characteristics. Defining those important characteristics is the major difficulty when selecting your sample. Nevertheless, one should not abandon common sense while doing research. If St. Hopeless were a hospital serving primarily middle-class white Americans, and if it had been designated "first class" by the American Hospital Association, then it might be logical to define the population to which the results of the study could be extrapolated as all white middle-class patients who were admitted to first-class hospitals in the United States in the early 1990s. As the details of the study develop, other limitations on population description may emerge.

One could also do a study in which the sample of five people was identical to the total population of five people, the five people being staff therapists in a given department. It could be a descriptive study, designed to answer the question, How do therapists spend their time? The behavior observed could be everything performed on the job during 1 week's time. It could be recorded through a task description by a trained observer. The results might prove very beneficial to patient care by suggesting better use of the therapists' time. The results might not be applicable to a hospital across the street, which may have a totally different approach to organization and management. Thus, the characteristics of the sample and the population from which it is taken are crucial. The researcher must first identify his goals and purposes, then define the question, and finally, polish a hypothesis. He can then address himself to the questions of what population is appropriate and how a sample can be correctly chosen from that population.

The population and the sample must have the same scope and limitations. Most studies specify criteria of inclusion—for example, all patients between the ages of 18 and 64 with a diagnosis of deltoid bursitis. Many authors also specifically state a number of characteristics that would exclude many subjects from their study (criteria of exclusion). If characteristics such as mental retardation and cerebral palsy were excluded from the sample, then obviously they would be excluded from the population to which the conclusions may be extrapolated. If the question concerns the motor development of children during the first year of life after premature birth, then obviously neither population nor sample would include 2-year-olds or infants who were delivered after a normal-term pregnancy. Mistakes in this area are perhaps more frequently made by readers than by writers. As you learn to read scientific literature, it is wise to keep this issue in mind so that you do not extrapolate the findings of the study to a population beyond that intended by the author or, more importantly, beyond that justified by the sample and data collected. In deciding whether or not the results of a study should be applied to your patients, ask yourself these questions: If my patients had been available to the researcher, would they have been included in the sample? Are my patients in the population of this study?

IDEALIZED SAMPLING PROCEDURES

In this section we discuss how to select a fair and representative sample from a population and avoid a selection bias. The theoretical and mathematical ideals governing the concept of sampling are described. A later section deals with the application of these models to clinical research.

Theoretically, every individual in a population is identified and listed. This list is sometimes called a *frame*. A nonmedical example with a fixed and known population will be used to illustrate the basic concepts. If the population under study were every registered Republican in the state of Virginia, it should be possible to make a frame listing the names and addresses of every single person in the population. Since this number would be in the thousands, it might be logistically and economically impractical to examine each individual in that population. Therefore, the researcher could decide to choose a sample of 300 from the described population. If one wished to infer values or characteristics of the population from those values or characteristics observed in the sample, then it is important that the sample be representative of the population.

In the theory of **probability sampling** it is important that each and every member of the population have an equal opportunity to be in the sample. There are several ways to draw such a sample. The simplest and most direct is to put each person's name or an identifying number on a slip of paper, thoroughly jumble up all of the names, and then randomly draw from the box until 300 names are drawn. The purist would also shake the box up between each of the 300 draws and replace each slip of paper after it had been drawn.

Figure 2–1 is taken from a table of random numbers. To use this table you close your eyes and put your finger anywhere on the table. The number you have located in this way is your beginning point; you then proceed down the list taking every number between 1 and 45,000 until you have selected 300. You would then have randomly selected a sample of 300 (n) from your population of 45,000 (N). Most tables of random numbers go only to 9999, so some variation like systematic sampling illustrated below would be more practical.

Another method of obtaining a sample would be to randomly choose 30 counties in the state and then randomly choose 10 subjects from the lists of the registered Republicans in each of the 30 counties in order to reach the desired n for your sample. Some people would contend that in this procedure the population has been redefined as those registered Republicans in the 30 selected counties. However, if both the 30 counties and the 10 representatives were selected in random fashion, there is little reason to believe that the redefined population is not also representative of the theoretically larger population of the whole state.

Since our defined population is registered Republicans in the state, and our sample has been chosen from registered Republicans in the state, we have clearly met the criterion for appropriate subjects, but are they representative? The most powerful tool for assuring representativeness is that of randomization, which is based on the law of chance. If the sample is randomly chosen from the population, then the law of chance dictates that the sample is almost always representative of the population. However, since "almost always" is not an absolute guarantee, it is wise to double-check whenever possible, for example, with a second sample.

Stratified Random Sampling

Going back to the method using 10 subjects from each of 30 counties, suppose that just by chance none of the 30 counties chosen included any of the large cities in the state. The sample has then been biased, by chance, in favor of the rural areas. A technique for correcting this error is called **stratified random sampling.** For example, if you have reason to believe that dwellers in the large city complexes are different in some of the important parameters that you wish to measure from those who dwell in rural areas, then you would take steps to make sure that both subgroups,

Random Numbers

1368	9621	9151	2066	1208	2664	9822	6599	6911	5112
5953	5936	2541	4011	0408	3593	3679	1378	5936	2651
7226	9466	9553	7671	8599	2119	5337	5953	6355	6889
8883	3454	6773	8207	5576	6386	7487	0190	0867	1298
7022	5281	1168	4099	8069	8721	8353	9952	8006	9045
4576	1853	7884	2451	3488	1286	4842	7719	5795	3953
8715	1416	7028	4616	3470	9938	5703	0196	3465	0034
4011	0408	2224	7626	0643	1149	8834	6429	8691	0143
1400	3694	4482	3608	1238	8221	5129	6105	5314	8385
6370	1884	0820	4854	9161	6509	7123	4070	6759	6113
4522	5749	8084	3932	7678	3549	0051	6761	6952	7041
7195	6234	6426	7148	9945	0358	3242	0519	6550	1327
0054	0810	2937	2040	2299	4198	0846	3937	3986	1019
5166	5433	0381	9686	5670	5129	2103	1125	3404	8785
1247	3793	7415	7819	1783	0506	4878	7673	9840	6629
8529	7842	7203	1844	8619	7404	4215	9969	6948	5643
8973	3440	4366	9242	2151	0244	0922	5887	4883	1177
9307	2959	5904	9012	4951	3695	4529	7197	7179	3239
2923	4276	9467	9868	2257	1925	3382	7244	1781	8037
6372	2808	1238	8098	5509	4617	4099	6705	2386	2830
6922	1807	4900	5306	0411	1828	8634	2331	7247	3230
9862	8336	6453	0545	6127	2741	5967	8447	3017	5709
3371	1530	5104	3076	5506	3101	4143	5845	2095	6127
6712	9402	9588	7019	9248	9192	4223	6555	7947	2474
3071	8782	7157	5941	8830	8563	2252	8109	5880	9912
4022	9734	7852	9096	0051	7387	7056	9331	1317	7833
9682	8892	3577	0326	5306	0050	8517	4376	0788	5443
6705	2175	9904	3743	1902	5393	3032	8432	0612	7972
1872	8292	2366	8603	4288	6809	4357	1072	6822	5611
2559	7534	2281	7351	2064	0611	9613	2000	0327	6145
4399	3751	9783	5399	5175	8894	0296	9483	0400	2272
6074	8827	2195	2532	7680	4288	6807	3101	6850	6410
5155	7186	4722	6721	0838	3632	5355	9369	2006	7681
3193	2800	6184	7891	9838	6123	9397	4019	8389	9508
8610	1880	7423	3384	4625	6653	2900	6290	9286	2396
4778	8818	2992	6300	4239	9595	4384	0611	7687	2088
3987	1619	4164	2542	4042	7799	9084	0278	8422	4330
2977	0248	2793	3351	4922	8878	5703	7421	2054	4391
1312	2919	8220	7285	5902	7882	1403	5354	9913	7109
3890	7193	7799	9190	3275	7840	1872	6232	5295	3148
0793	3468	8762	2492	5854	8430	8472	2264	9279	2128
2139	4552	3444	6462	2524	8601	3372	1848	1472	9667
8277	9153	2880	9053	6880	4284	5044	8931	0861	1517
2236	4778	6639	0862	9509	2141	0208	1450	1222	5281
8837	7686	1771	3374	2894	7314	6856	0440	3766	6047
6605	6380	4599	3333	0713	8401	7146	8940	2629	2006
8399	8175	3525	1646	4019	8390	4344	8975	4489	3423
8053	3046	9102	4515	2944	9763	3003	3408	1199	2791
9837	9378	3237	7016	7593	5958	0068	3114	0456	6840
2557	6395	9496	1884	0612	8102	4402	5498	0422	3335

FIGURE 2–1 Part of a table of random numbers. (From Owen, DB: Handbook of Statistical Tables. Addison-Wesley, Reading, MA, 1962, with permission.)

N = 45,000 Registered Republicans in Virginia
n = 300 sample

	Urban	Rural	
Male 156	62	94	
Female 144	58	86	
	120	180	300

FIGURE 2–2 Number of individuals in each of four classifications (cells) based on a two-way stratification of a sample.

urban and rural, are represented in your sample. One approach would be to identify all Republicans in the state as either city dwellers or urban dwellers and then draw an equal number of individuals from each group. Or, if you know from other sources that 40 percent of the state's population lives in major cities and 60 percent in rural areas and small towns, you could draw a proportional stratified sample: 120 people from the urban list (40 percent of 300) and 180 (the other 60 percent) from the rural list.

Stratification can be used as long as the number of individuals in each stratified sample does not drop too low. (As a rule of thumb, no fewer than five in each "cell.") For example, you might want to further stratify both the urban and rural populations into male (52 percent of the population) and female (48 percent of the population), if you had good reason to believe that this was an important differentiation for your study (Fig. 2–2). The guiding principle is that the method of sampling chosen must be the one that offers the best possibility of giving you a sample that is truly representative of the population you wish to make inferences about.

Systematic Sampling

Yet another option is known as **systematic sampling.** If you had a list of all 45,000 registered Republicans in the state of Virginia and you wanted a sample of 5 percent, 2250, you could enter a table of random numbers until you located a number from one to 20. If that procedure gave you the number 13, then you would begin with the 13th person on the list of the population as your first subject. You would then take every 20th person on the list until you had 2250.

Cluster Sampling

Another procedure is called **cluster sampling.** Using this technique you would select (by either drawing out of a hat or using a table of random numbers) every 10th county in the state. You would then use *all* of the registered Republicans in that county as a part of your sample. This procedure is sometimes used when the population is composed of students and they are collected in clusters in schools. For example, you might randomly select 10 of the physical or occupational therapy schools in the United States, and then test all of the students in the schools thus selected (or all of the junior students, or all of the first-year female graduate students, or all of the faculty, and so forth). An example of another method of cluster sampling would be to randomly select 15 states, then randomly select 10 hospitals in each state, then randomly select two therapists from each hospital to answer your questionnaires. In a similar vein, Madigan[2] described her sample as, "All freshmen and sophomore OTA students ($n = 163$) and junior and senior occupational therapy students ($n = 100$) enrolled in four occupational therapy educational programs in Illinois."

Double Sampling

The last form of sampling to be illustrated is **double sampling.**

To continue with our hypothetical sample of registered Republicans in the state of Virginia, you might send a questionnaire to the 300 selected individuals and ask them 10 preliminary questions. One of these might be, "Did you vote in the last general election?" Let us say, for the sake of illustration, that 122 of the respondents indicated that they did vote in the last general election. You could then send these 122 people a longer and more detailed questionnaire, pursuing the issues pertinent to the objectives of your study. This is an example of double sampling. It is most useful in descriptive survey types of research. Some of the problems and limitations of survey samples are discussed in Chapter 5.

As noted earlier, randomization is the most powerful tool we have for imposing control on the process of sampling to prevent bias and to assure a representative sample. Obviously, a biased or nonrepresentative sample will not permit inference to the population.

Wherever possible, randomization should be used not only to obtain a sample from a population but also to divide the sample into different groups or to assign different treatments. If two or more groups are to be formed from the sample, the purpose of random assignment of subjects to different conditions or treatment groups is to form groups that are equivalent to each other in as many pre-experimental variables as possible. Only then can differences be attributed to the treatment procedures. In both instances, sampling and group assignment, the process of chance is fundamental.

It should be noted here that chance in research does not imply haphazardness. Chance is used in research as part of a carefully planned and executed technique, just as the table of random numbers has been carefully compiled.

NONPROBABILITY SAMPLING PROCEDURES

Nonprobability samples refer to those samples taken from a population for which there is no frame, for example, osteoarthritic patients. We cannot identify all osteoarthritics in any given age group or geographic region; therefore, we cannot give each one a chance to be in a research project. This category of nonprobability samples includes most clinical studies done by health care professionals. However, even under these circumstances, the researcher does the best she can with randomization. For example, Falconer[3] collected "a proportionally stratified, clustered sample of telephone numbers in California; private household numbers were selected using a random-digit dialing procedure. Telephone interviews were conducted with 5,614 persons." From those interviews, "data [were gathered] representing impairment and physical and social disability...from...2,350 working-aged adults who reported a musculoskeletal disorder." Since people who report their problems may be different from those who do not, Falconer's population would be so defined. Her sample was limited to a geographic area of the nation. How far do you believe you should extrapolate?

Given the practical impossibility of obtaining a truly representative sample, the clinical researcher takes a **sample of convenience.** Examples include all osteoarthritic clients admitted to a therapy in-service program during the months of January through March; the first 50 clients with right hemiplegia admitted to a therapy in-service program who met specified criteria for admission to a study; and so on. No one knows for sure how much bias this introduces into a sample. The best the researcher can do is to be as clear and objective as possible in describing the sample so that readers can compare their own patients to the researcher's sample. Samples of convenience pose a threat to external validity; this is discussed in Chapter 4. The less sure the reader is that the sample is truly representative of a population, the more cautious must be the interpretation and use of the data obtained. Data obtained from samples of convenience may often be best considered as pilot studies, which suggest fruitful avenues to explore further.

GROUP ASSIGNMENT

Once a representative sample has been chosen from a defined population, the researcher often needs to divide the sample into two or more groups, for example, experimental and control or comparison groups. The ideal way to do this is by randomization. For example, Carlton[4] proceeded as follows. "Subjects in this study were food service employees at a small liberal arts university located in the Pacific Northwest. . . . From a list of all food service personnel, a random sample of 36 subjects and 18 alternates were selected. Subjects were randomly placed into one of two groups."

If samples cannot be chosen and group assignments made all at once, as indicated in the ideal sampling procedures noted earlier, then the experimenter must assign individuals from a sample of convenience in a sequential fashion over a period of time rather than at the beginning of the experiment. In sequential assignment to groups, a modification of the hat technique can be used. If, for example, you are forming three treatment groups and you want n equal to 30 (10 people in each group), then you can write the number 1, for treatment group 1, on 10 pieces of paper, the number 2, for group 2, on 10 pieces of paper, and the number 3, for group 3, on 10 pieces of paper; shuffle them thoroughly in the hat; and draw them out, writing the numbers down one at a time as they are drawn. Say the resulting sequence begins 3, 1, 1, 3, 2, 1. Then the first person to enter your experiment would go into group 3, the second and third persons would go into group 1, the fourth person to group 3, and so on. You can also enter a table of random numbers, and record in sequence each time you come upon a 1, 2, or 3, and then assign subjects according to that sequence. Clients may also be assigned alternately to experimental or control groups as they are identified and admitted to the study. An example of serial admission may be found in Wingate.[5] "After approval of this study by the Human Rights Committees at three area hospitals, all patients admitted to these institutions over a 13-month period for a breast biopsy were requested to participate in the study, but only those whose biopsies were found to be malignant and who subsequently underwent modified radical mastectomies were retained."

Once your experimental and control groups have been formed, you should check to make sure that your randomization has produced homogenous groups. There are statistical methods for doing this, and occasionally you will see these "tests of homogeneity" reported in articles, attesting to the fact that the groups observed were reasonably similar to each other. For example, Connolly and Michael[6] formed two groups of retarded children, one group with and the other without Down syndrome. To ensure that the two groups were comparable on the variables of age and IQ, they used a t-test to demonstrate no significant differences between the two groups on those variables. Look at Table 2 in the Giannini article in Appendix C. This table exemplifies tests of homogeneity demonstrating no significant differences in experimental and control groups on the variables of age and body surface area. For other tests of homogeneity, see paragraph 9 in the Magill-Evans article in Appendix C.

ASSIGNMENT BY MATCHING

Sometimes it is not possible to control a sample through randomization; at other times the sample may be so small that randomization is unlikely to operate effectively to evenly distribute critical variables between groups. In such cases an alternate procedure, which is called **matching,** may be used. With this technique the researcher imposes his own criteria and attempts to force the groups into equivalency along dimensions or characteristics which the researcher believes to be important. Tests of homogeneity illustrated earlier are intended to demonstrate that randomization did for the samples what the researcher does in the matching procedure.

The first step in assignment by matching is to identify the important characteristic to be controlled by the researcher. Let us say that age is considered to be a confounding variable if not controlled; that is, it will weaken any conclusions drawn if it is not properly controlled. Using matching, you can impose this restriction on your sample so that both groups have the same average (mean) age and the same age variation. (A statistical measure of variation called *variance* is defined in Chapter 5.) The concern here is that the mean ages and variances of the two groups are equal, or nearly so. This technique might be used to equate a senior physical therapy class and a senior occupational therapy class. Individuals may sometimes be moved from one group to another to ensure this balance in age—for example, in a study to compare two halves of a senior class in school, each group receiving different educational "treatments."

If you match individual pairs, you find two individuals who are very similar to each other with regard to crucial variables that you want to control. You then randomly assign each individual to one of the two groups. Let us say, again, that age is an important factor in the criteria that identify your sample. When you find two 31-year-old people who meet the criteria for admission into your sample, you randomly assign one to the first group and the other to the second group. You then may find two people 23 years old and randomly assign one to each group, and so on.

Notice that matching on critical variables is used for control, as a substitute for the control of chance. Chance still plays a minor part in selecting which one of each pair goes to each group. If you have three or more groups, you must find three or more individuals who are alike with regard to the crucial variable that you want to control. You may also match on more than one variable; for example, you might match two 30-year-old white females. In both group and individual matching procedures it is important to have strong evidence of a significant relationship between the matched variable and the experimental task.

A major limitation of matching is that once you get beyond two variables it becomes extremely difficult to find matching pairs. If you are matching triplets it is even more difficult. On a practical level, then, one is often limited to two groups matched on one or two critical variables, and therein lie the major flaws of this technique. First of all, it is difficult to identify all of the critical variables that you need to control. Secondly, there is a possibility that by matching individuals you introduce a systematic bias. Especially when you are working with human beings whose characteristics are very complex, it is practically impossible to control all relevant factors except through randomization. For these reasons many researchers say that matching should never be used as a substitute for randomization, and most would agree that you should never use matching if randomization is possible. Usually it is better to introduce controlling variables in the definition of the population and sample, for example, white females between 20 and 40 years of age who are not on any anti-inflammatory drugs.

Individuals are sometimes matched at the beginning of an experimental task that involves repeated measures. Let us say that you plan to take three measures of shoulder range of motion: at the beginning, in the middle, and at the end of your experimental treatment. It might be possible to match individuals on the actual performance level of the task itself so that a person with 100 degrees of active flexion of the shoulder would be matched with another person with 100 ± 5 degrees of active flexion of the shoulder. These two would then be randomly assigned to two treatment protocols. In like manner two patients with only 15 degrees of active flexion would be randomly assigned to the same two treatment groups. *All other factors being equal,* it would then be reasonable to assume that differences between the individuals of a pair in your second and third measures of range of motion could be attributed to treatment technique, since both individuals started out at the same level. However, with this procedure we also run into the problem of compounding variables such as length of time the tightness has existed in the shoulder, severity of the disease process, motivation, and other factors that may tend to destroy the equality between a pair. Thus, matching should be avoided whenever other sampling methods are possible. In reviewing the physical and occupational therapy literature of the past several years, in preparation for revising this text, I found very few examples of studies using a matching design.

A variation on matching is called **quota sampling** wherein the researcher specifies that the sample of convenience will contain certain quotas or proportions. For example, to represent the community served by the hospital, a sample may be required to include 52 percent male, 48 percent female, 25 percent African Americans, and 10 percent Latinos. These quotas are achieved by matching as the groups are formed.[7]

Look at some research articles in the literature and decide how the authors selected their samples and how each sample was divided into groups. In Appendix C, how did Giannini and McClain get their samples? How did Magill-Evans divide her sample into groups (paragraphs 8 and 9)? An example of matched pairs may be found in Howard,[8] who found her sample in a child care center and a women's support shelter. She divided her sample into 12 physically abused children and 12 nonabused children and paired the groups according to each child's age and family income. Her review of literature indicated that race was not an important consideration to her question, so her groups were not matched on race.

Figure 2–3 illustrates some of the basic ideas of research design that we have discussed so far in this chapter. A population is identified as carefully as possible. It is all the people, objects, or events to which the results of a study might be relevant. From that population a sample is drawn. Ideally, complete **randomization,** which uses the laws of chance, will produce a truly representative sample of the population. As a researcher you are going to "do something" with or to that sample. You may treat the entire sample as one group, or you may divide it (hopefully by randomization) into several treatment groups. The treatment may consist merely of observation in a natural setting, or it may require experimental manipulation and measurement.

The question of how many groups constitute the sample is an important issue in later chapters, which deal more specifically with research designs. It is important at this point to realize that the criterion measures or data collections discussed in Chapter 3 may be taken once, twice, or many times on each group. Unfortunately, the taking of criterion measures is sometimes called data sampling, and it is not to be confused with the topic of this chapter, population sampling. Three data collections, one from

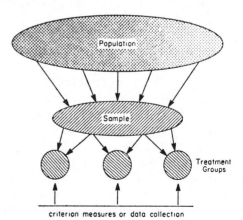

FIGURE 2–3 Diagram of population, sample, and treatment groups.

each of three treatment groups within a sample, are illustrated in Figure 2–3.

Sample Size

One of the most common questions asked by beginning researchers is, "How large a sample do I need?" There is no clear-cut answer to that question. A rule of thumb, which does not offer much help, is that the larger the sample, the better. A more helpful rule is that the greater the variation in the population (and sample) on the variable you plan to measure, the larger the number needed in the sample. The larger the sample, the greater the probability that randomness and chance are operating as expected. Larger numbers reduce the chance of sampling error.

The requirements of your chosen statistical tools must also be considered in the question of sample size. Some statistical tests require a minimum number in each group, usually at least five. If you cannot increase the sample size, you may have to settle for a greater probability of error in drawing conclusions from your data.

Statistical formulas can help to determine the appropriate sample size for a given set of criteria with probability samples and metric levels of measurement (discussed in the next chapter). These formulae are less helpful with samples of convenience, but they may still be useful.[9] Hulley and Cummings[10] provide several tables in their appendices that set minimum sample sizes for different statistical tests, depending on how sure you want to be that you are correct in your interpretation of your data. For example, for the familiar t-test, they recommend a sample size anywhere from 12 to 3563, depending on the desired power and probability of your tests; these topics are discussed further in Chapter 8. Whenever possible, it is wise to consult someone familiar with these statistical methods and/or textbooks such as those listed in Appendix D.

Types of Research

No classification of research types is universally accepted. In this text we divide all research into three major types: descriptive, correlational, and predictive (experimental). Chapters 5 through 9 discuss these types individually and identify their various subclasses and component parts. For now, a quick overview of their similarities and differences will suffice.

First, let us look at the similarities. All three involve a question to be answered, but the questions themselves are different. All three have a population, and all three look at a sample taken from the population. (In cases of very small populations, the sample may be the total population.)

All three collect data from the sample; they differ in the kinds of data they collect and the way they go about collecting data. Finally, all three interpret their data in an attempt to find the most likely and reasonable answer to the question. As Leedy[11] has so clearly pointed out, no amount of data collection, fact finding, or fact transcribing "can be dignified by the term research.... The mind of the researcher must do battle with the observed fact ... until the fact reveals its inner significance," that is, its relation to the question being asked. So all types of research ask a specific question, search for the answer in an organized and planned way, and answer the question through interpretation of the data collected.

How do these three basic types of research differ? In general, they differ (1) in the kind of question asked, (2) in the degree to which the sample is manipulated by the experimenter, (3) in the statistical tools used to summarize and/or interpret the data, and (4) in the formal properties of the predictions made on the basis of the data.

For **descriptive research** the generic question is, What are the existing characteristics of the real world relative to the specific question? More popularly expressed, "let's tell it like it is." The descriptive researcher rarely manipulates any aspect of the sample; rather she looks at it in its natural setting in planned, controlled ways and records her observations. On the basis of these observations the researcher then proceeds to describe the characteristics of interest in the population on the basis of the observed characteristics in the sample. For example, if 80 percent of this representative sample has characteristic A, then by extrapolation approximately 80 percent of the population has the same characteristic. We will examine descriptive research in more detail in Chapter 5.

In most **correlational** research the generic question is, To what extent do two (or more) characteristics tend to occur together? As characteristic A increases, does characteristic B increase, decrease, or remain the same? To what extent are these two variables *associated* with each other? Occasionally, a researcher will manipulate one characteristic and then see whether characteristic B increases or decreased as a result of the manipulation of characteristic A. But most correlations are between measures of observed phenomena in their natural state. Here are two examples: To what extent do high GPAs occur in college freshmen with high SAT scores? To what extent does joint inflammation occur together with (correlate with) a decrease in that joint's range of motion? There is no implication of causality in correlation, yet the typical interpretation is that if these two factors have correlated repeatedly in a sample, then they will probably correlate in the rest of the population. The issue of causality is discussed further in Chapter 6.

In **predictive research** the generic question is generally one of comparison: Is treatment A different from treatment B? If they are different, is it an important difference or a minor one? If sample data suggest that the two treatments are different, which treatment is better? If the first group receives treatment A, how will that change their scores on the criterion measure in comparison to those in the second group who get treatment B? The interpretation of predictive research is almost always in terms of probability. Here is a typical answer to a predictive research question: The probability is 1 in 100 of being wrong when I say that treatment B is better than treatment A, and if that is true for the individuals in this representative sample, then by extrapolation it will be true of the individuals in the population. In predictive research one usually manipulates a single variable (identified as the independent or research variable) and then observes what happens to another variable (the dependent variable).

Manipulation is so common in predictive research that it is often identified with it, but it is also possible to manipulate variables in descriptive and correlational research.

The above descriptions of research types are generalities based on relatively pure definitions of the three approaches. As we study each type in detail and look at examples from the literature, it will become clear that many published reports are mixtures of two or even all three types, and that within types there are mixtures of various designs. These facts have proven to be a source of frequent confusion to beginning students, but that is the way the literature is written, so the student has to master it. In this text we will first establish general models for each type and subtype and then look in the literature to see how individual researchers have modified and altered the designs to meet the demands of their particular question and the exigencies of their environment.

Research Design in Health Care Environments

The biggest compromise that health care workers generally make with the ideals stated earlier involves the identification of the population and the random selection of a sample from that population. If one's population is all registered Republicans in the United States, or all fourth-grade females in public schools in the state of Tennessee, it is possible to compile a list (frame) of the names and addresses of the entire population. With adequate time and financing, it would also be possible to do certain kinds of research on samples from those populations, such as mail survey questionnaires, which are typical of much descriptive research. In the case of the population in the public schools in one state, it might even be possible to do predictive research with cluster sampling followed by random assignment to experimental and control or comparison groups. However, when one's population is all individuals with right-sided hemiplegia in the United States whose disabilities resulted from cerebral aneurysms, it is not practically possible to identify with any precision all of the individuals who belong to that population. Given the time and financial constraints of most clinical health workers, a representative sample from that national population of hemiplegic patients is not feasible. Nevertheless, with most research on hemiplegic patients, it is highly desirable to extrapolate the interpretations of one's study to the broad population. To what extent can we reasonably do that?

Almost every research article in any health science journal will demonstrate established criteria by which individuals were admitted to the study. As patients who meet the criteria for the study come through a clinical service, they are included in the sample and assigned to treatment groups. For an example, look at paragraphs 5, 6, and 7 in the article by Giannini in Appendix C. Data are collected, probability statements made, and interpretations done. Often the sample is all patients who met the criteria for admission to the study who were admitted to the hospital or department within a given time span, like 6 months or a year. What is the population for such a study? As indicated earlier in this chapter, the most defensible answer is that their population is all patients or potential patients of that type who, by reason of their geographic location, have the potential to be admitted to that service over an extended time span—say, 5 years. The most critical question that the reader must answer is, "To what extent is the writer's sample representative of the patients I treat?" In answering the question, the reader must consider psychological and social factors as well as physiological and pathological similarities. To the extent that you can logically defend the thesis that the writer's sample is representative of your population, you are justified in extrapolating the results of that study to your own patients. As noted earlier, the author's conclusions must be drawn convincingly before the clinician will be willing to apply them to clients. In this way a clinician can learn from the literature and hopefully increase his professional competence, as long as he is aware of the assumptions underlying the scientific process and the application of statistical tests.

Basic and Applied Research

One often sees these terms, and they appear to have a very clear-cut meaning. Yet when you look at the literature and attempt to classify research into these two areas, it becomes evident that it is not a real dichotomy (two mutually exclusive classes). These terms are really the two ends of a spectrum, with innumerable variations in between. This variation is explored further in Chapter 11, but for now let it suffice to briefly define the two extremes.

"Pure" or **basic research** is interested in the acquisition of knowledge for its own sake without any concern for the utility of that knowledge. For example, a researcher might be interested in the effects of different types of heat on the microcirculation of muscular and connective tissue. She could pursue this topic from several points of view by performing a number of experiments without ever knowing of the existence of the field of physical therapy or giving any thought to the medicinal uses of the information that she is gathering. Basic research tends to test theory and establish general laws; applied research then tests the application of the theories and laws to specific circumstances.

Applied research (sometimes called action research, and occasionally even, mistakenly, clinical research) is concerned with the solution of immediate problems without any concern for the basic reason as to why the solution works. For example, a physical therapist might be interested in the influence of shortwave diathermy on muscle spasm in acute, idiopathic low-back pain. He might study that question and find answers and never give a thought to the possible explanation of how it works in terms of the influence of heat on microcirculation of the tissues or an influence on nervous tissue. Quality assurance research, as it is described by the Parentes,[12] fits under the rubric of applied research. Quality assurance research may be descriptive, correlational, or predictive. One common descriptive form, according to the Parentes, is to compare practice to published norms; for example, if there are published norms stating that no more than 5 percent of the patients in a nursing home should have decubiti, the researcher would collect data on the actual percent of decubiti in the facility and compare that data to the norm. Goldstein[13] discussed followup studies and program evaluation research that are similar to quality assurance studies. More will be said about normative research in Chapter 5.

Obviously, there are a number of gradations in between these two extremes, and frequently the classification of research into these two categories is of academic interest only. An example from the literature of an in-between study is the article by Brown and Baker.[14] They are obviously interested in the clinical implications of their study of the effect of shortwave diathermy on healing muscle injury in rabbits. Equally obviously, more research is needed to see if the modality will have similar or different effects in humans. One important question relating to this issue is the following: "Can I apply what I learned from this research study directly to patient care, or are there other questions that must be answered first?" For example, are the results of Hagbarth's study of the effects of vibration on neuromuscular responses in cats directly applicable to patient care? Or would it be important to first examine the results of intervening studies, which deal with the influence of vibration on normal humans and on humans with neuromuscular pathologies? These questions are discussed further in Chapter 11.

Human Rights

One of the problems we have in clinical research is that of protecting individual human rights in the research process. This is a problem of medical ethics. In recent years there have been several well-publicized incidents where researchers did not protect the rights or interests of individual human beings. The public reaction to these reports has been an increased awareness of and demand for open accountability of researchers on ethical matters. An excellent two-part summary of the issues surrounding human rights in research has been written by Michels.[15] Okolo[16] has written a very brief history of medical ethics from the fifth century B.C.E. to our present age. The professional codes of ethics of the American Occupational Therapy Association[17] and the American Physical Therapy Association[18] are concerned more with patient care than with research, per se. Nevertheless, the student and clinician should be very familiar with these documents and how they have been interpreted by the judicial committees of their respective associations.

Bruckner[19] has given a brief, clear statement of the basic schools of ethics; consequentialism, nonconsequentialism, and utilitarianism. More details may be found in Purtilo's[20] writings, for example, *Ethical Dimensions in the Health Professions*. Davis[21] has summarized the basic principles contained in most ethical systems. Under "duties," Davis lists the principles (1) do no harm, (2) be faithful to contracts, and (3) do all one can for the patient. Under "rights," she lists (1) rights of patients, (2) rights of health professionals, and (3) rights of society. Under "responsibilities," she includes the responsibilities of (1) health professionals, (2) patients, and (3) society. Under the topic of "justice," she discusses seeking a fair distribution of resources and compensating for injuries.

Okolo[22] considers the principle of beneficence (do no harm) as the most fundamental principle of ethics in health care. She also emphasizes the principles of autonomy and justice. These three principles suggest three questions for the researcher to ask concerning each research project: Am I trying to do good to the patients? Am I respecting the freedom of choice that each patient possesses by right? Am I being fair to everyone concerned with this project?

Drew[23] has identified ethical issues in three major categories: subjects, research designs, and professionalism. Informed consent is synonymous with written consent; legal consent must be voluntary and based on adequate information, and the patient must have the mental capacity to consent. While details will vary from institution to institution, the patient should be told the purpose of the study, the procedures to be used, any known physical or psychological risks, possible benefits the patient may expect from participation (cost-benefit ratio), alternate treatments available, and a statement acknowledging that the patient may withdraw at any time without prejudice to the subject, and that privacy will be maintained.[3, 24-26]

Ethical issues related to design often concern single-blind (subject does not know what treatment is being administered) or double-blind (neither subject nor researcher knows what treatment each subject is getting) designs where full knowledge of the design might bias the results. Although research committees may occasionally give different permissions, usually the subject must be told what the different treatments are and the risks and benefits of each. Deception must always be justified, and full disclosure usually follows at the end of the experiment.

Control groups may also create ethical issues. When dealing with patients it usually is not ethical to divide your sample into experimental and control groups where the control group receives no treatment. Sometimes it is possible, when there is no clear evidence that a treatment will help, to give all subjects good treatment according to present knowledge and then add on the unknown quantity to see if it makes a difference. Researchers will also sometimes provide free treatment at a later date to subjects who consent to be in a no-treatment group for a time for research purposes. Most institutions now have a human research committee; checking with them early in the planning stages of a study can save the clinician much time and frustration. A good overview of the functioning of these boards and of the issue of informed consent can be found in Mitcham and Steadman.[27]

Review Questions

A Preliminary Research Protocol   All patients admitted to a large metropolitan inpatient arthritis clinic during 1993 are initially screened by an activities of daily living (ADL) test. Those with low scores in self-care are further evaluated. All patients with more than 30 percent but less than 60 percent of normal passive range of motion in the elbow of the dominant arm and whose active elbow range of motion is 90 percent of passive range or more, are admitted to the study. All subjects are put on the same medication, diet, and general routine. All subjects are given identical therapy programs except for the length of time they spend in daily, bilateral, rhythmic, upper-extremity active exercises that emphasize maximal range of shoulder and elbow joints. Using a table of random numbers, the therapists divide the research subjects into three groups. One group spends 1 hour daily (in three 20-minute sessions) on the rhythmic exercises. One group spent 2 hours daily (in six 20-minute sessions) on the rhythmic exercises. The third group rests while the other groups are exercising. Range of motion is recorded at the beginning of the study (pretest) and again in 3 weeks (posttest). The pretest and posttest range of motion scores for the elbow of the dominant arm are compared for significant differences among the three groups. The purpose of this study is to determine which group (1-hour, 2-hour, or resting) will show the greatest gain in elbow range of motion.

1 Is this basic or applied research?

2 Is it primarily descriptive, correlational, or predictive? Could it be more than one? How?

3 What is the population of this study?

4 What is the sample of this study?

5 What are the controls?

6 How is sampling done?

7 Could other forms of sampling have been used? What changes in design would be required to use different sampling techniques?

Additional Readings

Brink, PJ, and Wood, MJ: Basic Steps in Planning Nursing Research; From Question to Proposal, Chapter 10. Wadsworth, Monterey, CA, 1983.

Bulpitt, CJ: Randomized Controlled Clinical Trials, Chapters 3, 6, 7. Martinus Nijhoff, Boston, 1983.

Drew, CJ, and Hardman, ML: Designing and Conducting Behavioral Research, Chapters 2, 3, 8. Pergamon, New York, 1985.

Goldstein, G: A Clinician's Guide to Research Design, Chapters 5, 8. Nelson-Hall, Chicago, 1980.

Pavalon, EI: Human Rights and Health Care Law. American Journal of Nursing Company, New York, 1980.

Pocock, SJ: Clinical Trials: A Practical Approach, Chapters 4 to 7. John Wiley & Sons, New York, 1983.

Prentice, ED, and Purtillo, RB: The use and protection of human and animal subjects. In Bork, CE (ed): Research in Physical Therapy. Lippincott, Philadelphia, 1993.

References

1. Travers, RMW: An Introduction to Educational Research, ed 3. Macmillan, London, 1969.
2. Madigan, MJ: Characteristics of students in occupational therapy educational programs. AJOT 39:41, 1985.

3. Falconer, J: Toward validation of constructs for classifying human performance dysfunction. OTJ Res 6:329, 1986.
4. Carlton, RS: The effects of body mechanics instruction on work performance. AJOT 41:16, 1987.
5. Wingate, L: Efficacy of physical therapy for patients who have undergone mastectomies. Phys Ther 65:896, 1985.
6. Connolly, BH, and Michael, BT: Performance of retarded children, with and without Down syndrome, on the Bruininks-Oseretsky Test of Motor Proficiency. Phys Ther 66:344, 1986.
7. Brink, PJ, and Wood, MJ: Basic Steps in Planning Nursing Research, from Question to Proposal, ed 2. Wadsworth, Monterey, CA, 1983, p 144.
8. Howard, AC: Developmental play ages of physically abused and nonabused children. AJOT 40:691, 1986.
9. Francis, K: Computer communication: Determination of sample size. Phys Ther 66:104, 1986.
10. Hulley, SB, and Cummings SR (eds): Designing Clinical Research. Williams & Wilkins, Baltimore, 1988, pp 215–220.
11. Leedy, PD: Practical Research: Planning and Design. Macmillan, New York, 1974.
12. Parente, R, and Parente, JA: Alternative research strategies for occupational therapy, Part 2: Ideographic and quality assurance research. AJOT 40:428, 1986.
13. Goldstein, G: A Clinician's Guide to Research Design. Nelson-Hall, Chicago, 1980, pp 213–223.
14. Brown, M, and Baker, RD: Effect of pulsed Shortwave diathermy on skeletal muscle injury in rabbits. Phys Ther 67:208, 1987.
15. Michels, E: Research and human rights, Parts 1 and 2. Phys Ther 56:407, 56:546, 1976.
16. Okolo, EN (ed): Health Research Design and Methodology. CRC Press, Ann Arbor, 1990, pp 82 ff.
17. American Occupational Therapy Association: Occupational Therapy Code of Ethics. Rockville, MD, 1988.
18. American Physical Therapy Association: Code of Ethics and Guide for Professional Conduct. Alexandria, VA, 1987.
19. Bruckner, J: Physical therapists as double agents: Ethical dilemmas of divided loyalties. Phys Ther 67:383, 1987.
20. Purtilo, RB, and Cassel, CK: Ethical Dimensions in the Health Professions. WB Saunders, Philadelphia, 1981.
21. Davis, CM: The influence of values on patient care. In Payton, OD (ed): Psychosocial Aspects of Clinical Practice. Churchill Livingstone, New York, 1986.
22. Okolo, EN: op. cit.
23. Drew, CJ, and Hardman, ML: Designing and Conducting Behavioral Research. Pergamon, New York, 1985, p. 30ff
24. Goldstein, G: op. cit.
25. Okolo, EN: op. cit., pp. 84–86.
26. Hulley, SB, and Cummings, SR (eds): op. cit., p 223.
27. Mitcham, MD, and Steadman, CD: The institutional review board and human subjects research: An overview. OTJ Res 4:253, 1984.

3

Measurement

OBJECTIVES

1   Define measurement; nominal, ordinal, and metric (interval and ratio) measurements; criterion measures. Illustrate each as they relate to professional practice.
2   Identify levels of measurement reported in research studies.
3   Exemplify parameter and statistic and define parametric and nonparametric as they relate to measurement and statistics.

Basic Terms

According to Rothstein,[1]

Without a scientific basis for the assessment (and measurement) process, we face the future as independent practitioners unable to communicate with one another, unable to document treatment efficacy, and unable to claim scientific credibility for our profession. Physical therapy, like medicine and law, will always remain partially an art, but without measurement it can be nothing more than an art.

Gillette[2] has made a similar observation for occupational therapy: "Neither the research process itself nor good clinical practice can succeed without good measurement devices."

Measurement is the process of quantifying people, objects, events, or their characteristics. As Stevens[3] observed in his classic paper, "Measurement ... is defined as the assignment of numerals to objects or events according to rules. The fact that numerals can be assigned under different rules leads to different kinds of scales and different kinds of measurement." A standardized measure is a measure in which the procedure for performing it has been described in detail in a protocol, enabling others to follow the same protocol.

Theoretically, we can measure anything if the appropriate rules are used. As Hasselkus and Safrit[4] have noted, "A substantial portion of any occupational therapist's workday is inevitably spent 'measuring' behaviors." The same can be said of physical therapists. Therapists measure strength, range of motion (ROM), motor functions such as gait or activities of daily living, temperature, pulse, blood pressure, sensory integrative behaviors, developmental level, the level of cooperation between family members, and so forth. They also measure performance levels of employees under their supervision, the efficiency of the department in terms of patients treated per therapist hour, costs per unit of treatment time, and so on. In order to study any of these phenomena we collect information about them and record that information as a measurement of the phenomena observed.

Some measurements are straightforward: the number of steps an amputee can walk before stopping, the time in minutes that it takes a hemiplegic patient to put on a shirt, the degree of motion in an arthritic wrist. These are concrete, observable, biological phenomena related to frequency, weight, height, time, and length. However, therapists must also measure phenomena in the psychosocial and other functional areas where precise measurement is not possible. Such phenomena cannot be defined by specific measures such as inches or pounds; they are given, instead, a rating system of some sort. To measure a patient's independence in daily living, Hasselkus and Safrit[5] used this measure:

> Numbers are assigned (for example, 0, independent; 1, minimal assistance; 2, moderate assistance; 3, total dependence) to the behavioral indicators and inferences are drawn with regard to the underlying property: independence.

We use similar measures with phenomena such as spasticity, motivation, cooperation, and sensation. Learning in the classroom and in the clinic is another phenomenon that cannot be measured directly; we measure something else and then infer from that measure the underlying property of learning.

In an interesting article about problems and issues in measurement research in occupational therapy. Smith[6] discusses three significant problems:

1   The same tools often cannot be used to assess (measure) functional outcomes and dysfunctional diagnostic information; for example, goniometry may tell you more about dysfunction than

    it does about function, but we have tended to use the same tool to define both interests.

2 Extreme variance in both populations and samples works against a need for assessment tools than can be used by all therapists and be understood within and across professions.

3 Measurement scales and traditional measurement methodologies themselves create problems in developing clinically meaningful assessment tools.

Smith felt a need to develop assessment tools that were stronger than the ordinal scale, which is discussed later in the chapter.

As stated in Chapter 1, research is designed to answer a question on the basis of collected data. The data that are collected form the **criterion.** The criterion to be measured must be defined in operational terms, because "without an operational definition, no measurement can be made."[7] The **criterion measure** is that which quantifies the criterion. For example, read Stern, paragraphs 6 and 9, in Appendix C. The criterion is hand volume; the measurement tool is a commercial hand volumeter set. The criterion measure is the reading on the measurement tool in milliliters (see Table 2, p. 330).

It is important to be sure that the criterion measure is truly relevant to the phenomenon under study. This may seem obvious; however, Hamilton[8] points out that we may be fooled into measuring the wrong thing.

An example from general medicine will illustrate what I mean about the problems of the relevance of criterion. When anticoagulant drugs were first introduced as a "treatment" for coronary thrombosis, they roused tremendous interest. A great spate of research followed. . . . Nevertheless I often wondered if all that effort had been somewhat displaced. It seemed to me that the real criterion was not the maintenance of a low coagulability of the blood, but the incidence of recurrence of thrombosis and ultimately the death rate or expectation of life. In due course, researches were published which had used these criteria, and unfortunately, the results were shown to be much less good . . . than had been hoped for.

In addition to choosing the right things to measure, we need measurement tools that allow us to (1) measure performance, (2) distinguish transient from permanent, (3) identify observable traits associated with performance, and (4) identify conditions under which change occurs.

The attributes of interest in a particular research project must, at some level, be observable, or countable. Sometimes several possible measures are available, in which case every possible measure should be evaluated with respect to (1) the specificity of its relationship to the phenomenon under investigation, (2) how well that measurement communicates accurately to others, and (3) the sensitivity of the measure. For example, inches are more specific to a measurement of stature than are pounds; the concept of inches communicates effectively to the general population of Americans, and the inch is a more precise measure than the foot. On the other hand, millimeters would communicate more effectively to the scientific community and are more sensitive to change in length than inches.

Four types or levels of measurement are generally discussed in connection with research design: nominal, ordinal, interval, and ratio.[9] Interval and ratio measures will be discussed together as metric measures. Not everyone agrees with the importance of these classifications,[10] but most accept them as important, and they are used in many statistics texts.

Levels of Measurement

NOMINAL MEASUREMENT

The **nominal scale of measurement** is the weakest level of measurement. The data are placed into broad categories, and each category is operationally defined. Numbers may be used in this scale, but they can be replaced with any other system of symbols, such as the alphabet, without changing the measurement. For example, on questionnaires where the responses were either "yes" or "no" the data are divided, and thus measured, into those two categories, which might be numbered 1 and 2. If there are only two categories, the measurement is often referred to as *dichotomous.* In another instance, patients in a sample might be measured as belonging to class A, osteoarthritic; class B, rheumatoid arthritic; class C, traumatic arthritic; or class D, combinations and other. The categories of data measured at the nominal level are mutually exclusive, independent, and exhaustive; that is, each person, event, or characteristic should fit into one—and only one—category and the categories should be independent of each other.

Other examples of nominal classes are male or female; spastic, athetoid, or other; left-handed or right-handed; inpatient or outpatient. There is no limit to the number of such categories. It is important to note that although numbers may be used to mark the categories—for example, class 1, class 2, class 3—no mathematic value has been assigned to the numbers. One *can* count the number of people or events in each category and then state the percentage of the total sample that may be found in each category or classification. It is easy to get confused at this point; the categories themselves (class 1, class 2, class 3) are nominal. However, the frequency counts or percentages within each category are often (frequency counts) or always (percentages) considered metric. In a study of diagnostic categories the basic measurement occurs in the assignment of individuals into the categories, a nominal measurement.

For example, Harrison and Kielhofner[11] provide a table giving the frequency count of subjects, by age, under four headings: cerebral palsy, mental retardation, developmental delay, and other. These are nominal headings (age is metric), and the only thing done with the data is a frequency count. They provide another table with frequency counts of the number of times each of 16 types of play was observed; this is nominal data with no suggestion of order or sequence to the observations. Many descriptive studies provide frequency counts on the variables of interest; see, for example, Parham.[12] Neistadt[13] studied the evaluations written by 22 occupational therapists containing 608 treatment goals. The goals were classified as either remedial or adaptive, categories that were exclusive, independent, and exhaustive as she defined them. And finally, Gose,[14] looked at several variables through a retrospective chart review in order to study the effects of continuous passive motion (CPM) in the postoperative management of patients with total knee replacements. He collected data on a nominal frequency count of postoperative complications in his sample. Patients who received CPM had significantly fewer postoperative complications.

ORDINAL MEASUREMENT

The **ordinal scale of measurement** is sometimes called the ranking scale. At this level not only is there a distribution of data into independent, mutually exclusive, and exhaustive categories; there is also a qualitative relationship between categories. For example, if 20 students in a class hand in a term paper and the professor rank-orders the papers from 1 (best) to 20 (worst), then not only are there 20 categories, but there is a better-than, poorer-than relationship between any two categories. In the same illustration, it is important to note that there is no equality of difference between categories; in other words, the best paper in the class may be much better than the second best, whereas there could be only a small difference between the second- and the third-best papers.

Clinicians use many ordinal scales. One example is the manual muscle test, where muscle strength is graded zero, trace, poor, fair, good, or normal, with possible subgrades denoted by + or − in between. Sometimes numbers are used in manual muscle testing; 1 to 5 or 0 to 100. However, we must not be deceived by this numbering system into thinking that there is the same difference between muscles graded 10 and 15 as there is between muscles graded 95 and 100. It is still an ordinal scale whose "scores" reflect greater-than or less-than relationships; there is no equality of difference between grades. Activities of daily living scales are another example of ordinal ranking. It is also important to note that the ordinal scale implies an underlying continuous gradation between minimum and maximum, whereas the categories in the nominal scale are discrete.

Many questionnaires, attitude scales, personality inventories, and other measurement tools use a Likert scale, which is generally a 5-point scale: for example, highly agree, 1; agree, 2; indifferent, 3; disagree, 4; and highly disagree, 5. These scales represent an underlying continuum of opinion broken into five subcategories. The same continuum could be broken into a limitless number of categories, or merely divided: agree or disagree. Not only is there no objective measure of difference between numbers 1 and 2; it is also possible that one person may highly agree and mark number 1, yet feel very differently from another person who also marks the questionnaire 1, highly agree. (A few writers say there are occasions when a Likert scale of measurement can be treated as interval data. For example, see Okolo in the references.)

It is important to note that in both nominal and ordinal measurement you cannot perform arithmetic operations (add, subtract, multiply, divide, square) on numbers associated with those scales; you can only count the responses in each rank. Most of the measures taken in the behavioral and social sciences, including education, are at the ordinal level of measurement. This fact is too frequently overlooked by researchers. The prevalence of ordinal measurement in occupational therapy assessment has been decried by Smith.[15]

Delitto and Rose[16] used an ordinal scale, the Visual Analog Scale, to measure pain and then rank-ordered their subjects' comfort levels according to the waveform used (waveform is nominal data). Dickstein and her associates[17] formed three independent groups, treated each group with a different exercise approach, and assessed the outcomes with four measures: (1) functional independence as measured by the Barthel index (ordinal); (2) muscle tone measured on a 5-point scale (ordinal); (3) isolated motor control on three measurement tools (range [metric], manual muscle testing [ordinal], and strain gauge [metric]); and (4) ambulatory status, measured on an ordinal scale.

METRIC MEASUREMENT

The **metric scale of measurement** has a very important characteristic; the distances between any two numbers on the scale are of known and equal size. With a constant unit of measurement it is possible to assign real numbers to our observations, and the data resulting from such measurement may be properly treated with arithmetical procedures. Thus, the difference between 3°C and 4°C is the same as the difference between 20°C and 21°C. Therapists use metric scales daily to measure time, length, distance, weight, and temperature. It should be noted that the same phenomena may be measured on more than one scale. For example, we may measure the strength of a muscle on the ordinal scale of manual muscle testing, or we may measure it on a metric scale using a strain gauge. Frequency counts are called "ordered discrete data" by some writers and considered to be continuous metric data when the number of possible values is high, for example, the number of steps walked may be valued in the hundreds.[18]

Metric measurement has generally been divided into two categories: the **interval scale** and the **ratio scale.** The difference between these two scales relates to a zero point. In the interval scale both the unit of measurement and the zero point are arbitrary. For example, consider the Fahrenheit and centigrade scales in measuring temperature. The unit of measurement is arbitrary; it is different between the two scales, yet both scales measure the same thing and they are equivalent to each other—there are formulae for translating one into the other. They are linearly related, but the size of the unit is arbitrary. Also, in both of these scales the zero point is arbitrary. In one scale, 0 has been arbitrarily defined as the freezing point, while on the other scale 0 is considerably below freezing. In the ratio scale, only the unit of measurement is arbitrary; there is an absolute zero. For example, in inches and centimeters the size of the unit is arbitrary although they measure the same thing. In both systems of measurement, 0 (no length) has the same value and is not arbitrary. On the interval scale, arithmetic may be applied to the differences between the numbers; in the ratio scale arithmetical operations may be applied to the numbers themselves. Perhaps the most important point is that one cannot form a ratio with interval data.

Dickstein (cited above) uses both metric and ordinal measures. Gose (cited above) uses metric measures of ROM, length of stay in hospital, and postoperative days, as well as the nominal measure of frequency of complications. Finally, Howard's data[19] on chronological and play ages of two groups of children are metric.

Differentiating Levels of Measurement

To summarize, nominal data have the property of identity; this scale identifies real differences between and among data and assigns numbers or symbols to events, objects, or people in order to *classify* them. Ordinal data have the property of identity and order; the data can be put in some kind of semiquantitative sequence. The ordinal scale assigns numbers or symbols to events, objects, or people in order to *rank* them. Metric data have the properties of identity, order, and additivity. That is, they are strictly quantitative and admit the arithmetic operations. The metric scales assign numbers to events, objects, or people in order to *quantify* them; absolute zero may (ratio) or may not (interval) be identifiable.

When we are measuring strength with metric data, it is on the interval scale because although there may be no exertion on the various mechanical devices, this does not necessarily mean that there is no contraction of the muscle; in other words, a 0 on the strain gauge or weights does not indicate absolute 0 in strength. The same is true for isokinetic devices.[20] On the other hand, when we are measuring how much weight a person can lift against gravity and it is expressed in terms of weight lifted rather than in terms of muscle strength, then we are using a ratio scale. It is possible that the person is not able to lift any weight at all against gravity; that is, a real zero point exists, regardless of muscular activity.

Most of the time it is not necessary to distinguish between interval and ratio data; therefore, throughout the rest of this book we will refer to three levels of measurement: nominal, ordinal, and metric. The level of measurement becomes quite important when we get to the process of data reduction and also when we consider hypothesis testing through statistical tools. The level of measurement is important both for descriptive and predictive statistics.

Parameters and Statistics

In the previous chapter we defined the population as all of the individuals to whom our study could reasonably refer, and we defined a sample as those individuals we are going to study who have been drawn from the population. It is clear that we intend to extrapolate what we find from the *sample* to the *population*. It is necessary to give these two definitions something of a mathematical slant in order to understand some of the important implications of levels of measurement.

When we are dealing with data collection—that is, with the measurement of observations—we can define a population as a collection of all potential observations identifiable by a set of rules. For example, the rules might state that our population is all ROMs we could potentially observe in adults who have rheumatoid arthritis. The sample, then, is a subset of actual observations or measurements taken from the population. A **parameter** is a measure computed for all potential observations in a population. For example, we speak of the mean or average age of all people in the United States. This arithmetic mean is a parameter of our population. We do not actually go out and measure it even though it exists. A *statistic* is a measure computed from actual observations on a sample; for example, if we take a sample of 1000 people from the population of the United States, and we ascertain their ages and derive an arithmetic mean, this arithmetic mean is a statistic. From that statistic we extrapolate the parameter for the population.

Many statistical tests and measures, such as mean, standard deviation, t-test, and F test (each of these terms will be defined more carefully later on), make a number of assumptions about the nature of the parameters of the population. For example, if you want to apply a t-test to a given sample of data, you can only do that legitimately if the parameters of the population from which your sample is drawn meet certain criteria, to be discussed in Chapter 8. These tests are therefore called **parametric.** Tests and measures that do not make those assumptions about the parameters of the population from which the sample is drawn are called **nonparametric** measures and statistics. Therefore, in general, all statistical descriptions or summaries of data and all statistical tests of hypotheses can be divided into parametric (those that make specific assumptions about the parameters of the population from which the sample is drawn) and nonparametric (those that do not make those assumptions).

Parametric statistics require metric measurement. Nonparametric statistics are appropriate for nominal and ordinal levels of measurement. As we explore different research designs in subsequent chapters, we will refer again and again to the appropriate parametric and nonparametric statistics and tests. Nonparametric tests are often very appropriate in clinical studies involving relatively small numbers of subjects, so they need to be understood by clinical researchers. Whenever you see these two terms, you should automatically think nominal and ordinal level of measurement for a nonparametric statistic, and metric level of measurement for a parametric statistic. Nonparametric statistics *can* be applied to metric data, although a considerable amount of information is discarded in the process. Applying parametric statistics to nonparametric data is a more controversial matter among researchers. Some say that it is frequently permissible; others disagree. No attempt is made to resolve this issue here, but students should be aware of the controversy when reading the literature. The conservative approach, however, is to use nonparametric tools for nominal and ordinal data and parametric tools for metric data. Parametric and nonparametric designs will be illustrated in Chapter 8.

Here are two examples. Witt and MacKinnon[21] state:

"We chose nonparametric correlation and statistical testing because we could not ensure that the underlying assumptions of the parametric analysis of variance for repeated measures would be upheld. We used an intact existing group of people from the respiratory health club and, therefore, did not have a random sample from a larger population. This group may not represent the larger population."

Deitz and colleagues[22] declare, "Because the assumptions for the use of parametric statistics were not met, the relationships were examined using Spearman's rank correlation coefficients." The Spearman is used with ordinal data.

Review Questions

1 Review the article by Giannini in Appendix C. What criterion measures are used? What levels of measurement are employed? What are their data? The answers to these questions are somewhat complex, so read carefully.

2 Review the article by Beattie in Appendix C. What criterion measures are used? What levels of measurement are employed? What are their data?

3 Classify the following data as (1) nominal, ordinal, or metric, and (2) appropriate for parametric or nonparametric statistical treatment.
   a Shoulder ROM measured by goniometry
   b Hamstring strength measured by strain gauge
   c Grades on an anatomy quiz
   d SAT scores of an entering therapy class
   e Diagnoses on a neurologic ward
   f Number of therapists in each state

Additional Readings

Ghiselli, EE, Campbell, JP, and Zedeck, S: Measurement Theory for the Behavioral Sciences. WH Freeman, San Francisco, 1981.

Rothstein, JM: Measurement in Physical Therapy. Churchill Livingstone, New York, 1985.

Drew, CJ and Hardman, ML: Designing and Conducting Behavioral Research. Pergamon Press, New York, 1985, Chapters 9 and 10.

References

1. Rothstein, JM: Measurement in Physical Therapy. Churchill Livingstone, New York, 1985, Chapter 1.
2. Gillette, N: The challenge of research in occupational therapy. AJOT 45:660, 1991.
3. Stevens, SS: On the theory of scales of measurement. Science 103(2684):677, 1946.
4. Hasselkus, BR and Safrit, MJ: Measurement in occupational therapy. AJOT 30:429, 1976.
5. Ibid.
6. Smith, RO: The science of occupational therapy assessment. OTJR 12:3, 1992.
7. Rothstein, op cit, p 47.
8. Hamilton, M: Lectures on the Methodology of Clinical Research, ed 2. Churchill Livingstone, London, 1974, p 124.
9. Stevens, op cit.
10. Gaito, J: Measurement scales and statistics: Resurgence of an old misconception. Psychol Bull 87:564, 1980.
11. Harrison, H and Kielhofner, G: Examining reliability and validity of the preschool play scale with handicapped children. AJOT 40:167, 1986.

12. Parham, D: Academic reward structures and occupational therapy faculty, Part 1: Characteristics of faculty. OTJ Res 5:83, 1985.
13. Neistadt, ME: Occupational therapy treatment goals for adults with developmental disabilities. AJOT 40:672, 1985.
14. Gose, JC: Continuous passive motion in the postoperative treatment of patients with total knee replacement. Phys Ther 67:39, 1987.
15. Smith, op cit.
16. Delitto, A and Rose, SJ: Comparative comfort of three waveforms used in electrically eliciting quadriceps femoris muscle contractions. Phys Ther 66:1704, 1986.
17. Dickstein, R, et al: Stroke rehabilitation: Three exercise therapy approaches. Phys Ther 66:1233, 1986.
18. Hulley, SB and Cummings, SR: Designing Clinical Research. Williams & Wilkins, Baltimore, 1988, p 33.
19. Howard, AC: Developmental play ages of physically abused and nonabused children. AJOT 40:691, 1986.
20. Rothstein, op cit, p 36.
21. Witt, PL and MacKinnon, J: Trager psychophysical integration: A method to improve chest mobility of patients with chronic lung disease. Phys Ther 66:214, 1986, p 216.
22. Deitz, JC, Crowe, TK, and Harris, SR: Relationship between infant neuromotor assessment and preschool motor measures. Phys Ther 67:14, 1987, p 15.

*The work of science is
to substitute facts for
appearances, and
demonstrations for
impressions.*

JOHN RUSKIN, *STONES
OF VENICE*

Reliability and Validity

Reliability

Reliability is most important when criterion measures and measurement tools are concerned. If a measuring tape is made of highly elastic
material, it will be highly unreliable as a measurement tool: for example,
every time you measure a table, you will get a different length. An accurate
measurement tool—that is, a *reliable* tool—will provide the same answer

67

every time. Hence, if a table is 3 feet wide, 100 different people should be able to measure it with the same tape measure and come out with exactly the same answer each time. Any variability in 100 such measurements should be attributable to human error rather than error in the measuring device. If the anatomy quiz is reliable, then the students should make exactly the same score on the quiz the second time they take it as they did the first time, assuming that they learn or forget nothing during the period between the two tests or learn nothing from taking the test the first time. If a personality test is reliable, then changes in scores over time should indicate a change in the personality. The less reliable the test, the less you can depend on the results as a guide to action.

By way of example, let us suppose that a marksman fires 100 rounds at a target. If every bullet hits the target, but in 100 different places scattered all over, the marksman's aim is valid (he did what he was supposed to do, i.e., hit the target) but not reliable. If all 100 bullets enter a circle 3 inches in diameter (the same as the bull's-eye), but that circle is in the upper left-hand corner of the target, the marksman's aim is reliable but not valid. If all 100 bullets enter the bull's-eye, the marksman's aim has both validity and reliability. The point here is that it is possible to have one without the other.

Three types of reliability are of interest in dealing with clinical measurements: intrarater reliability, interrater reliability, and the reliability of parallel forms.[1] A fourth type, internal consistency, is of interest mostly in educational and psychological paper-and-pencil tests.

Intrarater reliability tests the reliability of one rater in repeated measurements or the stability of a measure over time. If Jane Doe, therapist, is going to use any measurement tool to record patient progress, then measured variability should be true variance, not error variance in the tester or the instrument. So the rater needs to be reliable within ("intra") herself. If the rater is reliable, then tests of intrarater reliability will also tell us if the variable or characteristic being measured or the measurement tool itself is stable over time; that is, if there is variability and it is not in the rater, then it is either in the variable (characteristic) or the instrument. Repeated measures by the same rater can demonstrate those kinds of variability. If your purpose is to test a variable for stability, then you must deal with the possible compounding variable of time.

Interrater reliability refers to consistency of measurement between two or more raters. If more then one therapist is going to record data on a patient, or if you are to use a test on your patient because someone else has used it successfully, then it is important that all therapists concerned apply the tool consistently and reliably. Otherwise, the data are meaningless. Again, if time changes the variable, then interrater reliability data may be meaningless.

The **reliability of parallel forms** refers to obtaining the same results from two versions of the same test. It is especially important in paper-and-pencil tests such as the PES licensing examination, the SAT, personality tests, and so on. It could also be important if one were using two different activity of daily living (ADL) tests or manual muscle tests. The important question is this: Are the two forms equal (parallel) to each other? For example, Robinson and colleagues[2] studied

the test-retest reliability of lumbar isometric strength testing in patients with chronic low-back pain (CLBP).... Isometric torque measurements were obtained from 89 patients with CLBP at seven different angles of lumbar flexion. Because previous studies have demonstrated significant strength differences between male and female subjects, separate data analyses were performed for each gender. Results indicate moderate to high reliability for patients' idiosyncratic range of motion.

The statistics used to test for reliability, with additional examples, are explained in Chapter 6.

Bhasin and Goodman[3] studied both the validity and reliability of an assessment tool called the Occupational Therapy Functional Assessment Compilation Tool (OT FACT). Concerning the reliability of the tool they stated:

Open-ended responses on activity configurations of 25 patients with multiple sclerosis were coded using categories from the (OT FACT), Level II—Functional Activities of Performance.... The inter-rater reliability for the five occupational therapists who coded the responses was .89. When the same categories were used by patients to code responses, there was complete agreement between therapist and patient in 94% of the activities coded.

Again, the statistics are discussed in Chapter 6. For now, it is important simply to grasp the concept of reliability and validity. Harrison and Kielhofner[4] looked at interrater reliability, test-retest (intrarater) reliability, and concurrent validity of a scale to measure developmental level of several diagnostic categories of children at different age levels. DiFabio[5] studied the interrater and intrarater reliability of three trained examiners and a computerized analysis system in determining the onset of muscular activity. DiFabio found that the computer was the most reliable. The examiners were more consistent with each other than they were with the computer, and intrarater reliabilities were higher than the interrater scores.

STANDARD ERROR

In taking a measure—for example, the heights of 50 people—there are three sources of variability: real variance in actual heights of the subjects, error variance in the measurement tool, and error on the part of the one doing the measuring. If the real variance is considered representative of the normal population, there is the possibility of a third type of error— namely, **sampling error**—if the sample is not truly representative of the population. **Variance** is a measure of variability or real differences in a characteristic of a sample or population. A reliable measurement tool is one in which the variance due to error is small in comparison to the variance due to real differences in the objects measured. The best test for reliability is repeated measures of the same object with the same instrument. This is relatively easy to do with physical and some biological measures. It is much more difficult to do with psychological measures, where the subject may change as a result of the testing procedure.

If you took many measures of one person's height, you would get a distribution of measures. At a practical level the true height can be defined as the mean or average of all of the heights measured. The standard deviation of all of those measures is called the *standard error* of measurement. In 19 times out of 20, the true score will lie within two standard errors of the mean of the sample. Note that standard error of measurement refers to measurements taken from one individual. In evaluating individual scores one should take account of the standard error.

Sampling error is concerned with the error of measurements on different individuals. In evaluating group data one should take account of the sampling error. Sampling errors may be of two kinds: **random error** and **systematic error**. Random error is due to chance; one just accidently chooses a nonrepresentative sample. Most often random error results from selecting too small a sample. Systematic error is due to bias, either conscious or unconscious. For example, a sample drawn from only one hospital may create unconscious bias because of the demographics of the people served by that hospital. Errors of measurement may also suffer from random or systematic error. All errors are threats to either internal or external validity (discussed below), so minimizing error is a very important part of research design.

Validity

Validity refers to the appropriateness, truthfulness, authenticity, or effectiveness of a study. The purpose of this chapter is to expand on this fundamental definition and discuss some of its major implications.

Crocker[6] defined validity as "the extent to which measurements are useful for making decisions relevant to a given purpose." A test in anatomy has a certain validity if it gives a true indication of the student's knowledge of anatomy; it has a more important validity if it successfully predicts future use of the anatomical information. A personality test is valid if it accurately reflects the extent to which a person possesses certain characteristics and/or predicts future behavior. Validity is concerned with the appropriateness of inferences based on a particular measurement.[7] A measurement tool is never merely valid; it is valid for making a particular measurement. A ruler is a valid instrument for measuring length, distance, or circumference; it is not a valid instrument for measuring weight. In exactly the same sense, a research design is never valid in itself; it is only valid for testing a particular question or kind of question.

Questions of validity are first and foremost questions of logic and rationality; there are many instances when mathematical tools can be brought to the assistance of reason, but they can never be substituted for it. The question of validity can be attached to every single item on the research protocol in Appendix B. Is each question a valid one? Will its answer give me useful information of the type that I want or need? Given a valid question, are the data that I plan to collect valid for answering that question? Is the criterion measure suitable for answering the question? Is the measurement tool chosen appropriate to the criterion? Is the statistical tool appropriate to the level of measurement and to the way the question is phrased? If any point in the research protocol is invalid, then the entire study is in jeopardy.

Types of Test Validity

Test makers in the psychosocial sciences, particularly psychology and education, often speak of several different types of validity. These types include face; content and construct validities, which are more cognitive in nature; and concurrent and predictive validities, which are more experimental. Most of these validities are also most relevant to clinical measures used in physical and occupational therapy. Defining the validity of a measurement tool as the extent to which that tool measures what it claims to measure addresses only construct validity; other issues must be dealt with, especially the uses to which the measured data will be put.[8] Valid data are useful in that they enable the experimenter to make some true inferences about the data or the sample from the results of using the measurement instrument; we will relate this use to content and construct validity. Another measured use of validity data is the prediction of some aspects of behavior in situations other than the one in which the measurements were taken; we will relate to this purpose in the discussion of concurrent and predictive validity. In general, validity is determined by comparing performance on the tests to other objective and independently observable facts about the behavior of interest.

FACE VALIDITY

Face validity relates to the subject's acceptance of the test. In some ways it is the public relations aspect of test giving. Patients will sometimes resist taking a test if it does not "make sense to them," that is, if it does not appear to be related to something they can understand and accept. For example, compare the vital capacity test as a measure of lung function and the (now outdated) frog test as a measure of pregnancy. The first test has clear face validity; blowing into a tube and measuring the amount of air that one can expire in one breath is clearly related to lung function. Only an endocrinologist, however, could immediately understand the validity of injecting a sample of a woman's urine under a frog's skin as a test for pregnancy; it therefore had no face validity for the average person. Face validity can be important in winning a patient's cooperation in a testing situation. On the other hand, there are times when experimenters may not want any face validity in the test because they may wish to disguise the purpose of the test (e.g., a questionnaire) in order not to bias the subjects' answers. In choosing a test, therefore, some thought should be given to the validity of its appearance and to the usefulness of that appearance.

CONSTRUCT VALIDITY

Construct validity is related to content validity, but it is at the same time more abstract and more basic. All the other types of validity depend on construct validity. It addresses these questions: What does the score on this test mean or signify? What does it tell us about the person, object, event, or characteristic being measured? Rothstein[9] cites the example of manual muscle testing (MMT), which has lost its original construct validity. MMT was originally intended to test muscular weakness resulting from damage to the anterior horn cell in the spinal cord; the intellectual construct or principle (see Chapter 1) was a relationship between that damage and that weakness. Today, attempts to infer functional performance from MMT scores implies a very different construct or principle.

Construct validity is related to the concept of hypothetical constructs, which is discussed in Chapter 11. The presence of construct validity in a test grounds that test behavior in theory. Construct validity is particularly important when we are measuring concepts that cannot be examined directly but can only be inferred from behavior (hypothetical constructs). Examples include intelligence, spacial relationships, verbal reasoning, concept formation, motor abilities, strength, tone, endurance, coordination, and figure-ground differentiation. Operational definitions are especially critical when dealing with hypothetical constructs. Because it is tied so clearly to behavior, construct validity shades into the experimental validities that are discussed below.

Construct validity of a new instrument for the Posture and Fine Motor Assessment of Infants (PFMAI) was studied by Case-Smith[10]

through an evaluation of how accurately the PFMAI discriminated between the (25) premature subjects and the (65) full-term subjects. . . . PFMI accurately classified 78% of the subjects as being either premature or full-term. . . . These results indicate that the PFMAI has the adequate . . . validity necessary for use as a clinical and a research instrument.

Van Deusen and Harlowe[11] worked on the construct validity of a CVA evaluation tool by demonstrating a high degree of agreement between two rather disparate tests: Brunnstrom's arm and hand stages and scores on Schenkenberg's Line Bisection Test of unilateral neglect.

CONTENT VALIDITY

While construct validity defines what we wish to measure, **content validity** regulates the *sampling* of that construct. Content validity raises the question, Does this measure truly sample the behavior that I want to study? For example, does an ADL test sample the behaviors that I am interested in testing? Content validity may deal with content in the usual sense of factual information, or it may deal with process, such as manual dexterity. The scope of a given test should be proportional and comprehensive. For example, a comprehensive test in anatomy should have a proper proportion of questions dealing with gross anatomy, neuroanatomy, and histology.

CONCURRENT VALIDITY

Concurrent validity refers to the relationship between test scores (or other measures) and either "criterion states" or measurements whose validity is known. The word "concurrent" implies clearly that this relationship exists at approximately the same time a test is given. We discussed criterion measures in Chapter 3. Here criterion refers to an external standard that is either met or not met. For example, either students can correctly test the strength of the biceps muscle or they cannot; if the paper-and-pencil functional anatomy test is concurrently valid for that criterion, then those students who pass the anatomy test can *at the same time* meet the criterion of strength testing. Concurrently valid tests imply that anyone who passes this test will be able to do this other thing *right now.* Either the two are comparable or they are not. Tests of concurrent validity express the extent to which one is comparable to the other.

Most frequently, concurrent validation is used to establish the validity of a new test in comparison to an older test for which the validity is known. For example, a new IQ test that is quick and inexpensive could be compared to the well-established Stanford-Binet or Wechsler-Bellevue tests. A paper-and-pencil personality test could be compared to the Rorschach inkblot test; the Bennett manual dexterity test could be compared to a current job performance test.

Concurrent validity may sometimes be used as a stepping stone to the development of predictive validity. If George's score on the Bennett manual dexterity test is comparable to his score on the Barthel index of ADL functioning (concurrent), can we predict that George will become more functionally independent at home as his dexterity scores increase (predictive)?

Earlier in this chapter we reviewed the reliability of the OT FACT assessment tool, as reported by Bhasin and Goodman. Let us now look at their test of concurrent validity for the same tool.

In a separate study of eight patients, 86 percent of the OT FACT categories reported on a "typical day" were also reported 10 days later when an "actual day" was recorded. These findings indicate that the OT FACT categories were a reliable and valid tool for coding activity configurations of patients with multiple sclerosis.[12]

The "what I actually did on one day" and "what I usually do" data were considered as parallel data sets. Since they were very similar (86 percent agreement) the actual data were interpreted to be concurrent validation for the more general data from the assessment tool. Percentage was the statistic used.

Earlier in this chapter we looked at a study by Case-Smith and her work on the construct validity of the PFMAI. In her study, Case-Smith[13] observed:

Concurrent validity was investigated through administration of the Peabody Developmental Motor Scales . . . and the PFMAI ($n = 25$). Strong positive correlations resulted between the Peabody Gross Motor scale and PFMAI Posture scale and between the Peabody Fine Motor scale and PFMAI Fine Motor scale. Concurrent validity was also measured through correlation scores on the Bayley Scales of Infant Development . . . with scores on the PFMAI.

Results supported the validity of the new test (PFMAI) by comparing it to the widely accepted Peabody test.

Bundy and coworkers[14] tested the concurrent validity of six measures of equilibrium, including the Bruininks-Oseretsky Balance subtest, the tilt board tip, and parts of the Southern California Sensory Integration Test. They found that the tests were not comparable, in other words, they measure different things and are not, therefore, concurrently valid. Such information is important. It is not really negative information, but it does say that these tests measure different things.

By contrast, Agnew and Maas[15] demonstrated concurrent validity between an expensive instrument and one that is readily available in most clinics. Two instruments for measuring grip strength, the Jamar dynamometer and an adapted sphygmomanometer, were compared in 88 subjects with rheumatoid arthritis. Correlations of 0.83 for the right hand and 0.84 for the left hand were found between instrument measurements. Because these correlations were found to be high and linear, regression tables for predicting grip strength from one instrument to the other were provided. As norms for the Jamar dynamometer already exist, clinicians and researchers now have a standard for comparing patients and subjects and the normal population for grip strength.

PREDICTIVE VALIDITY

Predictive validity is a future-oriented prediction based on a measure made today. Does the score on the ADL test today predict the patient's future functional ability? Predictive validity is also criterion-related—that is, it is related to outside objective criteria or direct measures of performance. As in the discussion of criterion measures in Chapter 3, it is important to be sure that the criterion to which the test is correlated is the correct one. If a test or measure is predictively valid, then we can say that people who do well on this test have a high probability of later achievement in a given area. This does not carry any sense of causality, but only of association. (We will consider association and causation further in Chapter 6.) For example, students with scores above a certain level on the Graduate Record Examination (GRE) are much more likely to be successful in graduate school than those with lower scores.

Examples from the literature follow. Anacker and DiFabio[16] studied 47 community-dwelling elders between the ages of 65 and 96 years.

Subjects with two or more falls in the 6 months prior to study were assigned to a fall group ($n = 16$), whereas those with no history of falling during the same time interval were assigned to a no-fall group ($n = 31$). In order to remove any bias in the testing procedure, the tester was not aware of group assignments. Subjects were evaluated using a sensory organization test (SOT) for standing balance and a "get up and go" test (GUGT) for general mobility.... [Results indicated that] the SOT and GUGT may be useful [i.e., predictive] in the field to establish criteria for screening elders in a fall-prevention program.

Youdas and colleagues[17] "retrospectively examined the intertester reliability and predictive validity of judgments made by an admissions committee." These judgments were based on applicant essays, and predictions were made about the applicants' future success in a physical therapy academic program. Six members of the admissions committee and 52 student records were involved in this study. They concluded that the essay evaluations were not reliable and that the essays were not valid for predicting future success in physical therapy school. Such negative information is useful in that they can discard or change the essay and look for more useful information for the admissions process.

The purposes of a study by Titus and colleagues[18] were

(a) to determine to what extent a sample of 25 stroke patients would differ from normative samples on perceptual abilities, (b) to explore relationships between particular perceptual tests and performance of daily living tasks with the use of a comprehensive battery of standardized tests available to occupational therapists, and (c) to evaluate and compare the effectiveness of these assessments in identifying the deficits and abilities of this sample.

They concluded that six of the nine tests they administered were useful in predicting perceptual performance.

Internal and External Validity

In discussing internal and external validity in research design, most writers refer to Campbell and Stanley[19] as the standard text on this subject. According to Campbell and Stanley, internal validity is an absolutely minimum requirement without which the experiment cannot be interpreted. **Internal validity** refers to the relationship between the independent variables (the "treatment" you are studying) and the dependent variable (what you measure to see if the treatment made any difference). A study is *internally valid* when the differences that are measured in the dependent variable are accounted for by differences in the independent variables. Any threat to internal validity represents a loss of control over that relationship and a resultant loss of technical soundness in the study. The major means of maintaining internal validity are the controls discussed in Chapter 2. Threats to internal validity are threats to the conclusion that any change demonstrated in the dependent variable is accounted for by changes in the independent variable. A study has high internal validity when all factors that might influence the dependent variable are controlled except the variables under study.

External validity is concerned with generalization from the sample to the population; therefore, methods of sampling are crucial. The more externally valid the study, the more safely one can make predictive statements about the population on the basis of the results of the study. Hulley and colleagues[20] have likened internal and external validity to the physiology of a study and the structure or design of the study to its anatomy. Each is dependent on the other for the integrity of the whole.

THREATS TO INTERNAL VALIDITY

Campbell and Stanley[19] discussed eight threats to internal validity: history, maturation, repeat testing, instrumentation, statistical regression, sampling bias, experimental mortality, and selection interaction. Let us discuss each one of these briefly. The reader may need to return to this section after having mastered the basic designs discussed in Chapters 5 through 9.

History

History refers to the passage of time and/or concurrent experience that can change the outcome of a study. Several designs are particularly vulnerable to this problem: the before-and-after measurement design, repeated measures, and the time series designs. For example, if you use the before-and-after test design with no controls and you say that the patients got better as a result of your treatment, it could be that the natural history of the disease, not the treatment, caused them to get better, or that mere passage of time may have produced the changes seen. On the other hand, developmental studies are so designed that history *is* the independent variable.

Maturation

Maturation is a special form of history. In addition to age, it includes things like growing wiser or growing more tired. When dealing with human subjects and affective materials, even something as minor as a good or bad weekend experience may be a maturation experience that confounds your variables if your before-and-after tests are done on Friday and Monday. The two major controls for history and maturation are randomization and control groups. Control groups are particularly powerful against these two threats to internal validity. Randomization takes care of systematic influences by spreading the influences of history and maturation equally among all groups. In the time series design, the A-B-A-B design (see Chapter 7) is intended to help control for the variable of maturation or history.

Repeat Testing

Repeat testing is, obviously, a primary threat in repeated measures designs. People may learn something from the test-taking experience itself that enables them to get a better score when taking the test the second time, even though there has been no improvement in the characteristic being measured. The effects of learning how to do the test could easily influence the results when one is using manual muscle, vital capacity, and ADL tests. It may make sense to let your subjects practice a strain gauge or an unfamiliar functional test until they learn how to do it, and then ask for their maximum effort.

Instrumentation

Instrumentation refers to changes in calibration. Some instruments such as electromyogram (EMG) machines must be calibrated every time they are turned on. The same threat is present with observational measures if the observers change the way in which they observe and record their observations. This is a common source of internal invalidity when judgment on the part of the observer or subject is required, as in the analog pain scale or in MMT. Human observers are much more likely to get out of calibration than are mechanical contrivances or instruments. One useful control for this problem is replication—measuring several times and then averaging the results. Using multiple observers also provides another available control if one is dealing with human, rather than mechanical, measuring instruments. When human observers are rating data that has already been collected, an approach to dealing with rater bias is to shuffle the before-and-after test data so that the observer does not know where the data came from and therefore will not be biased.

Statistical Regression

Statistical regression is particularly threatening when groups have been formed on the basis of extreme scores. Regression here means movement toward the average or mean; it is likely to happen in repeated measures to those individuals who have atypically high or low scores on the first testing. For example, one might establish two experimental groups where one group is, by definition, individuals who score high on an IQ test and the second group is individuals who fall in the middle range of an IQ test. Statistical regression would almost guarantee in this case that the subjects with the extreme score would regress toward the middle on subsequent testing. In such cases changes on the second test are the result of statistical regression toward the mean rather than actual change in behavior.

Sampling Bias

Bias results from differential selection of group members. In true experimental designs, a sample is drawn from the population and individuals are randomly assigned to groups. However, in quasi-experimental designs it is often not possible to do this, and the groups are formed in some other way. For example, groups may be based on preexisting conditions, such as two therapy classes, designated as an experimental group and a control group. Under these conditions it is likely that bias has been introduced into the research. The same might be true if a certain ward in a hospital is designated as an experimental group and another ward as the control group. One way of dealing with this threat is to use matched pairs. However, as we have seen earlier, this is not always an effective method of control since it can introduce biases of its own. The Hawthorne effect, discussed in Chapter 7, might also be considered a threat to internal validity because the experimental group is made to feel special, and that perception alters their responses.

Experimental Mortality

Experimental mortality refers to a differential loss of subjects from the groups. Mortality here means dropping out of the experiment. Subjects may fail to show up the day that you are doing testing, and it may be that some extraneous factor is operating to differentially select the subjects who drop out of the study, for example, those who must use public transportation because they cannot afford a private car. This extraneous bias may influence your results. In discussing questionnaires and surveys in Chapter 5 we will see that subjects may differentially drop out of your study on the basis of their reaction to your questions. Follow-up investigations are particularly threatened by this problem.

Selection Interaction

Selection interaction is most likely to occur when there is no control group or when the control group is not equivalent to the experimental group. In such cases the factors that led to selection of the experimental group may interact with maturation or history or testing; this interaction, rather than your treatment, may cause change. For example, the experimental group is the junior occupational therapy class, the control group is the senior occupational therapy class. The dependent variable is a perceptual motor test administered repeatedly using a before-and-after test design. The independent variable could be training in a novel motor task. A greater improvement in the junior class could be attributed to an interaction between the selection process (junior versus senior) and maturation (the seniors have already completed the junior curriculum, which includes instruction in perceptual-motor disabilities). Training in the novel motor task may thus be biased between the two groups.

THREATS TO EXTERNAL VALIDITY

Campbell and Stanley[19] list four threats to external validity: reactive or interaction effects of testing, interaction effects of selection biases, experimental arrangement, and multiple treatment interference. Remember that according to our definition of external validity, these are threats to the representativeness of your sample, which in turn threatens the validity of inference or prediction to population characteristics or behavior.

Interaction Effects of Testing

Interaction effects of testing are related to the internal threat of repeat testing. However, here we are considering the possibility that in the process of taking and reacting to the tests, the sample may become different in some important way from the population which it is supposed to represent. This would be likely to occur when the test instrument is something that the subject must practice in order to give a reliable score. An example is vocational testing. This factor should always be considered when an experimenter is interpreting the results and projecting those results onto the population.

Interactive Effects of Selection Biases and Experimental Arrangement

These external threats are not often encountered in PT and OT research. They are, however, sometimes a problem in certain areas of psychological research. For example, there might be an interaction between the criteria for admission to a study and the treatment; subjects of the personality type chosen may respond differently to the treatment than the general population. In the second instance, the physical arrangement of the examination room may change some subjects' normal responses to psychological questions.

Multiple Treatment Inference

This threat to external validity refers to designs with more than one experimental or independent variable. In such cases the interaction between the experimental variables can confuse the results. For example, if you used two treatments and the subjects get better, what accounted for the results: treatment A, treatment B, or their interaction?

No experiment is ever so perfect that each internal and external threat to validity is totally avoided. In fact, quite frequently external validity and internal validity war against one another, and the researcher has to make trade-offs between the two in order to get the most feasible arrangement. At one point in the research, the experimenter may wish to emphasize the precision of the results and may therefore sacrifice some degree of external validity. For example, the population and sample may be so narrowly defined that not many clients are included—but it would strengthen the conclusions for *that* population. At another point in the study the researcher may wish to emphasize the applications of the experiment to the world beyond the laboratory and may therefore make some sacrifices of internal validity in order to achieve more predictability. For example, treatment may be a composite of methods and modalities. It helps a large number of clients but does not clarify the contribution of each component of the treatment. The researcher is faced with the practical decision of doing nothing because it cannot be done perfectly, or doing the best he or she can within the confines of the environment in which the research must be done. Again, practicality and careful thinking about what it is you are trying to accomplish are keys to good research.

Using Correlation Coefficients

Rothstein[21] has observed that "unless measurements are shown to be valid and reliable they do not yield *information,* but rather numbers or categories that give a false impression of meaningfulness." The primary tool for establishing both validity and reliability of tests and measurement tools is the technique of correlation, which is discussed in Chapter 6. Validity and reliability data are published and reported in the form of correlation coefficients, which vary between $+1.0$ and -1.0. These validity and reliability coefficients are given the same interpretation as are other correlation scores, as discussed in Chapter 6. Suffice it to say that the closer the validity or reliability coefficient is to $+1.0$, the more reliable and more valid is the instrument. We are speaking now of reliability, concurrent validity, and predictive validity. Content and construct validity are more frequently established descriptively by panels of appropriate experts. The same is true of the validity and reliability of research questions and research designs; these are established primarily by rational thinking.

You will probably never see a reliability or validity coefficient for any test exactly at the $+1.0$ level. On the other hand, if validity and reliability data fall below $+0.5$, one should be cautious about the interpretation of measurement results. As Bundy and colleagues[14] pointed out, low correlation coefficients indicated that the tests measured different things. Whether a coefficient between $+0.5$ and $+1.0$ is acceptable or not depends on what you are going to do with the data. The more important the decision, the higher validity and reliability should be.

Validity and reliability data of measurement tools have seldom been reported in journal articles in the past. One reason is space limitations. A second reason is that the writer frequently makes assumptions about the sophistication of the reader: if readers are truly interested in the material being reported, either they are already familiar with the measurement tools or will make the effort to become so. Writers should, as a minimum, give references to the test manual or other validity and reliability information; then readers not already familiar with the measurement tool can look up the relevant data. Most psychological tests have test manuals that describe the sample on which the test was validated, the population to which that sample belonged, the number of people involved, and the exact procedures used for establishing the validity and reliability coefficients, which are reported in tables in the manual. The situation has changed in recent years. Some journals, like *Physical Therapy,* are beginning to require statements about the validity and reliability of measurements. Look at Gianinni, paragraphs 13 through 17, in Appendix C. What kinds of data do they provide concerning reliability and validity? What types of reliability and validity do they work with?

For validity and reliability data on hundreds of different psychological, vocational, aptitude, and interest tests, see Buros.[22]

Review Questions

1 Reread the article by Gianinni in Appendix C. If you were going to replicate their study, what would you identify as your controls against internal invalidity? What controls might you establish for assuring the validity and reliability of the dependent variables?

2 As you proceed through the rest of this book, if you do all the review questions and work suggested, you will write several research protocols. As you do each one, try to identify any potential threats to internal and external validity. Ask yourself the following questions: What is the validity and reliability of your dependent variable? On what evidence do you know this? If you feel that you are lacking information on the reliability and validity of your criterion measure, how could you find information about it? Return to this question again after you have read Chapter 10.

Additional Readings

Bulpitt, CJ: Randomised Controlled Clinical Trials. Martinus Nijhoff, Boston, 1983, Chapters 5 and 9.

Campbell, DT and Stanley, JC: Experimental and Quasi-Experimental Designs for Research. Rand McNally, Chicago, 1963.

Ghiselli, EE, Campbell, JP, and Zedeck, S: Measurement Theory for the Behavioral Sciences. WH Freeman, San Francisco, 1981.

Goldstein, G: A Clinician's Guide to Research Design. Nelson-Hall, Chicago, 1980, Chapter 6.

Kerlinger, FN: Foundations of Behavioral Research, ed 2. Holt, Rinehart & Winston, New York, 1973.

Rothstein, JM: Measurement in Physical Therapy. Churchill Livingstone, New York, 1985, Chapter 1.

References

1. Rothstein, JM: Measurement in Physical Therapy. Churchill Livingstone, New York, 1985, Chapter 1.
2. Robinson, ME, et al: Reliability of lumbar isometric torque in patients with chronic low back pain. Phys Ther 72:186, 1992.
3. Bhasin, CA and Goodman, GD: The use of OT FACT categories to analyze activity configurations of individuals with multiple sclerosis. OTJR 12:67, 1992, p 67.
4. Harrison, H and Kielhofner, G: Examining reliability and validity of the Preschool Play Scale with handicapped children. AJOT 40:167, 1986.
5. DiFabio, RP: Reliability of computerized surface electromyography for determining the onset of muscle activity. Phys Ther 67:43, 1987.
6. Crocker, LM: Validity of criterion measures for occupational therapists. AJOT 30:229, 1976.
7. American Psychological Association: Standards for Educational and Psychological Tests. Washington, DC, 1974.
8. Sim, J and Arnell, P: Measurement validity in physical therapy research. Phys Ther 17:102, 1993.
9. Rothstein, op cit, p 19.
10. Case-Smith, J: A validity study of the Posture and Fine Motor Assessment of Infants. AJOT 46:597, 1992.
11. Van Deusen, J and Harlow, D: Continued construct validation of the St. Marys CVA evaluation: Brunnstrom arm and hand stage ratings. AJOT 40:561, 1986.
12. Bhasin, CA and Goodman, GD, op cit, p 67.
13. Case-Smith, J, op cit, p 597.
14. Bundy, AC, et al: Concurrent validity of equilibrium tests in boys with learning disabilities with and without vestibular dysfunction. AJOT 41:28, 1987.
15. Agnew, PJ and Maas, F: Jamar dynamometer and adapted sphygmomanometer for measuring grip strength in patients with rheumatoid arthritis. OTJR 11:259, 1991.
16. Anacker, SL and DiFabio, RP: Influence of sensory inputs on standing balance in community-dwelling elders with a recent history of falling. Phys Ther 72:575, 1992.
17. Youdas, JW, et al: Reliability and validity of judgments of applicant essays as a predictor of academic success in an entry-level physical therapy education program. JPTEd 6:15, 1992.
18. Titus, MND, et al: Correlation of perceptual performance and activities of daily living in stroke patients. AJOT 45:410, 1991.
19. Campbell, DT and Stanley, JC: Experimental and Quasi-Experimental Designs for Research. Rand-McNally, Chicago, 1963.
20. Hulley, SB, Newman, TB, and Cummings, SR: Getting started: The anatomy and physiology of research. In Hulley, SB, and Cummings, SR (eds): Designing Clinical Research. Williams & Wilkins, Baltimore, 1988.
21. Rothstein, op cit, p 2.
22. Buros, OK: Mental Measurements Yearbook. Gryphon Press, Highland Park, NJ, 1972.

*People in general have
no notion of the sort
and amount of evidence
often needed to prove
the simpliest matter of
fact.*

PETER M. LATHAM

Descriptive Research

OBJECTIVES

1   Define and illustrate each of the following descriptive
    research designs: qualitative, nominal, normative, historical,
    developmental, meta-analysis.

2   State at least one method for implementing each design
    above.

3   Identify and evaluate descriptive designs and methods in
    given studies.

4   Describe characteristics and uses of case study, intensive
    case study, and survey.

5   Identify major statistical concepts and methods used to
    summarize descriptive data.

6   Critique major methods of descriptive research.

Before we go any further into the analysis of descriptive, correlational,
and predictive research, let me suggest an overriding concept that the
student may profitably trace throughout this and the next several chapters.
It is the concept of the sequential development of a body of knowledge
through the sequential use of research types and designs. If nothing or
almost nothing is known about a topic, a general sequence of research
design proceeding from descriptive to correlational to predictive will be

efficient in developing reliable information. Descriptive research often proceeds from its qualitative or nominal forms to its normative forms; predictive research often proceeds from simple to complex designs and from nominal to ratio levels of measurement. This progression also relates to the development of theory discussed in Chapter 11.

The concept of sequence and progression within research designs is a general one and obviously there will be significant variations from one topic to another depending on many details of the nature of the topic and the level and reliability of what is already known. Nevertheless, it is suggested that the student keep this general sequence in mind as the particulars of each type and design are mastered. Content experts within the several practice areas in occupational and physical therapy should be able to help students to define where the techniques and theories within their area of expertise currently stand in relation to the sequence discussed above.

Definition

One of the major purposes of descriptive research is to discover some of the essential characteristics of a particular population as it exists in nature (in situ). It is assumed that this information is not readily available, and therefore the researcher needs to take a controlled look at a representative sample of the population in order to observe and describe what is there. Chapter 2 gives an overview of the nature of descriptive research. The student might be well served to review that portion of Chapter 2 now.

Another major function of descriptive research, which flows from the first purpose, is to provide some facts on which to base reasonable hypotheses for experimental research. Descriptive research provides a firm foundation for building new knowledge in almost any area of interest. All of the sciences that are today characterized by highly sophisticated experimental research began at some time in history with a simple and careful description of natural phenomena. Descriptive research begins the process of changing impressions into measurement and observations and interpretations into data.[1] The therapies are in need of a great deal of descriptive information on which to base useful hypotheses regarding the effectiveness of clinical practice.

The following are examples of descriptive questions.

- What topics in continuing education programs would therapists in Georgia like to see presented?

- How do people with spinal cord injuries feel about traveling in public in wheelchairs?

- What percentage of the patients admitted to hospitals in this state are referred to physical and occupational therapy?
- How was this unusual rheumatoid arthritic patient treated in this department, and what were the results?
- What were the most frequently used therapeutic modalities in the therapy clinics of stateside army hospitals during World War II?
- What is the typical sequence of events in the development of contractures in clients with juvenile rheumatoid arthritis from the first diagnosis of the disease to age 25?

Each of these questions is representative of one of the subclasses of descriptive research.

Two major methods for all subclasses of descriptive research are the survey and the case study. Survey tools include questionnaires and interviews, rating scales, and check lists. In looking at descriptive research, we will concentrate more on methods or tools than on designs. Descriptive studies *may* be organized so that some of the features of the classical designs discussed in Chapters 8 and 9 are visible in the study, but it is not necessary.

In "pure" descriptive research, nature assigns the treatment. However, many useful descriptive studies have *some* of the elements of predictive research, especially the manipulation of independent variables. Such studies are still within the realm of descriptive research because of what is done with the data. This point is often confusing to the beginning student. A given study may have elements of descriptive, correlational, and predictive research in it and be considered as predominantly one type, or one article may even be classified as all three.

Subclasses of Descriptive Research

QUALITATIVE RESEARCH

Let us start with a method that concentrates primarily on people and the meanings they attach to or derive from their experiences. According to Leiniger,[2] "the prevailing quantitative type of research ... reflects logical positivism and an emphasis on studying people as reducible to measurable objects independent of historical, cultural and social contexts" Conversely, the primary purpose of qualitative research is to study people, individually or collectively, *in their socialcultural context.* "Health and illness states are embedded in the cultural values, religious views, economic conditions, and social environments of human expressions. Indeed, the real meaning and quality of life, health, and care are best known from a holistic and social structure frame of reference."[3] The approach is holistic or gestaltic and puts an emphasis on the totality of experience and the *meaning* of that experience, such as health, illness, or permanent impairment, to people. Qualitative research has been called *holistic-inductive* because it is interested in rich verbal descriptions of people and phenomena that are based on direct observation. This is compared to **hypothetico-deductive research**, which places an emphasis on quantitative deductions based on data gathered in response to a specific hypothesis.[4] As Parse and colleagues[5] note, "the qualitative approach offers the researcher the opportunity to study the emergence of patterns in the whole configuration of man's lived experiences. It is an approach in which the researcher explicitly participates in uncovering the meaning of these experiences as humanly lived."

Qualitative research is a type of descriptive research; its methodological tools include philosophical analysis, grounded theory, ethnography, historical methods, participant observation, ethnoscience, life history and worldview approaches, and phenomenology.[6] Merrill[7] has suggested that ethnography and life histories are two qualitative methods of particular use in therapy. These methods are adapted from anthropology and psychology. Perhaps the most famous ethnographer known to most of us is the cultural anthropologist Margaret Mead. A classic in the field of qualitative research in psychology is Barker's study of a typical boy.[8] Examples of qualitative research have become common in the occupational therapy literature in recent years; it is less common in physical therapy.[8a] Krefting[9] has recently discussed the need for rigor in qualitative research in occupational therapy. Based on a review of literature she recommends four criteria for assessing qualitative research: true value, applicability, consistency, and neutrality. She then provides a good summary of strategies for increasing the trustworthiness of qualitative studies found in textbooks on methodology.

In a recent text, Strauss and Corbin[10] defined grounded theory research as a process of building theory "that is inductively derived from the study of the phenomenon it represents." Strauss and Corbin stress the *qualitative* analysis of data, and their data most often consists of pages and pages of narrative field notes, which are rich in detail, rather than data sets of measures of a few phenomena. Theory is discussed in detail in Chapter 11.

As an example of grounded theory research, Pierce[11] did a study whose purpose was

to generate a grounded theory of early object rule acquisition. The grounded theory approach and computer coding were used to analyze videotaped samples of an infant's and a toddler's independent object play, which produced the categories descriptive of three primary types of object rules: rules of object properties, rules of object action and rules of object affect. This occupational science theory offers potential for understanding the role of objects in human occupations, for development of instruments, and for applications in occupational therapy early intervention.

"In ethnographic description the researcher tries to render a 'true to life' picture of what people say and how they act; peoples words and actions are left to speak for themselves."[12] Such descriptive studies are often called "thick descriptions" and may be book-length reports or doctoral dissertations (see Barker[13] or Bogdan, Brown, and Foster[14]). Huttlinger and colleagues[15] have described an ethnographic study of

chronic diabetes among the Navajo people.... It focuses on the dominant metaphorical images that were used by the informants to describe their illness experiences. The data suggest that diabetes can be considered a metaphor for larger social changes in the life-style and traditions (e.g., away from sheepherding as a means of basic subsistence to obtaining urban-centered employment) of native Americans and their effects on the [Navajo]. Implications of our findings include the importance of metaphorical communication for perceptions of compliance, powerlessness, and patient and therapist satisfaction with the therapeutic relationship.

The interested reader may also want to see Krefting[16] and the March 1991 issue of the *American Journal of Occupational Therapy*.[17]

DeMars[18] has provided an interesting example of the use of information derived from ethnographic field research to improve practice. She used psychosocial clinical interviewing skills, principles of group dynamics, and "ethnographic interviewing techniques based on participant observation" to facilitate and revise a leisure skills and career development curriculum and a health promotion program for Native Americans.

Jensen and colleagues[19] reported a qualitative study whose purpose

was to further investigate the work of master and novice clinicians within the practice setting. The sample consisted of three master clinicians and three novice clinicians practicing in orthopedic outpatient physical therapy settings in three different regions of the United States. Data collection by three researchers included observation of each clinician treating at least three patients, audiotaping of all treatment sessions, interviews with clinicians and patients, and a review of patient records. Analysis of the data within and across cases revealed five attribute dimensions that distinguished the master clinician from the novice clinician. One attribute dimension [i.e., confidence in predicting patient outcomes] related to knowledge, and four attribute dimensions [i.e., ability to control the environment, evaluation and use of patient illness and disease data, focus of verbal and nonverbal communications with patients, and importance of teaching to hands-on care] related to improvisational performance. Further investigations are needed to confirm these findings and add to the body of knowledge concerning the parameters of physical therapy that may affect the efficacy and quality of patient care.

Note the relatively rare design element of three researchers in three locations.

In another example, which uses both ethnography and grounded theory, Yarbrough[20] did a study of the physical therapy department in a large metropolitan hospital. She worked in the department as a participant observer for several months and took copious field notes of activities and interpersonal interactions of the staff. She refined her questions and the concepts she wanted to study in response to what she saw and heard in the field. She also did some structured and semistructured interviews of people in the hospital who interacted with the therapists. Thus the concepts she studied were "grounded" in the observations made during the field experience.[21] The results are a detailed description of the hopes, attitudes, frustrations, values, frame of reference, and problems of a group of physical therapists and how others perceived them.

Life histories are another approach to qualitative research. Merrill[22] described a study she did on the life histories of four adolescents, two with juvenile rheumatoid arthritis. Data analysis was ongoing; in this it resembles clinical problem solving, as described in an earlier chapter. She collected approximately 100 pages of data on each subject, based on 10 to 14 hours of observation over a 2-week period and two intensive interviews. The data were summarized as case studies. Validity and reliability were established through a method called triangulation; that is, the data are confirmed by (i.e., triangulated with) at least two different methods of data collection, in this case through interview, time log, and observation. From the study Merrill developed 17 questions of importance to occupational therapy in the management of adolescents with juvenile rheumatoid arthritis.

Another qualitative technique is called **constant comparative analysis**. Taylor and Bogdan[23] describe this as a technique in which the researcher simultaneously codes and analyzes data *in order to develop concepts*. Niehues and colleagues[24] used constant comparative analysis to explore the nature of occupational therapy practice in the public schools.

Five expert school system practitioners participated in open-ended, in-depth interviews conducted by the principal investigator. These occupational therapists were asked to narrate a situation from their practice when they felt their interventions had made significant differences for students and in students' abilities to learn in school. Transcripts from the narrative interviews were analyzed for thematic content using a method of constant comparative analysis.... Three major themes emerged from this analysis: reframing, untold stories and situatedness, and ambivalence and paradox. The results of this study describe the practice of expert occupational therapists in public schools from a unique perspective. They also provide some insights into the ways in which educationally related occupational therapy services developed over time.

For another example of constant comparative analysis, see Llewellyn.[25] Mulcahey[26] has used a phenomenological appraoch "to explore the experience of returning to school following a spinal cord injury." Hasselkus[27] used participant observation to study the meaning of daily routines and activities to people with Alzheimer disease in an adult day-care center.

Somewhat surprisingly, computer programs are beginning to be developed by individual researchers to help in the analysis of qualitative data. Commercial software companies have yet to venture into this area, but individuals have developed packages for their own use and then offered them to others. Ten such programs are reviewed by Tesch.[28]

This has been a brief introduction to a methodology about which books have been written. The interested reader should pursue the additional readings and references listed at the end of the chapter. Can you think of some general topics in the "culture of disability" that could profitably be approached in an qualitative way? Such studies could lead to more specific questions, which could be answered through more traditional methods. The results could lead to the development of concepts and principles for improving the care of our patients.

NOMINAL DESCRIPTIVE RESEARCH

Nominal descriptive research (often called a case study) is the most general approach to controlled observation. It is appropriate when you know almost nothing about the topic of interest—when you do not know enough about the topic to ask more specific and answerable questions and when your sample is extremely small (usually one). The population for your sample may or may not be clearly defined in the beginning. The usual technique is to identify an interesting subject and the answerable questions that intrigue you about that individual or situation. The researcher then makes one or several preplanned observations of that sample. These observations are preplanned because you know what you are looking for, how you are going to look for it, and how you are going to record your observations. The latter includes an identification of the level of measurement and the measurement tool you are going to use. In some instances the only tools used in case studies are direct observation or interview; in that instance the case study technique resembles qualitative methods discussed earlier. For an example of a qualitative study of one case, see Dyck.[29] In other instances case studies report typical clinical measures such as range of motion, gait pattern, activities of daily living, or prevocational skills. Examples will be cited below.

A case study describes an interesting chain of events. Let us say, by way of example, that you have a patient who has a rare disease or an unusual injury about which you know very little. A survey of the literature, including standard textbooks, elicits very little additional meaningful information. Therefore, you decide to institute a nominal descriptive research project using the case study method. These are some possible research questions.

- What are the distinctive characteristics or the distinctive manifestations of this disease or injury as exemplified in this one patient?

- What are the functional outcomes of a specific treatment in this case?

You begin by observing the patient carefully and making notes (both mentally and in writing) of the patient's behavior, atypical as well as typical. You may note that sometimes the patient can maintain independent sitting balance and at other times she cannot. You may decide to begin to measure the patient's ability to sit independently by doing a frequency count of the number of times she can maintain balance when she is placed in the sitting position, and the number of times she does not. After a while you may decide to refine that observation by a metric measure of the number of seconds that she remained in independent sitting balance when placed in that position. Note that while the observational protocol is preplanned, it can change in response to what is observed.

A cumulative record of such observations is given in Table 5–1. The metric measurement of data (seconds) has been converted to nominal categories with a frequency count.

You may then decide to try to observe the patient further to see if you can determine what circumstances prevail when the patient is maintaining balance and what, if anything, occurs when she loses her balance. You might in time discover that rotation of the patient's head to either left or right immediately precedes the loss of balance. Thus the study continues, and in time you may have a very detailed description of the patient's motor behavior: what motor acts she can perform, in what ways they deviate from normal, a detailed description of abnormal movements, how they begin, how they proceed, how they end, and so forth. You have named (the meaning of the word "nominal") the essential characteristics of this particular patient; this is an example of nominal descriptive research using the case study. A case report by Walde and colleagues[30] is an example from the literature.

TABLE 5–1   **OBSERVATIONS ON A PATIENT'S SITTING BALANCE AFTER BEING PLACED IN A SITTING POSITION**

Independent Sitting (seconds)				
0–5	5–10	10–20	20–40	40+
IIII	IIHI III	III	I	I

This case report describes a patient in whom arthroscopic surgery of the temporomandibular joint (TMJ) was used to break up adhesions between the TMJ disc and the articular eminence and therefore improve mobility of the joint. Post-surgical physical therapy procedures used were high-voltage electrical stimulation, transcutaneous electrical nerve stimulation, moist heat, ultrasound, ice, mobilization and therapeutic exercises. Postsurgical goals included normalization of range of motion, elimination of pain, elimination of inflammation and mandibular function without restriction. Special emphasis is given to an unusually effective mobilization technique used to decrease tenderness in the TMJ. The conservative therapy described may be used for persons with similar symptoms and evaluation findings who do not require surgery.

A similar example may be found in Wieder.[31] Note that in Walde the effective treatment was a battery of therapeutic modalities, whereas in Wieder only one treatment is responsible for the observed results. Another example of a single treatment modality in a case study may be found in an article by McClure,[32] which

describes the management of a patient with limited shoulder range of motion (ROM) by use of an elevation splint. The limited ROM was believed to be due to structural changes in the tissues surrounding the glenohumeral joint following a Magnuson-Stack repair for anterior glenohumeral instability. The patient's ROM plateaued approximately 6 months postoperatively and did not improve with a variety of physical therapy techniques. Use of an inexpensive easily fabricated elevation splint was begun 8 months postoperatively, and subsequent improvements in ROM were observed. The rationale and suggestions for clinical use of the splint are discussed.

The time series designs discussed in Chapter 7 are also nominal, but they have the potential for being predictive in nature. Because of their potential importance in validating clinical practice, they have been given a separate chapter.

Read the Carter and Campbell article in Appendix C. This article is an example of both a nominal descriptive study and an **intensive case study**. What makes this an intensive case study is the number of repeated measures on the same individual with deliberate attempts to define the parameters measured in operational terms and to quantify observation at a level that is intellectually defensible. This kind of intensive study requires pre-planning and rigorous control, but since it does not have to meet any of the mathematical requirements of predictive research, the descriptive researcher is free to follow the responses of the patient and the therapists' own intuition and insight and still continue to record useful information. A change in treatment need not damage the research design, and could even enhance it. A series of intensive case studies, such as the one modeled by Carter and Campbell, could lead to a normative study of tremendous practical importance to the clinician. For an interesting discussion of case studies as models, see the editorial by Rothstein[33] in the October 1992 issue of *Physical Therapy*, as well as two examples published in the same issue.[34,35]

NORMATIVE DESCRIPTIVE RESEARCH

Let us continue with our hypothethical example above and assume that over the next 2 or 3 years you were referred nine more cases of the same disease. Let us further assume that for each of the subsequent nine cases you did a detailed case study using the same methods of observation that you used on the first one. You would then be in a position to publish a modest normative study based on the 10 cases.[36] In this context the word "norm" means "average" or "typical." **Normative descriptive research** defines average or typical characteristics of a given sample. Therefore, in our normative study you would report that on the basis of 10 cases you have data to substantiate the statement that 40 percent of these patients can maintain sitting balance for 40 seconds or longer if they can maintain their head in midposition during that time. You might further state that 20 percent of these patients lost their sitting balance when their heads rotated to the left, and 74 percent lost their balance when their heads rotated to the right. Your data might indicate that the average age of patients who manifested this disease was 14.62 years, and that the age range for your sample was 10 to 18 years. With your normative descriptive research you have begun to define some important characteristics that are typical of this patient population. The methodology you have used is that of case study: controlled observation that was preplanned in terms of what was to be observed and how it was to be measured and recorded.

An example from the literature is Campbell and Wilhelm.[37]

The purposes of this study were to 1) determine if a group of infants at high risk for later developmental abnormality could be selected on the basis of large numbers of serious neonatal problems, 2) ascertain how early developmental outcome could be predicted, and 3) document the development of the infants longitudinally during the first year of life. Fifteen infants were selected on the basis of high scores on a neonatal risk assessment scale. They were examined with a variety of developmental tests at regular intervals during their first year, at age 2 years, and at age 3 years. The results suggest that the selection process successfully identified a group of infants with developmental problems and that motor performance at 3 months was predictive of neurologic outcome at 3 years. Different patterns of neuromotor development in the first year were identified among those infants with severe cerebral palsy, those with milder neurologic problems, and those with apparently normal outcome.

This is a normative study. It appears to be an expansion of the nominal intensive case study of Carter and Campbell, which may be found in Appendix C. Campbell and her colleagues are demonstrating the progression mentioned at the beginning of this chapter.

For another modest normative study (11 subjects) see Winter,[38] who concluded that his "analyses demonstrate that the safe trajectory of the foot during swing is a precise end-point control task that is under the multi-segment motor control of both the stance and swing limbs." Cameron and Monroe[39] did a study whose purpose was

to determine the relative transmission of ultrasound by the media commonly used by physical therapists to apply phonophoresis. The relative transmission of ultrasound energy through various phonophoresis media was compared with that of degassed water, which is the ideal standard. Transmission was assessed by placing a thin layer of the test medium on the transducer of a therapeutic ultrasound unit and measuring delivery of ultrasound with an ultrasound power meter. The media evaluated produced two significantly different groups of transmission results: (1) transmission greater than 80% of that of water and (2) transmission less than 40% of that of water. Media that optimize the therapeutic efficacy of phonophoresis in both clinical and experimental settings are discussed.

Many of the things therapists do every day contain important nominative and normative information that is unavailable in the literature. It has been observed, for example, that criteria for precisely defining brain damage fall into this category.[40] Similar observations have been made about the need for very basic information on the effects of therapeutic procedures, and how these effects vary with different circumstances or patient characteristics.[41]

Earlier it was stated that two major methods of descriptive research are case study and survey. We have seen how the case study can lead to important information. Let us now consider the survey.[42] Probably the most common tool for survey research is the questionnaire; another tool is the interview. The major difference is that a questionnaire is self-administered, while the questions in an interview are administered by the researcher. For an example that combines both of these techniques, see Donohue, Payton, and Yarbrough.[43] We are all familiar with a number of surveys that describe people as they are. The national census is done every 10 years and describes a number of important characteristics of people living in the United States. The Gallup polls are also descriptive research, usually of the survey type.

Let us say you want to know what therapists in the state of California think about national health insurance and how they believe it might influence their practice. You could obtain this information by writing a series of good questions about that topic and mailing it to a representative (i.e., randomly chosen) sample of all the therapists registered in the state. Or you might choose to ask the same questions in person in structured interviews. On the basis of their answers you could then make normative statements. For example, you might discover that 40 percent of your sample believed that national health insurance would increase their caseload. You could then extrapolate this finding and hypothesize that 40 percent of all the therapists practicing in the state of California believed that national health insurance would increase their caseload.

Surveys have probably most often been used to study psychological and sociological attitudes, opinions, and behaviors; they can, however, be used to collect almost any kind of factual information as well, for example, the content taught in research courses in undergraduate occupational therapy curricula. Petersen[44] got a 60.3 percent return (which is very good) on surveys sent to program directors in occupational therapy schools. The data were presented in tables with actual numbers and in percentages, for example, percentages of programs offering a topic.

In essence, the survey exposes the sample to a predetermined set of questions, the answers to which can be quantified with descriptive statistics. When the answers are closed—true-false or multiple choice—it is important that the fixed responses provided are exhaustive and mutually exclusive; otherwise the one taking the questionnaire will be frustrated and disinclined to complete the instrument. Hurd and coworkers[45] have written an interesting program for training interviewers to do structured interviews. Hurd also gives examples of questionnaires on health practices in two African countries.

A checklist, which is similar to a questionnaire, is also used in descriptive research. For example, one might send out a checklist of all possible therapeutic modalities to a randomly selected sample of therapists and ask them simply to check off all of those modalities that they use at least once a week (nominal data), or they might be asked to use the same checklist and write in the average number of times that they use each therapeutic modality each week (a frequency count transformed into metric data). From such a survey one could conclude that the typical therapist uses modality A three times more frequently than modality B and twice as frequently as modality C.

Interviews, questionnaires, and checklists are also used in job analysis studies, which are designed to describe what people in certain occupational categories typically do, how they spend their time, and so forth. Such job analyses are done from time to time in both physical and occupational therapy and these data provide descriptive information that has a great many practical uses: justifying an increase in floor space for a department; increasing a department budget; increasing or decreasing the number of staff in a department; increasing salaries; changing job descriptions; changing curricula; improving function and safety of equipment, and so on. For example, Domenech and colleagues[46] studied the time utilization of therapists in a large hospital department; this lead to the realignment of some staff responsibilities.

Descriptive research is particularly amenable to *retrospective* studies, that is, gathering a data set from records already existing or looking for patterns in existing data. For example, see the Gose article reviewed in Chapter 3. Predictive research is usually *prospective*; data are gathered as the records are created for the purpose of research. Retrospective studies are more common in descriptive research. For example, Richert and Bergland[47] identified

> mental health rehabilitation services for patients with multiple personality disorder. Through the use of a literature review and a retrospective examination of 20 patients' records, the frequency of discipline-specific services is noted in occupational therapy, art therapy, movement therapy, vocational counseling, and recreational therapy. Recommendations for practice and program development include ongoing education about multiple personality disorder and continual assessment of the patient's functional level to identify subsequent treatment needs and services.

Practice   Go back to Chapter 1 and look at the example of the two therapists in St. Hopeless Hospital. Using the survey method of descriptive research, answer their first question: "What measurement tools and what therapeutic methods are currently being used by therapists in hospitals and clinics across the country? Now read the article by McClain, McKinney, and Ralston in Appendix C. Is it descriptive research? If so, what type? What elements from Appendix A can you find in this article on occupational therapists in private practice?

HISTORICAL DESCRIPTIVE RESEARCH

Historical research focuses on past events rather than present events; otherwise it is very much like other descriptive research. There is a research question, a method of data collection, analysis, and interpretation. The primary methodological tool of historical research is document analysis. The historical researcher must pay very careful attention to the validity and reliability of sources. Historical research is always flavored by inter- pretations: the original interpretation of an event recorded in historical documents (primary sources), and the successive interpretations of those documents made by other researchers (secondary sources). Demonstrating the validity or accuracy of primary sources of information is critical to useful historical research. Retrospective reviews are usually concerned with recent past events and are more likely to be used for predictive purposes than historical research. Retrospective reviews use data that have already been collected. Once the data are obtained, they may be subjected to predictive statistical analysis, as in the Gose article reviewed in Chapter 3.

The major difference between historical research and other classes of descriptive research is that it describes what *was* instead of what *is*. Since it has often been suggested that those who do not know history are doomed to repeat it, an examination of therapeutic procedures that have and have not worked in the past, for example, can be of benefit to today's patients. Historical reviews also help us to understand how we have arrived at out present circumstances on a given issue. For example, Reed[48] reviewed the history of federal legislation for persons with disabilities covering the time period from 1916 to 1990. Her conclusions involve interpretation that suggests a political dimension to clinical practice. Note how her historical review of literature is organized.

This paper discusses federal legislation relating to persons with disabilities and it divides into 13 areas. Several areas of legislation, such as education and basic education, have a long history beginning with World War I. Laws related to other areas, such as federal support for developing technology, have been adopted only within the past 5 years. The Americans with Disabilities Act of 1990 (ADA) (Public Law 101-336), which guarantees civil rights to Americans with disabilities, has five titles, and each is summarized. Although the ADA provides for Americans with disabilities to be included in American society, it has some major limitations, including the lack of an affirmative action requirement and of provisions for the education and training of persons with disabilities so that they can qualify for employment. Several of the federal laws related to persons with disabilities have affected the field of occupational therapy either favorably or adversely. The conclusion is drawn that occupational therapists need to be alert to pending legislation to promote the role of occupational therapy in serving persons with disabilities.

Levine[49] and Harvey-Krefting[50] provide two more examples in the occupational therapy literature.

DEVELOPMENTAL DESCRIPTIVE RESEARCH

Developmental research describes a sequence of events over a long period of time. Classic examples are the studies of Gesell and McGraw on the normal developmental sequence of human infants. Their method employed direct observations and repeated measurements of many characteristics in many infants over a considerable period of time. The article by Carter and Campbell in Appendix C might be classified as developmental because of the rapid change that occurred in their subject over a short period of time. In fact, the article may be classified in several different ways: it is descriptive research; it is a case study; and in a somewhat limited time frame, it is a developmental study of one child. The level of measurement for most of the parameters is ordinal, from 0 (no response) to 4 or 5 (fully developed response). Table 1 contains raw data—ordinal measurement based on repeated observations. The article cited above by Campbell and Wilhelm may also be classified from several points of view: it is descriptive and normative (though with a somewhat limited sample), and within a 3-year time frame, it is a longitudinal developmental study of 15 infants. It demonstrates nominal (frequency count of medical conditions in the sample), ordinal (neurologic and cognitive outcome categories), and metric (normalized mean scores on a psychomotor test) data. A series of case studies or survey instruments are often the measurement tools used in developmental descriptive studies.

Developmental studies may also be done on adults. For example, a therapist could mail a questionnaire to all newly graduated therapists in a designated geographic area and repeat the same questionnaire to the same therapists each year for a 10-year period. Such a sample is often called a **cohort**, that is, a sample followed over a period of time. The questionnaire could query the development of a number of characteristics, such as management skills and responsibilities, educational development, and so on. That would be a **longitudinal study**. Longitudinal studies are expensive and fraught with difficulties. Good reasons for doing a cohort study include accurately describing the incidence and natural history of a variable, documenting temporal sequence of a variable, and studying multiple-outcome variables.[51]

If the questionnaire described in the previous paragraph is administered once to postgraduate therapists with different lengths of experience, it would be part of a **cross-sectional study**. In a cross-sectional study, data are taken at one point in time from a sample stratified on some important characteristic—frequently age. Establishing causal relationships is more difficult in cross-sectional studies than in longitudinal studies. For a recent example of this technique see Branholm and Fugl-Meyer[52] or Levinson.[53] Perhaps the classic example of the developmental literature is Erikson's[54] study of childhood and society. More recent examples are Vaillant[55] or Sheehy,[56] written for the popular market.

REVIEW OF THE LITERATURE AND META-ANALYSIS

Almost every published article in the professional literature contains a review of the literature, with a summary and, usually, an integration or interpretation of the literature. For example, Huebner[57] reviewed 81 articles on autism and condensed that literature into 10 pages of text with three large tables and a summary diagram. Huebner's tables summarize the essential components of each article reviewed: number of subjects, research design, results, and so on. Other examples may be found in Elias and Murphy,[58] DiFabio,[59] or the entire December 1985 issue of *Physical Therapy*, which is a special issue devoted to cardiac rehabilitation. Reviews of the literature serve a very important function in continuing professional education. Experts in a given field have read, understood, integrated, and summarized for the busy reader a significant body of literature. Such reviews demonstrate some of the elements of descriptive research, in that the author had a guiding question: What does the literature say about _____? The authors searched systematically in the library for answers. Because no new data are gathered, this format by itself, is not generally regarded as research. As indicated in Chapter 1, review of the literature is but one step in the research process. However, as the authors struggle intellectually with the literature to find the implications of the data presented on a given problem, it takes on some of the qualities of historical research.

Meta-analysis goes a step beyond an interpretative review of literature in that the reviewer established criteria for evaluating the *quality*, or the validity, of the studies reviewed. Beckerman and her colleagues[60] "decided to focus on the methodological quality of the studies. In this way, conclusions about the efficacy of laser therapy can be drawn from the best methodological studies only."

The efficacy of laser therapy for musculoskeletal and skin disorders has been assessed on the basis of the results of 36 randomized clinical trials (RCTs) involving 1,704 patients. . . . The studies with a positive outcome were generally of a better quality than the studies with a negative outcome. No clear relationship could be demonstrated between the laser dosage applied and the efficacy of laser therapy, or between the dosage and the methodological score. In general, the methodological quality of these studies appeared to be rather low. Consequently, no definite conclusions can be drawn about the efficacy of laser therapy for skin disorders. The efficacy of laser therapy for musculoskeletal disorders seems, on average, to be larger than the efficacy of a placebo treatment. More specifically, for rheumatoid arthritis, posttraumatic joint disorders, and myofascial pain, laser therapy seems to have a substantial specific therapeutic effect. Further RCTs, avoiding the most prevalent methodological errors, are needed in order to enable the benefits of laser therapy to be more precisely and validly evaluated.[61]

Twenty-four criteria were selected by Beckerman and her colleagues, with an emphasis on internal validity. A table in the article shows how each of the 36 randomized clinical trials were rated on each of these criteria.

Summary Statements of Descriptive Data

A mass of raw data is often so unwieldy that it is difficult to see its important implications. Therefore, it usually becomes necessary to make some sort of summary statement about the observations made on the sample. This can be done using statistics. Table 5–2 summarizes the most common descriptive statistics for the various levels of measurement. Descriptive statistics usually summarize the data in two ways: central tendency and variability or dispersion. Statistics of central tendency tell you what the average or typical score looks like, and statistics of variability tell you how far from that average the scores spread.

If the series of numbers in Table 5–3 were conceived as a nominal

TABLE 5-2 **DESCRIPTIVE STATISTICS**

Level of Measurement	Central Tendency	Spread or Variability	Other
Nominal	Mode	Range	Frequency counts and percentages in categories
Ordinal	Median	Range	Frequency counts and percentages at levels (percentile)
Metric	Mean	Range; variance; standard deviation	Frequency counts and percentages at levels

list, the *range* would be 0 to 3. There are two 0s, seven 1s, two 2s, and five 3s; therefore, the *mode* would be 1 because there are more 1s than any other number. The mode is a measure of central tendency for nominal data. A sample may be bimodal if two frequencies are equal in number. The frequency counts can be transformed into percentages. For example, the 0s make up 12.5 percent (1/8) of the total list; percentages should, however, be used with caution when the sample (n) is small.

The *median* is the statistic of central tendency of a set of ordinal data; it is the middle of the range of recorded measurements, listed in order. For example, take all of the ratings of spontaneous activity in the supine position from the table in the article by Carter and Campbell. Sixteen ratings were made on one subject performing one activity. In Table 5–3 these 16 ratings are arranged from left to right in sequence from 0 to 3. Remember that this is not the sequence in which the measurements were recorded. A heavy line, dividing the series in half, represents the median of these ordinal data. Since there is an even number of measurements, no number falls at the median; in this case the average of the two numbers on either side of the line is the median. The *range* is 0 to 3.

Let us now take a more detailed look at the descriptive statistics for metric data. Say a class is given two separate exams and the class average on both exams is 75. On one exam the highest score is 100 and the lowest is 50, whereas on the other exam the highest score is 90 and the lowest is 67. (See Table 5–4.) In both sets of data, $n = 13$; that is, there are 13 bits of data in each set. To get the arithmetic *mean*, the set of scores is summed and divided by n; in Table 5–4, 976 was divided by 13 to obtain the mean of 75 (rounded off). Since the means are equal, in order to

TABLE 5-3 **ILLUSTRATION OF THE MEDIAN OF A SERIES OF MEASURES (DATA SUPPLIED FROM THE WORK OF CARTER AND CAMPBELL IN APPENDIX C)**

0	0	1	1	1	1	1	1	1	2	2	3	3	3	3	3

TABLE 5–4   **ILLUSTRATION OF DESCRIPTIVE STATISTICS FOR METRIC DATA**

Data Set A	Data Set B
100	90
97	88
95	77
95	77
86	77
82	76
71	75
66	72
63	71
58	70
57	69
56	67
50	67
976	976
n = 13	n = 13
$\bar{x}$ = 75	$\bar{x}$ = 75
sd = 18.07	sd =

compare the two sets of scores we need some measure of the spread or variability.

A common measure of variability for all three levels of measurement is the range. For data set A the range is 100 to 50; what is the range for data set B? Metric data can be analyzed with two other measures of spread or variability; these are known as variance (s) and standard deviation (sd). The formula for variance is:

$$\frac{(x - \bar{x})^2}{n - 1}$$

For data set A, this is worked out in Table 5–5. The standard deviation of data set A is the square root of the variance. Common symbols often used include:

x = datum for sample
$\bar{x}$ = mean for sample
s or sd = standard deviation for the sample
X = datum for population
$\bar{X}$ (μ) = mean for population
SD = standard deviation for the population

Further calculation of variance is illustrated in Chapter 9.

Remember that a statistic is a numerical statement that summarizes a number of real observations in a known group (your sample). A parameter

TABLE 5–5 **ILLUSTRATION OF STATISTICS OF VARIABILITY FOR DATA SET A FROM TABLE 5–4**

Score	Deviation from the Mean $(x - \bar{x})$	Square of the Deviation $(x - \bar{x})^2$
100	25	625
97	22	484
95	20	400
95	20	400
86	11	121
82	7	49
71	−4	16
66	−9	81
63	−12	144
58	−17	289
57	−18	324
56	−19	361
50	−25	625
	Sum of squares	3919

Sum of squares divided by $n - 1$ = mean square (variance) = 326.58
Square root of variance = standard deviation = 18.07

is a numerical statement about a population that has not been observed; the parameter is *estimated* on the basis of an observed statistic of a representative sample of a population. For example, if you measure the age of a representative sample of physical therapy students in the United States, you could calculate the mean age (statistics) for that group of students; you could then estimate the mean age (parameter) for *all* physical therapy students in the United States based on your observed sample. The branch of mathematics called *statistics* is concerned with making various numerical statements about samples and populations.

A statistical procedure that is seldom seen in the literature of physical and occupational therapy is that of establishing confidence intervals. If we pursued the example in the previous paragraph we might determine, on the basis of a representative sample of 100 physical therapy students, that their mean age was 24.7 years. If we took another representative sample of 100 other therapists, the mean age of that sample might be 25.2 years. The sample mean is only an estimate or an approximation of the average age of the population. By appropriate mathematical procedures (see Shott[62]) one could make a statement; for example, "we can be 95 percent certain that the true mean age of all physical therapy students in the United States is between 23.4 and 26.6 years." The ages 23.4 to 26.6 are called confidence intervals; note that there is still a 5 percent chance of being wrong.

The right-hand column in Table 5–2 is self-explanatory. In both Tables 5–1 and 5–3 it is possible to do a frequency count of the number of observations in each category, and it is possible to convert (transform) each of these frequency counts into a percentage of the total number. Each researcher must consider the nature of his or her data and the nature of the question being asked in order to decide when it is appropriate and useful to report frequency counts and percentages. Percentages are often useful in normative studies. Frequency counts or frequency distributions are often presented in the familiar bar graphs, often called histograms, and pie graphs, to facilitate understanding. These may be drawn with raw data or with percentages.

Many hand-held calculators will do mean and standard deviation; follow the instruction manual for each model. Most major statistical software packages, such as SPSS, SPSS/PC, and SAS, do descriptive statistics either independently or as a part of a larger statistical operation. These programs are discussed further in Chapters 8 and 9.

Practice   Using the formulas provided in Table 5–5, figure the variance and standard deviation for data set B from Table 5–4. What is the mode, median, and mean for the data in Table 5–1? What percentage of the data in Table 5–1 is in the category of 5 to 10 seconds?

Critique of Descriptive Methods

There are several sources of error that may invalidate a descriptive methodology. The most obvious are those that were discussed in Chapter 2; improper sampling, asking the wrong questions, collecting data inappropriate to the questions, and making incorrect inferences.

Another major source of trouble is bias (unconscious bias, not deliberate fraud) in selecting parameters to be observed in case studies or in selecting questions to be asked in interviews and on questionnaires or checklists. It is easy for the researcher to subconsciously bias the data in directions compatible with the expected or desired results. This problem is obviously compounded if several observers are working together on a project and observing different subjects. With multiple observers great care must be taken to be sure that all observers discriminate between one phenomenon and another in the same way, that they respond to the same cues, and that they agree on the definitions of what is to be recorded and how it is to be recorded.

Another source of bias is respondents who answer questions the way they think they "should be answered" or in ways which they think will please the researcher. In some kinds of questionnaires respondents may be inclined to answer in ways that are socially desirable rather than according to how they actually feel or think. People may also respond differently because they are consciously aware that they are being observed (the Hawthorne effect; see Chapter 8). It may not be possible to completely remove bias from descriptive research, particularly interviews and questionnaires. However, the careful researcher can apply as many constraints as possible, such as defining terms and methods of measurement and observation and writing interviews and questionnaire questions in unambiguous, well-defined terms that will incline everyone to read the questions the same way. Before developing a questionnaire or rating scale, one should refer to a good textbook on the subject, such as those provided by Jacobs[63] or Labaw.[64] In general, be precise, avoid loaded questions, avoid emotion-laden words, and, if possible, provide a series of graded choices from which the subjects may select an answer. Open-ended answers are open to subjective interpretation and are difficult to tabulate. Be sure that the questions are ones that the respondents are qualified to answer.

Most researchers consider a 40 percent return on questionnaires conducted by mail a very good response. Suppose that you mailed a questionnaire that dealt with attitudes toward social issues in medicine. Nonrespondents might be very conservative in their views; they may not have answered because they did not like your questions. Your sample would then be composed of those whose views were more liberal. It may also be that certain personality types are more inclined to answer questionnaires than are other types, and this will bias your sample. It may be that only people who feel that their answers are the socially correct ones will respond.

We have only touched on the possible sources of error in using questionnaires and other descriptive research techniques. However, the preceding information should be enough to make the reader alert to the scope and limitations of classic descriptive methodologies and studies using them.

Review Questions

1 Match the following questions — taken from the fifth paragraph of this chapter — with the design most suited to answering them.

What topics in continuing education programs would therapists in Georgia like to see presented?	a. Historical
How do people with spinal cord injuries feel about traveling in public in wheelchairs?	b. Developmental
What percentage of the patients admitted to hospitals in this state are referred to physical and occupational therapy?	c. Qualitative
How was this unusual client with rheumatoid arthritis treated in this department, and what were the results?	d. Nominal

| What were the most frequently used therapeutic modalities in the therapy clinics of stateside army hospitals during World War II? | e. Case Study |
| What is the typical sequence of events in the development of contractures in clients with juvenile rheumatoid arthritis from the first diagnosis of the disease to age 25? | f. Normative |

2 For *each* question listed above, what form would you expect the data to be in (i.e., words or numbers)? What level of measurement would be involved? What descriptive statistics, if any, would be appropriate?

3 Outline the essentials of a cross-sectional and a longitudinal study to answer the question: What are the long-term effects of polio?

4 Using Appendix A, identify as many features of a research protocol as are applicable in the article by Carter and Campbell in Appendix C.

Additional Readings

Berdie, DR and Anderson, JF: Questionnaires: Designs and Use. Scarecrow Press, Metuchen, NJ, 1974.

Brogan, DR: Nonresponse to sampling surveys: The problem and some solutions. Phys Ther 60:1026, 1980.

Cummings, SR, et al: Planning the measurements: Questionnaires. In Hulley, SB and Cummings, SR (eds): Designing Clinical Research. Williams & Wilkins, Baltimore, 1988, Chapter 5.

Dempsey, PA and Dempsey, AD: The Research Process in Nursing, ed 2. Jones & Bartlett, Boston, 1986.

Drew, CJ and Hardman, ML: Designing and Conducting Behavioral Research. Pergamon, New York, 1985, Chapter 6.

Field, PA and Morse, JM: Nursing Research: The Application of Qualitative Approaches. Croom Helm, London, 1985.

Goetz, JP and LeCompte, MD: Ethnography and Qualitative Design in Educational Research. Academic Press, San Diego, 1984.

Klein, HE (Ed): Case Method Research and Application. WACRA, Needham, MA, 1989.

Leedy, PD: Practical Research: Planning and Design, ed 2. Macmillan, New York, 1980, Chapters 8 and 9.

Linstone, A and Murray, T (eds): The Delphi Method: Techniques and Applications. Addison-Wesley, Reading, MA, 1975.

Magnussen, D and Bergman, LR: Data Quality in Longitudinal Research. Cambridge University Press, Cambridge, 1990.

Parse, RR, Coyne, AB, and Smith, MJ (eds): Nursing Research: Qualitative Methods. Brady Communications, Bowie, MD, 1985.

Shepard, KF: Questionnaire design and use. In Bork, CE (ed): Research in Physical Therapy. Lippincott, Philadelphia, 1993.

Stahl, SM and Hennes, JD: Reading and Understanding Applied Statistics. CV Mosby, St. Louis, 1980.

Strauss, A and Corbin, J: Basics of Qualitative Research: Grounded Theory Procedures and Techniques. Sage, London, 1991.

Taylor, SJ and Bogdan, R: Introduction to Qualitative Research Methods: The Search for Meanings, ed 2. John Wiley & Sons, New York, 1984.

References

1. Rothstein, JM (ed): Measurement in Physical Therapy. Churchill Livingstone, New York, 1985, Chapter 1.
2. Leiniger, MM (ed): Qualitative Methods in Nursing. Grune & Stratton, New York, 1985, p xi.
3. Ibid., p 2.
4. Okolo, EN (ed): Health Research Design and Methodology. CRC Press, Ann Arbor, 1990, p 82.
5. Parse, RR, Coyne, AB, and Smith, MJ (eds): Nursing Research: Qualitative Methods. Brady Communications, Bowie, MD, 1985, p 3.
6. Leininger, op. cit.
7. Merrill, SC: Qualitative methods in occupational therapy research: An application. OTJ of Res 5:209, 1985.
8. Barker, RG: One Boy's Day: A Specimen of Behavior. Archon Books, Hamden, CN, 1966.
8a. Shepard, KF, et al: Alternative approaches to research in physical therapy: Positivism and phenomenology. Phys Ther 73:88, 1993.
9. Krefting, L: Rigor in qualitative research: The assessment of trustworthiness. AJOT 45:214, 1991.
10. Strauss, A and Corbin, J: Basics of Qualitative Research: Grounded Theory Procedures and Techniques. Sage, London, 1991, p 23.
11. Pierce, DE: Early object rule acquistion. AJOT 45:438, 1991.
12. Taylor, SJ, and Bogdan, R: Introduction to Qualitative Research Methods: The Search for Meanings, ed 2. John Wiley & Sons, New York, 1984, p 124.
13. Barker, RG, op cit.
14. Bogdan, R, Brown, MA, and Foster, SB: Be honest but not cruel: Staff/parent communication on a neonatal unit. In Taylor, SJ, and Bogdan, R (eds): Introduction to Qualitative Research Methods: The Search for Meanings. John Wiley & Sons, New York, 1984, pp 170–194.
15. Huttlinger, K, et al: "Doing battle": A metaphorical analysis of diabetes mellitus among Navajo people. AJOT 46:706, 1992.
16. Krefting, L and Krefting, D: Leisure activities after a stroke: An ethnographic appraoch. AJOT 45:429, 1991.
17. There are several ethnographic studies in AJOT. 45:3, 1991.
18. DeMars, PA: An occupational therapy life skills curriculum model for a Native American tribe: A health promotion program based on ethnographic field research. AJOT 46:727, 1992.
19. Jensen, GM, et al: Attribute dimensions that distinguish master and novice physical therapy clinicians in orthopedic settings. Phys Ther 72:711, 1992.
20. Yarbrough, P: An Ethnography of Physical Therapy Practice: A Source for Curriculum Development. Unpublished doctoral dissertation, Georgia State University, 1980.
21. Glaser, BG and Strauss, Al: The Discovery of Grounded Theory: Strategies for Qualitative Research. Aldine, New York, 1967.
22. Merrill, op cit.
23. Taylor, SJ and Bogdan, R: op cit, p 126.
24. Niehues, AN, et al: Making a difference: Occupational therapy in the public schools. OTJR 11:195, 1991.

25. Llewellyn, G: Adults with an intellectual disability: Australian practitioners' perspectives. OTJR 11:323, 1991.
26. Mulcahey, MJ: Returning to school after a spinal cord injury: Perspectives from four adolescents. AJOT 46:305, 1992.
27. Hasselkus, BR: The meaning of activity: Day care for persons with Alzheimer disease. AJOT 46:199, 1992.
28. Tesch, R: Computer programs that assist in the analysis of qualitative data: An overview. Qual Health Res 1:309, 1991.
29. Dyck, I: Managing chronic illness: An immigrant woman's acquisition and use of health care knowledge. AJOT 46:696, 1992.
30. Walde, FL, et al: Clinical management of a patient following temporomandibular joint arthroscopy. Phys Ther 72:355, 1992.
31. Wieder, DL: Treatment of traumatic myositis ossificans with acetic acid iontophoresis. Phys Ther 72:133, 1992.
32. McClure, PW and Flowers, KR: Treatment of limited shoulder motion using an elevation splint. Phys Ther 72:57, 1992.
33. Rothstein, JM: Making models more attractive. Phys Ther 72:689, 1992.
34. Strickland, EM, et al: In vivo acetabular contact pressures during rehabilitation, Part 1: Acute phase. Phys Ther 72:691, 1992.
35. Givens-Heiss, DL, et al: In vivo acetabular contact pressures during rehabilitation, Part 2: Postacute phase. Phys Ther 72:700, 1992.
36. Parente, R and Parente, JA: Alternative research strategies for occupational therapy, Part 1: Experimental and individual difference research. AJOT:365, 1986.
37. Campbell, SK and Wilhelm, IJ: Development from birth to 3 years of age of 15 children at high risk for central nervous system dysfunction: Interim report. Phys Ther 65:463, 1985.
38. Winter, DA: Foot trajectory in human gait: A precise and multifactorial motor control task. Phys Ther 72:45, 1992.
39. Cameron, MH and Monroe, LG: Relative transmission of ultrasound by media customarily used for phonophoresis. Phys Ther 72:142, 1992.
40. Michels, E: Research Needs and Classical Applications: Neurological Disorders. Paper presented at the American Physical Therapy Association, Houston, Texas, June 27, 1973.
41. Gonnella, C: Designs for clinical research. Phys Ther 53:1276, 1973.
42. Mann, WC: Survey methods. AJOT 39:640, 1985.
43. Donohue, N, Payton, OD, and Yarbrough, P: Considerations for physical therapy recruitment and admissions. JPTEd 3:40, 1989.
44. Petersen, P, et al: Research education in undergraduate occupational therapy programs. OTJR 12:131, 1992.
45. Hurd, P: Research design and data collection methods. In Okolo, EN (Ed): Health Research Design and Methodology. CRC Press, Ann Arbor, 1990, Chapter 3.
46. Domenech, MA, et al: Utilization of physical therapy personnel in one hospital: A work sampling study. Phys Ther 63:1108, 1983.
47. Richert, GZ and Bergland, C: Treatment choices: Rehabilitation services used by patients with multiple personality disorder. AJOT 46:634, 1992.
48. Reed, KL: History of federal legislation for persons with disabilities. AJOT 46:397, 1992.
49. Levine, RE: Historical research: Ordering the past to chart our future. OTJ of Res 6:259, 1986.
50. Harvey-Krefting, L: The concept of work in occupational therapy: A historical review. AJOT 39:301, 1985.
51. Cummings, SR, Ernster, V, and Hulley, SB: Designing a new study: I. Cohort studies. In Hulley, SB, and Cummings, SR (Eds): Designing Clinical Research. Williams & Wilkins, Baltimore, 1988.

52. Branholm, IB and Fugl-Meyer, AR: Occupational role preferences and life satisfaction. OTJR 12:159, 1992.
53. Levinson, DJ: The Seasons of a Man's Life. Knopf, New York, 1978.
54. Erikson, EH: Childhood and Society. Norton, New York, 1963.
55. Vaillant, GE: Adaptation to Life. Little, Brown & Co, Boston, MA, 1977.
56. Sheehy, G: Passages: Predictable Crises of Adult Life. Bantam, New York, 1977.
57. Huebner, RA: Autistic disorder: A neuropsychological enigma. AJOT 46:487, 1992.
58. Elias, WS and Murphy, RJ: The case for health promotion programs containing health care costs: A review of the literature. AJOT 40:759, 1986.
59. DiFabio, RP: Clinical assessment of manipulation and mobilization of the lumbar spine: A critical review of the literature. Phys Ther 66:51, 1986.
60. Beckerman, H, et al: The efficacy of laser therapy for musculoskeletal and skin disorders: A criteria-based meta-analysis of randomized clinical trials. Phys Ther 72:483, 1992.
61. Beckerman, H, et al: op cit, p 483.
62. Shott, S: Statistics for Health Professionals. WB Saunders, Philadelphia, 1990, Chapter 6.
63. Jacobs, TO: A Guide for Developing Questionnaire Items. Human Resources Research Organization, Banning, GA, 1970.
64. Labaw, P: Advanced Questionnaire Design. Abt Books, Cambridge, MA, 1980.

Correlation Research

Definition

Descriptive research looks at variables one at a time, while descriptive statistics examines the variability and central tendency of one variable at a time (univariate analysis). Any relationships seen among variables are developed verbally and logically. In this chapter we begin to relate two or more variables to each other mathematically as well as logically (bivariate or multivariate analysis).

Simply stated, a **correlation coefficient** is a mathematical measure of the extent to which two or more paired phenomena or events tend to occur together. Ghiselli and colleagues[1] define a correlation coefficient as

an index of the degree of association between two variables or the extent to which the order of individuals on one variable is similar to the order of individuals on a second variable. This quantitative description of the relationship between two

111

variables indicates the accuracy with which scores on one variable can be predicted from scores on another as well as the extent to which individual differences on two variables can be attributed to the same determining factor.

For example, erythema (redness of the skin) and elevated skin temperature tend to occur together; these two phenomena have a positive correlation—they are associated. On the other hand, general body relaxation and a high environmental noise level do not occur together; these phenomena have a negative correlation—they are unlikely to be associated. Thus, a positive correlation implies that where you see one, you tend to see the other; a negative correlation implies that where you see one, you tend not to see the other.

Figure 6–1 illustrates several possible relationships between two hypothetical tests; each graph may be called a scattergram of a bivariate distribution. It is very important to note that two scores are *paired* in some way; they are either taken from the same individual or they are logically paired: for example, mother-daughter. They may be two scores on the same test or scores on two different tests. Let us say that they are two new tests

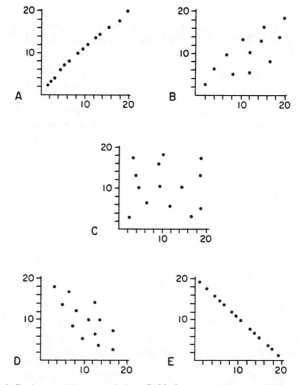

FIGURE 6–1 *A*, Perfect positive correlation. *B*, Moderate positive correlation. *C*, No correlation. *D*, Moderate negative correlation. *E*, Perfect negative correlation.

of sensory motor integration. You want to know (your research question) to what extent these two tests measure the same thing. It should be noted that the question is phrased so that it has nothing to do with whether or not either of these tests are, indeed, valid tests of sensory motor integration. The question only asks if they test the same thing, whatever that may be. To find out, we administer these tests to a random sample of 30 subjects chosen from the population of nursery school children in a given county. The testing results in two sets of data: scores on test A and scores on test B. By consulting a book on statistical methods we can derive a correlation coefficient from these two sets of data. Do subjects who have high scores on test A also have high scores on test B? Do subjects who have low scores on test A have low scores on test B? If so, the tests tend to test the same thing. As will be discussed below, the size of the correlation coefficient will indicate the *extent* to which they measure the same thing.

There is a range of possible correlations between a perfect positive correlation coefficient ($+1.00$) and a perfect negative correlation coefficient (-1.00); only three of these are illustrated in Figure 6–1, which also shows the two perfect extremes. In each of the graphs in this figure, the numerical scores for test A are represented on the vertical line and the numerical scores for test B on the horizontal line; a perfect score for both tests is 20. Graph A is what your data would look like if you had a perfect positive correlation, that is, if each student scored the same on each of the two tests: one student scores 20 on both tests; another student scores 8 on both tests, and so on. Mathematically, this is expressed as a $+1.00$ correlation.

Graph B is what your data would look like if there was a moderate positive correlation. Perhaps one student scored 9 on test A and 7 on test B, and another student scored 18 on test A and 19 on test B. Each point, then, represents one individual's two scores. You can see that these scores form a line that runs more or less from lower left to upper right, with some scatter. The correlation coefficient here is somewhere in the vicinity of $+.7$. Generally speaking, a correlation of .9 or more is considered high, a correlation of .8 moderately high, .7 moderate, and .6 and below is usually considered low.

Graph C illustrates no correlation between the two tests; one student made an 18 on test A and a 17 on test B, while another student made 18 on test A and 6 on test B. This distribution would produce a correlation coefficient of 0.0.

Graph D illustrates a modest negative correlation, wherein the students who score high on test A tend to score low on test B. A modest negative correlation coefficient would be $-.7$.

Graph E shows a perfect negative correlation; those who score high on test A score low on test B. Thus one person scores 20 on A and 0 on

TABLE 6-1 **SET OF ASSOCIATED PAIRED SCORES**

10	90
20	100
30	110
40	120
50	130
60	140

B, another person with a 19 on A gets a 1 on B, and so on. A perfect negative correlation is expressed as −1.0.

Graphs A and E have been presented as perfect linear regression lines; however, a correlation coefficient *by itself* without an associated equation for linear regression does not imply that the paired scores are identical—only that they co-relate perfectly.[2] The set of pairs in Table 6-1 would produce a correlation of +1.0 because they *vary* at exactly the same interval (in this case 10); they would not produce the same regression line as two identical lists.

Limitations of Correlation

Before we look at the uses of correlation, it would be well to take a look at its major limitation. One must never automatically infer a causal relationship between any elements in a correlation. For example, one could collect data to demonstrate a very high positive correlation between the increase of cancer in the United States and the increase in the use of aluminum cookware. It would be totally unjustified, however, to infer from this correlation that aluminum cookware causes cancer. Hamilton[3] points out that there is a high correlation between the occurrence of coronary thrombosis and the consumption of fat. There is a corresponding correlation between the increase in coronary thrombosis and an increase in the number of radios in use. A valid interpretation of these two correlations would require considerable knowledge about coronary thrombosis. A high correlation coefficient can result from random or systematic error (bias); or both variables could be caused by a third, unknown, factor; or one factor could really cause the other. With these possible pitfalls in mind, let us proceed to a discussion of the possible uses of correlation.

Uses of Correlation

Frequently there *is* a causal relationship between two phenomena. When there is a theoretical or logical relationship, then we can begin to think about predicting one variable from another. In this case a correlation coefficient may be conceptualized as "the ratio of the amount of information that two variables measure jointly, compared with the average amount of information measured individually by each of the two variables."[4] For example, if we were taking a correlation between intelligence test scores and grade-point average in college, we would get a fairly high positive correlation, and reason would support the idea that there was a causal relationship between IQ and achievement in college. Nevertheless, the correlation between these two variables would not be perfect; this suggests that factors other than intelligence have an influence on grade-point average and, conversely, that grade-point average does not necessarily reflect a student's IQ. For the clinician, correlational questions are more likely to be concerned with the extent to which symptoms occur together, the extent to which certain responses occur with certain diagnoses, or the association of given therapeutic procedures with measured outcomes.

One should be careful not to interpret correlation coefficients in terms of percentage. A correlation of .64 does not mean that when one factor varies, the other one varies 64 percent of the time. In order to approach that kind of information you need to square the correlation coefficient (r^2); this is called a coefficient of determination. For example, if the correlation coefficient of two factors is .60, one may say that 36 percent (.60 squared) of one variable is accounted for by the other one; that is, 36 percent of the information contained in variable A is shared by variable B, provided that one can demonstrate in theory a relationship between A and B. Conversely, 64 percent ($100 - 36$) of the information contained in variable A is not shared by B.

On the other hand, let us say we obtained a high positive correlation between social background and grade-point average. We probably would not conclude that one causes the other, but rather that they are both caused by other factors, such as family economic status, family attitude toward education, education of the parents, and the degree of parental motivation for the children's education. As was pointed out in Chatper 1, the researcher must produce a rational and defensible interpretation of the data. Thus, a knowledge of the subject under study is important for an appropriate interpretation of correlational data. In correlating factors A and B, at least four possible interpretations exist: A may have caused B; B may have caused A; both A and B may be caused by another or other variables; or there is no relationship between A and B (i.e., they are associated but not related).

Correlational research is similar to descriptive research in that it can be used as a rather broad, relatively nonspecific search for postulates or principles upon which more specific experimental research can be built. Early in your mastery of a subject matter area you may not be able to think of questions more specific than, What things tend to happen together and to what extent?

At other times correlation may be used with a very specific and definitive question. Many educational and psychological tests are validated by correlational studies, particularly in comparing an older, well-established test to a new one. For example, test A is a well-established but expensive and time-consuming test for functional abilities. Test B is a new, quick, easy, inexpensive test of functional abilities. If it could be shown that scores on test B had a very high correlation with scores on test A, then one might conclude that they tested the same thing and that test B could be substitutes for test A. One might further conclude that test B *is as valid as* test A for functional ability. A teacher might use correlation to establish the parallel equivalence of one examination with another, to compare the equivalency of a written test with a practical test. Conversely, one might like to demonstrate that there is little or no correlation between a written and a practical exam in order to demonstrate that these two tests sample different behaviors relevant to the same topic.

Correlation is also used to establish the test-retest reliability of tests of all kinds. Here are some examples of questions in this area. What is the correlation between repeated applications of the same test on the same patient by the same therapist (intratester reliability)? What is the correlation between repeated applications of the same test on the same patient by two different therapists (intertester reliability)? In these instances one hopes for very high correlations. Our recent professional literature has been rich with reliability studies. For example, see DiFabio[5] and Harrison and Kielhofner,[6] which were outlined in Chapter 4. See also other examples of validity and reliability studies in Chapter 4 that use correlational statistics.

Statistical Approaches

The perfect correlations illustrated in Figure 6–1 (A and E) are sometimes called lines of perfect linear regression. In graphs B and D one could draw a line that would "best fit" all the individual dots on the chart; this is called a line of best fit, or a regression line. In general, **regression** establishes a mathematical relationship between two or more variables that best describes the total group. Metric data are required for statistical treatment by regression. It is also possible for two sets of data to be associated in a nonlinear or curvilinear manner (e.g., measures of motivation).[7] However, these possibilities will not be explored in this text.

The general formula for a (straight) regression line is

$$Y = a + bX$$

where a is the point where the line intercepts the Y axis, and b is the slope of the line. "The correlation coefficient provides a quantitative description of how well the regression line fits the actual data."[8] The correlational measure of association is really a descriptive statistic, and the measure of the significance of that association is an inferential statistic.[9]

The correlational question concerns the degree of association between two variables in a given population, and the predictive question asks how accurately one can predict score A on the basis of score B. Regression analysis allows one to make such predictions. When regression is used for predictive purposes, it is proper to speak of one variable as the independent variable and the other variable as the dependent, or criterion, variable. At other times, when one is only asking an associational question, the variables do not have an independent-dependent relationship; they are then only the variables to be tested for association.

Most correlational techniques are designed to seek the relationship between two variables; there are at least a dozen different statistical tools designed for bivariate data. There are also correlational techniques for multivariate data.[10] Which technique is appropriate in any given study will depend on the nature of the data, specifically the level of measurement (whether it is nominal, ordinal, or metric), and whether the nature of each variable is continuous or discrete.

The two methods that are seen most frequently in the literature are the Pearson Product-Moment Correlation (r), which is appropriate for metric variables that are continuous, and the Spearman rank order correlation (ρ), which is appropriate for two variables that are measured at the ordinal level. Other techniques include: Cronbach's coefficient α for dichotomous or discrete data, for example, a Likert scale of strongly agree, agree, indifferent, disagree, strongly disagree,[11] a π coefficient for ordinal data,[12] Kendall's τ for small samples of ordinal data,[10] Kendall's coefficient of concordance (W) for three or more sets of ranked (ordinal) data,[13] Yule's Q for two nominal scale measures and κ for two or more nominal classifications.[14]

The κ coefficient is being used more frequently in the therapy journals in recent years. Its basic formula is:

$$\kappa = \frac{p_o - p_c}{1 - p_c}$$

where p_o = proportion of observed agreements, and p_c = proportion of agreements expected due to chance.[15] κ values higher than .7 are considered excellent; values between .4 and .7 are fair to good. O'Neil and her colleagues[16] used the κ statistic

to determine the amount of agreement between two therapists' assessments and treatment plans, thereby establishing the interrater reliability of both the evaluation form and the treatment model. The κ statistic was chosen because it is applicable to categorical [discrete] variables and because it assesses agreement beyond what would be expected based on chance alone.... The kappa values for patient assessments ranged from .45 to .94, except for the impaired balance category, which had a low Kappa value of .05. All the percentages of agreement for the assessments were 75% or better. The Kappa values for patient treatment ranged from .42 to .91, except for the postural training category in which the Kappa value was .11 and the balance training category in which the Kappa value could not be calculated. All percentages of agreement for the treatments were also 75% or better.

Other examples of the use of κ were cited in Chapter 4.[17,18]

There are numerous other formulae for different types of data. For examples of the use of Chronbach's α see Case-Smith[19] or Hayes[20]; for τ, see Harrison and Kielhofner[21]; for a multiple regression analysis, see McInerney and McInerney[22]; for the use of Kendall's W, see Corb[23] and Filiatrault and colleagues.[24] In Chapter 4 an article by Bhasin and Goodman was quoted that used Krippendorff's statistic to establish reliability.[25] Galski, Burno, and Eble used a combination of the Pearson correlation, point-biserial correlation, and multiple linear regressions to show that 93 percent of the driving outcomes of brain-damaged patients driving in traffic could be predicted by an assessment battery.[26]

Table 6–2 provides an example of the calculation of the Pearson cor-

TABLE 6–2 **CALCULATION OF THE PEARSON PRODUCT-MOMENT CORRELATION COEFFICIENT**

Subject	x	y	x^2	y^2	xy
1	30	32	900	1,024	960
2	80	77	6,400	5,929	6,160
3	68	75	4,624	5,625	5,100
4	100	99	10,000	9,801	9,900
5	110	116	12,100	13,456	12,760
6	50	55	2,500	3,025	2,740
7	95	96	9,025	9,216	9,120
8	75	75	9,625	9,625	9,625
9	72	70	5,184	4,900	5,040
10	85	85	7,225	7,225	7,225
Σ	765	780	67,583	69,826	68,630

$$r_{xy} = \frac{n\Sigma xy - \Sigma x\Sigma y}{\sqrt{[n\Sigma x^2 - (\Sigma x)^2][n\Sigma y^2 - (\Sigma y)^2]}}$$

$$= \frac{10 \cdot 68,630 - 765 \cdot 780}{\sqrt{(10 \cdot 67,583 - 585,225)(10 \cdot 69,826 - 608,400)}}$$

$$= \frac{49,700}{50,231.118} = 0.98$$

relation using hypothetical data. The Pearson is a generalized measure of linear association.[27] Suppose that you wanted to know how reliable you are in measuring flexibility at the elbow (intrarater reliability). Goniometry provides metric data, so the Pearson is appropriate. You ask a question of association concerning a bivariate distribution: What is the degree of association between two measures taken by one therapist on one sample? Select a sample of convenience: the first 10 patients with symptoms involving an elbow who consent to be subjects in your study. The decision is made to take only two measurements from each subject, so you may use the Pearson. You defend against bias by covering one side of the goniometer and having a colleague read the other side and record the data after each measurement. Separate the measurements by 15 minutes. Are there other considerations listed in Appendix A that you should consider before you proceed?

The conceptual model for the Pearson Product-Moment Correlation coefficient is:

$$r_{xy} = \frac{\Sigma (x - \bar{x}) (y - \bar{y})}{ns_x s_y}$$

where x = the first score,
    $\bar{x}$ = the mean of all first scores,
    y = the paired second score,
    $\bar{y}$ = the mean of all second scores,
  s_x and s_y = the standard deviations of the respective data sets.

Study the relationships that enter into this formula. Critical factors are the deviation of each score from the mean of its data set, $x - \bar{x}$ and $y - \bar{y}$, the sample size, n, and the standard deviation (a measure of variability) within each of the two data sets, s_x and s_y.[9]

Table 6–2 uses an easier formula using raw data; x represents your first measurement and y the second. We will use a goniometric system where full extension is 0 degrees. To simplify the illustration, only measures of maximum voluntary flexion will be used.

Congratulations, you are very reliable with a goniometer on the elbow, if these two samples of your performance are representative of your usual behavior. Of course, most statistical analyses can now be done on computers using any one of several statistical software packages, but it is sometimes helpful to see the basic format when one is first learning a new technique.

Case-Smith used the Pearson to demonstrate "low correlations between scores on tactile defensiveness and tactile discrimination." She used subtests of the Southern California Sensory Integration tests and concluded that "these two aspects of tactile function are separate but related phenomena."[28] For other examples of the use of the Pearson, see DiFabio,[29] Bundy and colleagues,[30] Robinson and colleagues,[31] and Agnew and Maas.[32]

Table 6–3 illustrates the computation of the Spearman, which may be used for data that are ordinal or higher.[33] Let us suppose that a suitable research protocol has been written and that we have scores on a teacher-made practical laboratory examination in a course requiring manual skills (score A) and scores given by clinical educators on "clinical efficiency" (score B) for 10 students. These are ordinal data. The maximum for score A is 50 and for score B is 10. Each score is ranked within its own data set. Be sure you understand how these ranking figures were derived for the table. Also notice how tied scores are ranked; for example, in column A, two subjects have a score of 45 for ranks 4 and 5; both are given a rank of 4.5. The difference between the ranks of each pair is recorded (D) and squared (D^2).

For examples of the use of the Spearman, see Van Deusen and Harlow,[34] Titus,[35] Deitz,[36] and Filiatrault.[37]

A third statistical technique that has been gaining increasing recognition in recent years is the intraclass correlation (ICC) for metric data.[38]

TABLE 6–3　**ILLUSTRATION OF THE SPEARMAN RANK-ORDER CORRELATION COEFFICIENT**

Subject	A	A Rank	B	B Rank	D	D^2
1	45	4.5	10	1.5	3	9.0
2	50	1	9	3.5	− 2.5	6.25
3	35	7	7	7.5	− .5	.25
4	30	9.5	5	10	− .5	.25
5	45	4.5	8	5.5	− 1.0	1.0
6	46	3	9	3.5	− .5	.25
7	30	9.5	6	9	.5	.25
8	32	8	7	7.5	.5	.25
9	48	2	10	1.5	.5	.25
10	37	6	8	5.5	.5	.25
					Σ	18.0

$$= 1 - \frac{6\Sigma D^2}{n(n^2 - 1)}$$

$$= 1 - \frac{6 \cdot 18}{10(100 - 1)}$$

$$= 1 - .109$$

$$= .891$$

This is a moderately high association.

There are several advantages to this procedure, especially in reliability studies. The first advantage is that the ICC measures agreement rather than association. The data in Table 6–1 would produce a perfect $+1.0$ using the Pearson but something less than that using an ICC formula. A second advantage of the ICC is that it is useful when more than two sets of data are produced, as in repeated measures. Partial correlation and multiple correlation techniques examine the association between three or more variables, for example, scores on tests of functional skills, flexibility, and strength. The ICC examines two or more sets of scores on the same variable, for example, four sets of scores produced by repeatedly measuring range of hip motion in the *same* group of subjects. The ICC formulas do not produce negative numbers like the Pearson or the Spearman. With the ICC, "no agreement" produces a 0.

Table 6–4 provides an illustration of the use of intraclass correlation using data from a study published by Riddle, Rothstein, and Lamb,[39] based on Riddle's master's thesis. The study was multifaceted; for illustrative purposes, Table 6–4 uses the data for intrarater reliability on two therapists.

TABLE 6–4 **ILLUSTRATION OF CALCULATION OF AN INTRACLASS CORRELATION**

Subject	Measure 1	Measure 2
1	44°	61°
2	27°	27°
3	39°	44°
4	46°	45°
•		
•		
•		
99	89°	87°
100	76°	67°

Analysis of Variance

Source of Variation	SS	df	MS	F
Between people	55217.52	99	557.75	
Within people	1728.00	100	17.28	32.277
Trials	50.00	1	50.00	
Residual	56945.520	99	16.949	

$$\text{ICC} = \frac{\text{BMS} - \text{WMS}}{\text{BMS} + (k - 1)\text{WMS}}$$

$$= \frac{557.75 - 17.28}{557.75 + 1 \cdot 17.28}$$

$$= .94$$

Each therapist gathered two data sets from 50 subjects for a total of 100 paired measurements of shoulder extension using a small goniometer. Riddle provided the raw data and analyses for Table 6–4.

Shrout and Fleiss[41] provide six different formulas for ICC depending on whether (1) one-way or two-way analysis of variance is desirable (analysis of variance will be discussed in Chapter 9); (2) differences between raters' mean scores are of interest; and (3) individual or mean ratings will be used. Analysis of variance (ANOVA) is used in the ICC only to produce the mean squares (MS) data to factor out variance. (In Chapter 9 analysis of variance will be used to generate a statistic called an F ratio.) The ANOVA was done by computer and only the results are available; a formula will be illustrated in Chapter 9. In the ICC formula:

k = the number of raters (two in this case)
SS = sum of squares
df = degrees of freedom
MS = mean squares
BMS = between mean squares
WMS = within mean squares

Effgen and Brown[42] used both the Pearson and the ICC to analyze their data. Note the almost identical results of the two tests.

The long-term stability of hand-held dynamometric measurements was assessed in 30 muscle groups of 12 children with myelomeningocele, before and after a 23-day interval. Measurements from a majority of the muscle groups had excellent stability, based on statistical indicators of association (Pearson Product-Moment Correlation Coefficients, r = .76 − .98) and agreement (intraclass correlation coefficients, ICC = .75 − .99). Muscle groups with lower long-term stability were the right and left wrist extensors and flexors, the left hip adductors and extensors, the left knee flexors, and the right and left knee extensors. Upper-extremity muscle groups had higher long-term stability than did lower-extremity muscle groups. The results indicate that the dynamometric measurements were highly reliable when the test-retest interval was 23 days. Other researchers have previously shown high reliability for these measurements over shorter periods of time. Improved reliability might be obtained by supporting the lower extremity during hip extension tests, padding the dynamometer end pieces, especially when testing over bony prominences, and using a smaller, digital dynamometer. The hand-held dynamometer appears to warrant use and further investigation with pediatric populations.

For other examples of the use of the ICC in physical and occupational therapy literature, see DiFabio,[43] Harrison and Kielhofner,[44] Griegel-Morris,[45] and Shields and Cook.[46]

It is also possible to apply a statistical test that will determine the probability that certain variables are unrelated in a population when one has obtained a given correlation as large as the one observed in the sample. (Probability tests will be discussed further in Chapter 8.) These tests determine the significance of a correlation coefficient, that is, your chances of being wrong if you said that a correlation as high as the one obtained would not occur by chance. For the Pearson, this probability test is a variation on the t-test to be discussed in Chapter 8. For example, checking the appropriate statistical table in Stahl and Hennes[47] reveals that the r = .98 in Table 6–2 is significant at or below $P = <.001$. This means that there is only 1 chance in 1000 of getting a correlation that high in your sample if in the population r = 0.

If two variables to be correlated have only a few values—for example, low, medium, or high pain to be correlated with mild, moderate, and vigorous exercise—the chi-square statistic can be used, and the chi-square produces an associated probability (p) value. The chi-square will be discussed and illustrated in Chapter 8; there you will be reminded that the test can also be used to test association.

Quite frequently one really wants to be able to use the statement of significance to predict one variable on the basis of another. If one can demonstrate a high correlation between preadmission SAT scores and grade-point average at graduation, and rationally defend a relationship between the two, then one should be able to predict that in next year's class the students with the highest entering SAT scores will have the highest GPA upon graduation. An expansion of the regression concept allows one to predict score B on the basis of score A.

Because it is possible to do a test of significance on a correlation statistic, and to use significant findings to make predictions, correlation is frequently considered to be a part of predictive statistics. However, many studies stop with the calculation of the correlation. Therefore, the author has chosen to discuss correlation as separate from both descriptive and predictive research designs. From yet another perspective, some writers separate research into observational (descriptive and correlational) and manipulative or experimental. Such distinctions are probably not of much importance, but the reader will see these terms used.

In some studies a **correlation matrix** will be found. A correlation matrix provides a table of all possible correlations among given data sets. Neeman[48] provides an example. Neeman administered the Purdue Perceptual-Motor Survey to 99 mentally retarded children and young adults. The test provides subscores for variables such as walking a board backward, rhythmic writing, and ocular pursuits. A table was created with 19 subscores listed on both the horizontal and the vertical; the correlation coefficient of each subscore with every other subscore is listed in the table— a total of 334 correlations. A computerized factor analysis produced seven factors—for example, laterality and ocular control—which were most associated with the scores of the subjects. Correlation matrices often appear with statistical tests of significance to define those associations in the table that are least likely to occur by chance.

Many factors affect the correlation coefficient. Wang has suggested that longer test instruments often have higher reliability than shorter ones, Likert scales often have higher reliability than dichotomous scales, and increasing the number of subjects will increase the reliability.[49]

Computer-assisted statistical analysis can greatly reduce the stress and strain of numbers crunching as well as the chances of human error. The SPSS, SPSS/PC, and SAS software packages discussed in Chapter 9 can be used to do regression and correlation studies. Many of the studies already cited mention computer use in their data analysis section.

Practice You have already reviewed paragraphs 13 through 19 in Giannini in Appendix C in conjunction with our discussion of reliability. Look at it now in terms of the correlations measured. What variables are tested for association? How are the correlations reported? What statistical tools were used? (Do not worry about the *p* values now, but come back to them after you have studied Chapter 8.) How were the correlational data interpreted? Can you think of some researchable questions that these correlations suggest? Also look at paragraph 17 in Magill-Evans and Restall in Appendix C. How have they used correlational data?

Review Questions

1 Turn to the review questions in Chapter 1. Question 2 states, ``What is the reliability of ``standard" manual goniometry as used by the therapists in the clinic?" Write a correlational research protocol for this question. Use as much of the model in Appendix A as you are familiar with and deem appropriate; define your variables, level of measurement, and so on. Make an educated guess as to the probable results. Interpret those results.

2 See question 6: ``Do goniometric measures of joint mobility predict the patient's level of functional ability?" Write a protocol as outlined above.

References

1. Ghiselli, EE, Campbell, JP, and Zedeck, S: Measurement Theory for the Behavioral Sciences. WH Freeman, San Francisco, 1981, p. 475.
2. Rothstein, JM (ed): Measurement in Physical Therapy. Churchill Livingstone, New York, 1985, Chapter 1.
3. Hamilton, M: Lectures on the Methodology of Clinical Research, ed 2. Churchill Livingstone, London, 1974, pp 34–35.

4. Malgady, RG and Krebs, DE: Understanding correlation coefficients and regression. Phys Ther 66:110, 1986.
5. DiFabio, RP: Reliability of computerized surface electromyography for determining the onset of muscle activity. Phys Ther 67:43, 1987.
6. Harrison, H and Kielhofner, G: Examining reliability and validity of the Preschool Play Scale with handicapped children. AJOT 40:167, 1986.
7. Ghiselli, op cit, p 80.
8. Malgady and Krebs, op cit.
9. Stahl, SM and Hennis, JD: Reading and Understanding Applied Statistics. CV Mosby, St. Louis, 1980, Chapter 11.
10. Leedy, PD: Practical Research: Planning and Design, ed 2. Macmillan, New York, 1980, pp 156–157.
11. Ghiselli, op cit, p 256.
12. Stahl and Hennis, op cit, Chapter 13.
13. Daniel, WW: Applied Nonparametric Statistics. Houghton Mifflin, Boston, 1978, pp 326–334.
14. Fleiss, JL: Measuring nominal scale agreement among many raters. Psychol Bull 76:378, 1971.
15. Cohen, J: A coefficient of agreement for nominal scales. Ed & Psychol Measure 20:37, 1960.
16. O'Neil, MB, et al: Physical therapy assessment and treatment protocol for nursing home residents. Phys Ther 72:596, 1992, pp 599–600.
17. Youdas, JW, et al: Reliability and validity of judgments of applicant essays as a predictor of academic success in an entry-level physical therapy education program. JPTEd 6:15, 1992.
18. Titus, MND, et al: Correlation of perceptual performance and activities of daily living in stroke patients. AJOT 45:410, 1991.
19. Case-Smith, J: A validity study of the posture and fine motor assessment of infants. AJOT 46:597, 1992.
20. Hayes, KW, et al: Computer-based patient management problems in an entry-level physical therapy program: Acceptance and cost. JPTEd 5:65, 1991.
21. Harrison and Kielhofner, op. cit.
22. McInerney, CA and McInerney, M: A mobility skills training program for adults with developmental disabilities. AJOT 46:233, 1992.
23. Corb, DF, et al: Changes in students' perceptions of the professional role. Phys Ther 67:226, 1987.
24. Filiatrault, J, et al: Motor function and activities of daily living assessments: A study of three tests for persons with hemiplegia. AJOT 45:806, 1991.
25. Bhasin, CA and Goodman, GD: The use of OT FACT categories to analyze activity configurations of individuals with multiple sclerosis. OTJR 12:67, 1992.
26. Galski, T, Bruno, RL, and Ehle, HT: Driving after cerebral damage: A model with implications for evaluation. AJOT 46:324, 1992.
27. Ghiselli, op cit.
28. Case-Smith, J: The effects of tactile defensiveness and tactile discrimination on in-hand manipulation. AJOT 45:811, 1991.
29. DiFabio, RP: Reliability of computerized surface electromyography for determining the onset of muscle activity. Phys Ther 67:43, 1987.
30. Bundy, AC, et al: Concurrent validity of equilibrium tests in boys with learning disabilities with and without vestibular dysfunction. AJOT 41:28, 1987.
31. Robinson, ME, et al: Reliability of lumbar isometric torque in patients with chronic low back pain. Phys Ther 72:186, 1992.
32. Agnew, PJ and Maas, F: Jamar dynamometer and adapted sphygmomanometer for measuring grip strength in patients with rheumatoid arthritis. OTJR 11:259, 1991.
33. Stahl and Hennes, op. cit.

34. Van Deusen, J and Harlowe, D: Continued construct validation of the St. Marys CVA evaluation: Brunnstrom arm and hand stage ratings. AJOT 40:561, 1986.
35. Titus, MND, et al: Correlation of perceptual performance and activities of daily living in stroke patients. AJOT 45:410, 1991.
36. Deitz, JC, Crowe, TK, and Harris, SR: Relationship between infant neuromotor assessment and preshcool motor measures. Phys Ther 67:14, 1987.
37. Filiatrault et al, op cit.
38. Rothstein, op cit.
39. Riddle, DL, Rothstein, JM, and Lamb, RL: Goniometric reliability in a clinical setting: Shoulder measurements. Phys Ther 67:668, 1987.
40. Riddle, DL: The Reliability of Shoulder Joint Range of Motion Measurements in a Clinical Setting. Unpublished master's thesis, Medical College of Virginia, Virginia Commonwealth University, 1985.
41. Shrout, PE and Fleiss, JL: Intraclass correlations: Uses in assessing rater reliability. Psychol Bull 86:420, 1979.
42. Effgen, SK and Brown, DA: Long-term stability of hand-held dynamometric measurements in children who have myelomeningocele. Phys Ther 72:458, 1992.
43. DiFabio, op cit.
44. Harrison and Kielhofner, op cit.
45. Griegel-Morris, P, et al: Incidence of common postural abnormalities in the cervical, shoulder, and thoracic regions and their association with pain in two age groups of healthy subjects. Phys Ther 72:425, 1992.
46. Shields, RK and Cook, TM: Lumbar support thickness: Effect on seated buttock pressure in individuals with and without spinal cord injury. Phys Ther 72:218, 1992.
47. Stall and Hennes, op. cit.
48. Neeman, RL: Perceptual-motor attributes of mental retardates: A factor analytic study. Percep and Mot Skills 33:927, 1971.
49. Wang, M, Airhihenbuwa, CO, and Okolo, EN: Data analysis and selection of statistical methods. In Okolo, EN (ed): Health Research Design and Methodology. CRC Press, Ann Arbor, 1990, Chapter 4.

*There is no average
individual; for that
matter, there is no
average rat.*

K. DUNLAP

7

*Single-Case
Experimental Designs*

Clinical Research

The difference between basic and applied research was discussed in
Chapter 2. In general, basic scientists are interested in working on theoretical problems, while clinical scientists are interested in clinical problems.[1] Basic research is usually done in laboratories by scientists who are
trained in the basic sciences such as chemistry, anatomy, physiology, and
so on. They are well educated in their discipline, in the scientific method,
and in research design, but they seldom have clinical experience or expertise. Clinical research is usually done in patient care settings by clinical
scientists who are trained in the professions such as medicine, nursing,
physical therapy or occupational therapy; they have clinical experience
but are often relatively less well trained in research methodology. As more
therapists are trained at the doctoral level, especially in the basic sciences,

the line between basic and clinical research is blurring in a few isolated instances, but it is generally true.

Goldstein[2] has defined clinical studies as any research "in which clinical judgment is used as either a dependent or an independent variable." The physical therapy diagnosis or occupational therapy diagnosis and many assessments of clinical outcomes are examples of clinical judgments. While Goldstein's definition could apply to any design, several designs are of special use to clinicians. This chapter and the section in Chapter 8 on sequential clinical trials are concerned particularly with the research needs of clinical scientists.

Since all of the research designs discussed in Chapters 5, 6, 8, and 9 are used in clinical research, why a separate emphasis here? There are two reasons, the first has to do with individual differences. Through an interesting quirk of history, the designs discussed in Chapter 8 were originally developed in a practice setting (agricultural field studies) but were later taken over by the laboratory scientists because they met their needs so well.[3] The problem is that Fisher's designs, such as the t-test for completely randomized block designs, were developed out of such questions as, Which treatment on two fields of corn produced the greatest yield *on the average?* He had no interest in what happened to individual stalks, heads, or grains of corn. Basic scientists found that approach compatible with their interests in basic questions about how things *generally* work.

By the middle of the 20th century psychologists and others who were concerned with the performance of individual human beings were becoming acutely aware of problems with group designs. A number of studies seemed to indicate that psychotherapy made no difference. However, when the data were analyzed carefully, it turned out that some patients got better and some got worse. The group design canceled out these effects because group designs are not sensitive to individual differences, only to group averages and variances. Clinical scientists are interested in individual patients, however, so new designs needed to be developed to respond to the need to document in a scientific way individual responses to therapeutic interventions.[4] Riddoch and Lennon[5] have made a similar point concerning physiotherapy. They did a meta-analysis of "40 core rehabilitation journals" and concluded that there were very few high-quality scientific studies of the outcomes of physiotherapy (see Chapter 5). They state that individual case studies relative to outcomes of therapy are clinically important, whereas general (group) studies are economically important. They cite a study in which 9 out of 10 patients had negative side effects from a therapeutic procedure, but it was good for the 10th patient. Both sets of data (patients 1 to 9 and patient 10) are clinically important, but the data from the 10th patient gets lost in a group study. "The problem here is that a particular therapy may only be effective in certain cases, and not others. If nonsignificant findings are obtained following a group study, it seems unlikely that further time will be spent investigating the effects of the therapy on a number of individual subjects. Thus, a particular therapy, potentially important for certain individuals, may be abandoned."[6] Single-subject designs document "a particular treatment *individualized* to the *individual* patient with the aim of producing significant changes in the *individual* patient's condition."[7]

It is often difficult to obtain equivalent groups of patients when the condition is characterized by wide variability, as, for example, in the case of people with cerebral palsy. For the same reason, it is often difficult to generalize from a group study to other groups or individuals. Barlow and Hersen have stated that, in fact, single-case designs produce greater generality than group designs do because they *account for* variability rather than averaging it out. "The more we learn about the effects of a treatment on different individuals, in different settings, and so on, the easier it will be to determine if that treatment will be effective with the next individual walking into the office."[8] Individual differences are considered something of a nuisance in group research, but they are important to the clinician who must treat such individuals. As suggested in the discussion of intensive case studies in Chapter 5, a single-case, time-series design repeated on a number of patients that gives consistent results can build strong support for the treatment applied. Intensive and experimental case studies may be the research tools most appropriate at the cutting edges of a discipline. They are also appropriate when large groups are not available for study.

The second reason for a special emphasis on clinical designs is the importance of clinical research in validating clinical practice. In occupational and physical therapy all research roads eventually lead to the central question, What difference does it make to the patient? Frequently the descriptive, correlational, and predictive designs discussed in other chapters are appropriate for answering this question. At other times, however, it is very difficult to apply traditional predictive designs to human subjects in a clinical setting because these designs make some assumptions about random assignment to treatment and control groups that are difficult or impossible to meet. Both the random selection of the sample from the population and random assignment of the sample to treatment groups may be very difficult. The creation of control groups also raises some ethical issues concerning optimum patient care. Unless you can truly say that you do not know whether the treatment will make a difference or not, it is difficult to defend withholding treatment for the sake of experimental design.

Single-case designs are useful in the evaluation of individual patients, both for the routine documentation of treatment effectiveness and in quality assurance studies. These designs may be easily utilized in a clinical setting without disrupting clinical routine. As in other forms of research it is important to define several factors carefully, including criteria for admission to the study (an important form of control), the independent variable, the dependent variable, the measurement tool, the time intervals between measurements, and other treatment variables. The designs in this chapter and in Chapter 8 have been developed to respond to just such concerns.

Single-Case Designs

Single-case designs address themselves primarily to questions of difference: Is there a difference between treatment A and treatment B? In single-case designs, treatment A is usually, but not necessarily, a no-treatment control.

Single-case experimental designs are also frequently called "interrupted time-series designs" because measurements are repeated at specific time intervals. They may also be called "intrasubject replication designs" because of the repeated measures taken of the dependent variable in one subject. "One subject" may mean one person, one department, or one hospital. Such designs are also called "ideographic designs."[9] Most of the designs discussed in the other chapters in this text are concerned primarily or exclusively with the end results of the experiment. Interrupted time-series designs lend themselves to the study of the *process* of treatment as well as the end results because repeated responses to treatment are examined individually, not just as group means. It is useful to consider time-series designs as a more experimental approach to the intensive case study design discussed in Chapter 5. In fact, single-case designs are called "intensive" because of the detailed look they take at one subject, in contrast to the extensive group designs of Chapters 8 and 9. Time-series designs are "not synonymous with the conventional case study in that single-subject research can have a formal experimental design, and data may be analyzed with quantitative measures,"[10] thus increasing the generalizability of the results.

Let us first consider the simplest time-series design, the A-B design.

A-B SINGLE-CASE DESIGN

Figure 7–1 illustrates the application of the A-B single-case design to a hypothetical clinical study. The question for this study is taken from the questions proposed in Chapter 1. Question 7 is, "Does heat applied prior to active exercise increase joint mobility more than active exercise alone?" (We shall see in Chapter 8 that this question can also be answered with a predictive research design.)

Let us say that we have one patient with limited joint mobility: full extension of the right elbow and limited flexion. On the first nine days of the experiment the patient receives only active exercise. On the 10th day

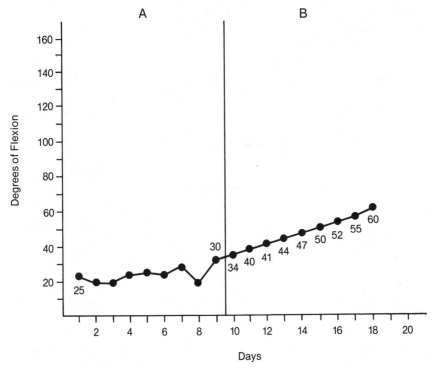

FIGURE 7–1   A-B single-case design.

a heat treatment is added to the routine before the same active-exercise program. The measured range of flexion at the end of each treatment is indicated on the vertical column of the graph. Phase A is called the baseline and phase B is called the treatment, even though the patient was receiving active exercise throughout the 18-day period. We are interested in the effects of the heat treatment. Figure 7–1 shows that although the patient showed a slight gain (5 degrees), the nine baseline days are best characterized as a straight horizontal line. During phase B there is steady improvement; over the second nine days of treatment the patient progressed from 34 to 60 degrees of active elbow flexion.

How can this data be interpreted? The heat seems to have made a difference. On the basis of this data the clinician would be encouraged to try again to see if indeed the combination of heat and active exercise is more effective than active exercise alone. However, on the basis of the data provided in Figure 7–1 the clinician must be cautious because there are several serious weaknesses in this design. Other influences occurring simultaneously with the heat treatment may have been responsible for the difference.

One of the things that encourages this alternate interpretation is the fact that the steady rise in range of motion actually began on day 8 rather than on day 10, and the largest change between any two days occurred between day 8 and day 9 during the baseline period. On the other hand, flexion on day 9 is barely above day 7, so day 8's flexion could also be the result of chance, or some transitory condition of increased pain, or some other uncontrolled, extraneous variable. Maturation or the healing effects of time may also account for changes seen in the A-B design. However, it does illustrate two very important criteria for the use of single-case, time-series designs: (1) the criterion measure is repeated very frequently, and (2) it is desirable for repeated measures to demonstrate a stable baseline before any treatment is begun. Repeated measures and a stable baseline are essential in most time-series designs. The ideal baseline is either stable or moving in a direction opposite to the one you expect the treatment to produce. As Riddoch and Lennon[11] note, "In order to counter the charge that the effects may simply be due to an extraneous variable and are not necessarily treatment-related, . . . small N designs may be employed. Here, the same therapeutic intervention is applied to a number of patients with similar aetiologies. Claims that changes are due to particular treatment interventions are justified if similar trends can be demonstrated across all the patients." By small N they mean 3 to 10.

For two examples of the A-B design see Dunbar, Jarvis, and Breyer[12] and Goodman and Bazyk.[13] Dunbar and her colleagues strengthened the A-B design by repeating the study on three children. Goodman and Bazyk strengthened their conclusions by studying the effects of their intervention on six tests related to hand use.

THE A-B-A SINGLE-CASE DESIGN

The A-B-A design is stronger because it decreases the chances of an extraneous variable being responsible for the graphed results. Figure 7–2 illustrates this design with hypothetical data. Let us assume another patient to whom heat is added (phase B) to active exercise of the elbow (phase A) as in the previous example. The second A phase is called the withdrawal or reversal phase because of what happens to the independent variable during this time. Laskas and her colleagues[14] used the A-B-A design to study the effects of four neurodevelopmental activities (NDT) on two dependent variables: heel contact on achieving a standing position and dorsiflexor response during a posterior equilibrium reaction. Results indicated that NDT had a positive influence on both target behaviors in a 2½-year-old quadriplegic male.

Given the data graphed in Figure 7–2, it would be difficult to argue against the effect of the treatment. Note that in this case the measured dependent variable only leveled off; it did not return to baseline in response

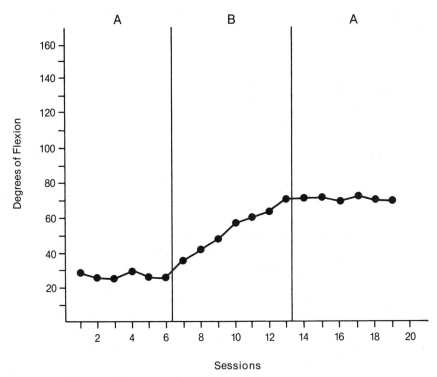

FIGURE 7–2   A-B-A single-case design.

to the withdrawal of the independent variable. This leveling off suggests that the gains made during the treatment phase are relatively stable. In other instances the dependent variable may regress toward the original baseline. An excellent example of A-B-A design is the study by Ostendorf and Wolf.[15] During the experimental phase B, a hemiplegic patient's intact upper extremity was restrained so that she used the affected arm of necessity. Frequency of use of the affected limb increased during phase B, but not the quality or efficiency of use as measured by several assessment tools. Ross used an A-B-A design with three subjects, each given three tests of visual scanning.[16] She concluded that the computer-assisted training program had no significant effect on the functional task.

B-A-B is a variation on this design wherein treatment is instituted, withdrawn, then reinstituted. Riddoch and Lennon have noted that the B-A-B design can be very effective when working with acutely ill patients for whom therapy must be instituted immediately.[17] After their condition stabilizes, the A phase can be tried in order to test the effects of the treatment. After a suitable withdrawal period has demonstrated a leveling off or a deterioration of the dependent variable, the second treatment (B) phase can be reinstituted.

THE A-B-A-B SINGLE-CASE DESIGN

Figure 7–3 illustrates the A-B-A-B design with hypothetical data. In this illustration, the A phases represent no treatment and the B phases represent biofeedback information on head position. The baseline is established in phase A_1, the treatment is applied during phase B_1, treatment is withdrawn during A_2, and treatment is reinstated during B_2. If the experiment is well planned, it will be extremely unlikely that the results here graphed could have happened in response to uncontrolled variables. The graphed data themselves argue strongly for the effect of the independent variable, positional biofeedback.

Unlike the data graphed in the A-B-A model above, the data in Figure 7–3 quickly returns to baseline when the treatment is withdrawn. This suggests that the treatment effect is temporary within the time span of phase B_1. In other motor learning studies this might not be so; once something is learned, forgetting is slower than shown here, depending on the nature of the material being learned and the abilities of the learner. Note that there is no overlap between phases; that is, the highest A score is lower than the lowest B score. We will return to this graph when we consider the analysis of time-series data.

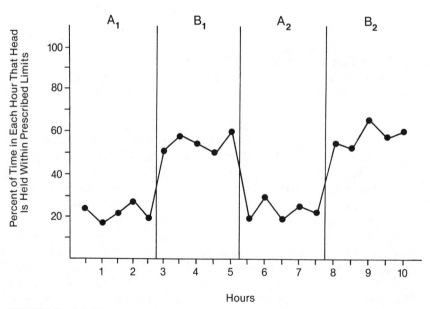

FIGURE 7–3   A-B-A-B single-case design.

A-B-C SINGLE-CASE DESIGNS

Up to this point we have been talking about experiments with one independent variable, that is, univariate designs, the A-B-A-B design and its variations. Let us now look at a single-case multivariate design. Phase A is baseline, phase B is treatment 1, and phase C is treatment 2. This applied research design permits the experimental analysis of behavior in an even more clinically typical format of more than one treatment modality. The design does not necessarily partial out the separate effects of the two treatments, and the graphed change may represent their interactive effects.[18] Figure 7–4 illustrates this design with hypothetical data. Note the overlap between some phases.

In designing and interpreting A-B-C models, one must be careful to avoid generating false impressions.[19] Goodisman has described a manipulation-free application of the A-B-C design without a baseline. His design permitted him to study the effects of four exercise variables on an independent measure of functional gait.[20] Another variation in A-B-C design— alternating treatments design—is detailed in Barlow and Hersen.[21] Riddoch and Lennon[22] have suggested the use of a neutral phase between different treatments—a B-A-C design. Figure 7–5 is reprinted from a study by the Neemans.[23] Their subject was a 22-year-old male with multiple impairments, including spastic quadriplegia. He demonstrated a stable IQ of 57 and was a client in a sheltered workship with a production record of 7.2 percent of estimated industrial norm. He performed upper-extremity activ-

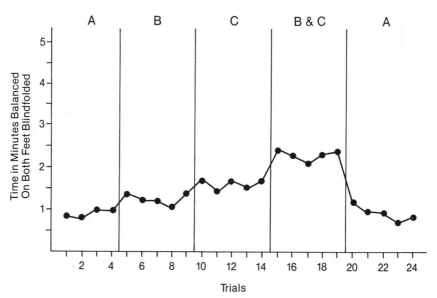

FIGURE 7–4   A-B-C design.

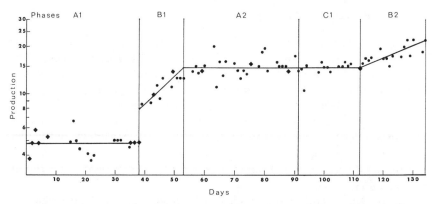

FIGURE 7–5   (Adapted from Neeman, RL, Neeman, HJ, and Neeman, M: A Single-Subject Study of Clinical Utility and Social Validity of Orthokinetics Treatment for Upper Extremity Dyskinesia in a Subject with Spastic Quadiplegia. Presented in part at the 9th International Congress of Physical Medicine and Rehabilitation of the International Federation of Physical Medicine and Rehabilitation, Jerusalem, Israel, May 1984, Abstract No. 204; with permission.)

ities very slowly because of spasticity. The experimental design was a time-series A_1-B_1-A_2-C-B_2 design, wherein A_1 was the pretreatment baseline phase and A_2 was the posttreatment control phase in which the subject worked at an industrial task without any therapeutic intervention. B_1 and B_2 represented treatment phases when the subject wore cuff-shaped orthokinetic orthoses on both arms; these orthoses were designed to control spasticity while the subject continued working. C was a placebo treatment phase (see p. 142) during which time the subject received personal attention while working and wore placebo cuffs made of plain elastic rubber bandage. During the B treatment phases three orthokinetic cuffs were placed to facilitate wrist and finger extension for functional grasp stabilization and grasp release. Daily production rates formed the dependent variable. The lines on Fig. 7–5 represent "lines of best fit" of the data, similar to regression lines discussed in the last chapter. However, here they are called celeration lines and are based on a statistical technique called the "split-middle procedure." Both visually and statistically, phases A and C produced no change. The B phases demonstrated change by acceleration in production, both visually and statistically. After autocorrelation was demonstrated to be nonsignificant (see statistical discussion, pp. 139–140), the Neemans used a t-test (see Chapter 8) to support significant differences in production rates pretreatment to posttreatment, treatment being phase B_1. Barlow and Hersen[24] defend this use of the t-test in cases where autocorrelation is not significant, as was found in the Neeman study. The Neemans inferred that this design protects against threats to internal validity and hence that the increase in production rate of the subject was an outcome of the orthokinetic treatment.

Sharpe[25] used an A-B-C design with contrasting results for the two treatments.

A single-subject rapidly alternating treatment design was used to compare the effectiveness of bilateral hand splints and an elbow orthosis in decreasing stereotypic hand behaviors and increasing toy play in 2 children with Rett syndrome. The subjects' responses were compared across three treatment conditions: no intervention, hand splints, and elbow orthosis. The order of the treatment phases was randomly selected for each subject. Data were collected in both a free-time condition and a toy-play condition; the outcome measures were stereotypic hand movements and hand-to-toy contact. Both subjects demonstrated a decrease in stereotypic hand movements and a corresponding increase in toy contact with the use of the elbow orthosis. The bilateral hand splints had no obvious treatment effect.

For an A-B-C-A design with five subjects aged 57 to 74, see Cermak et al.[26]

MULTIPLE-BASELINE DESIGNS

The ethical disadvantages of withdrawal of beneficial treatment may not be justifiable or acceptable in many situations. In order to achieve the strength of the A-B-A-B design without risking its disadvantages, the multiple-baseline design has been devised. A multiple-baseline study across behaviors is illustrated in Figure 7–6 with hypothetical data.

In this illustration the patient has limited ROM in three joints. Throughout the experiment all three joints receive active range of motion. However, the heat treatment is applied sequentially, first to the shoulder, then to the shoulder and elbow, and finally to the shoulder, elbow, and wrist. (An important assumption here is that the ranges of motion in the three joints are independent of one another.) The results graphed in Figure 7–6 give strong support to the idea that heat improved the treatment.

Martin and Epstein[27] indicate that this design may be used with a multiple baseline across behaviors, across subjects, or across settings. Redraw Figure 7–6 so that heat is applied to the elbow on three separate patients. Now redraw the figure to illustrate pain levels after exercise in physical therapy, in occupational therapy, and at home (multiple baselines across settings).

As an example from the literature, Barnes[28] used a multiple-baseline design across subjects with reversal phases (A-B-A-B-BC-B-BC) to study the prehension skills of three children with cerebral palsy. Two treatment procedures were used: weight bearing on extended arms and passive trunk rotation. Eight components of reach, grasp, and release were measured and graphed; Data were analyzed using a split-middle technique to evaluate trends.[29] Results indicated that weight bearing on extended arms improved prehension skills in all three children, but trunk rotation produced no

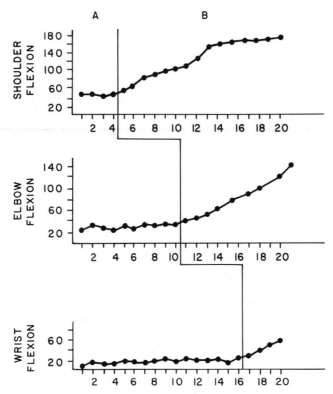

FIGURE 7–6   A multiple baseline study.

demonstrable change. For another study using multiple baseline across subjects, see Engel.[30]

ANALYSIS AND INTERPRETATION

The most typical, and perhaps the most useful, form of analysis of single-case interrupted time-series designs is through visual analysis of the graphed measurements of the dependent variable.[31,32] For graphic analysis to be effective, certain rules need to be observed. Measurement times are graphed on the horizontal, the dependent variable on the vertical. The spaces between points should be about the same on both vertical and horizontal; it is helpful to graph data on log paper. All possible points should be represented on the vertical; for example, if shoulder flexion is the dependent variable, the vertical should reflect degrees from 0 to 180. Baselines should be stable before treatment is initiated, and enough time and measurement points should be recorded in the treatment zones for change, or lack thereof, to be demonstrated. The target behavior should be observable and measurable, measurement tools should be reliable and valid, and all relevant terms should be operationally defined. Data collection plans should be specific and written. The graph should be drawn before data collection begins so that you are sure exactly what the data will look like.

In the visual interpretation of graphed data the following points should be considered.[33] How large is the mean (average) shift across phases? How great is the variability across phases? Is there a change in level between phases? Is there a change in slope across phases? Is there an overlap in range across phases? With visual inspection, if the baseline is not stable (level or going opposite to the desired direction) before treatment begins, interpretation may be in jeopardy; see, for example, the discussion of Figure 7–1. Riddoch and Lennon[34] offer one exception: they note that a slope in the desired direction may represent spontaneous recovery; if so, the treatment will need to change the rate of change in the slope significantly. Interpretation is based on

- Stability of all baselines.

- Variability of data in all phases.

- Changes in level within treatment phases. (Figure 7–6 illustrates a change in level with the initiation of treatment.)

- Changes in trends both within and between phases. (Trends may be upward or downward, sudden or gradual.)

Even when all of these rules are observed, there may still be problems with interpretations based on visual analysis alone. As Ottenbacher[35] has so clearly documented, visual inspection alone may lead to erroneous conclusions if the data are too dependent. Serial dependency or autocorrelation refer to the fact that two data points on a graph, as in Figure 7–1, may not be independent of each other. The second score may be dependent on the first, the third on the second, and so on. This is called a "lag 1 autocorrelation." If this autocorrelation is too high, visual inspection alone may give a false impression of change. Therefore, a test for autocorrelation is indicated.

Table 7–1 examines the lag 1 autocorrelation of data in phase B of Figure 7–1. The following steps were followed:[36]

1 Calculate the sum and mean of the nine scores.

2 Calculate the difference (d) between *each* score and the mean of *all* scores, that is, $x - \bar{x}$.

3 Multiply adjacent values: $(-13)(-7)$, $(-7)(-6)$, and so on.

4 Sum the values found in step 3.

5 Square the difference values from step 2.

TABLE 7–1 CALCULATION OF LAG 1 AUTOCORRELATION
COEFFICIENT FOR DATA FROM PHASE B OF FIGURE 7–1

Score	d	$x - \bar{x}$	d^2
34	-13	91	169
40	-7	42	49
41	-6	18	36
44	-3	0	9
47	0	0	0
50	3	15	9
52	5	40	25
55	8	104	64
60	13		169
Σ 423		310	530
$\bar{x}$ 47			

$$\text{Lag 1 autocorrelation coefficient} = \frac{310}{530} = .58$$

$$\text{Bartlett's value} = 2 \div \sqrt{n} = 2 \div \sqrt{9} = .66$$

6 Sum the values found in step 5.

7 Divide the sum from step 4 by the sum from step 6.

The result is the lag 1 autocorrelation coefficient for those data. Bartlett's value is $2 \div \sqrt{n}$, where n is the number of data points under analysis.[37] If the autocorrelation coefficient is *larger than* the associated Bartlett's value, then the autocorrelation is statistically significant. In Table 7–1 the autocorrelation of .58 is not statistically significant. This result supports the appropriateness of visual interpretation.

Although it is beyond the scope of this text, there are statistical methods for transforming the raw data to improve the quality of visual inspection, or inferential statistics may be applied. Ottenbacher[38] has also documented the relatively low interrater reliability of visual analysis, which suggests that more statistical sophistication is needed to develop this method into its full potential in the validation of clinical practice. One easy way to increase the confidence consistency in the analysis is to draw trend lines on each phase.[39] The split-middle technique is easy to do; it is described clearly by Woolery and Harris.[40]

In single-subject designs, we are not interested in mean scores for groups but whether the effect of treatment is immediate or delayed, abrupt or gradual, temporary or permanent. In other words, we are interested in the unique patterns of response to treatment over time. According to Payton,[41]

A causal hypothesis is based on rejecting less likely explanations of the data. Statements of causality are based on the trends demonstrated in the data in response to time and to the introduction of the independent variable and its subsequent manipulation through withdrawal or multiple baseline mechanisms. One expects the manipulation of the independent variable to have a reliable effect on the trends, levels, stability and/or variability of the data. The evidence from replication in a situation where the subject has served as his own control contributes to the believ-ability of the data. One can conclude that the treatment has been effective if variation is minimal within the experimental phases, if level or trend or both change in response to treatment, and if the withdrawal and second treatment phases mimic the initial A B phases.

The threats to internal and external validity discussed in Chapter 4 are relevant here also.

Farrell[42] studied a patient who could perform two tasks only with maximum assistance during the baseline phase. When therapy was insti-tuted for one task, the patient rapidly achieved independence on that task but remained dependent in the other task. Subsequent initiation of treat-ment for the second task led to independence. Riddoch and Lennon[43] observe that

In this instance successful treatment of one lower limb task did not generalize to another. Improvement in the second task only occurred as a direct result of the physiotherapeutic intervention. It is not easy to account for this improvement in terms of other environmental factors or spontaneous recovery, because (1) the patient remained dependent in another task until treatment was specifically directed towards it and (2) the original baselines were stable. It may not be necessary to perform any further analysis on data of this sort.

Statistical analysis of single-case designs is also possible but far beyond the scope of this text. While a few procedures are relatively easy,[44,45] most require elaborate mathematical analyses where computer assistance is indicated.[46,47] "It is also worthwhile to note," says Aufdemkampe,[48] "that until now no general agreement on the statistical analysis of results from single cases has been reached."

Practice   Read the article by Beattie in Appendix C. How many items from Appendix A can you find in Beattie? Based on the data given, do you agree with Beattie's conclusions? Analyze the internal and external validity of this study. How could you increase the external validity of this report?

Issues in Behavioral and Applied Research

Several critical issues have already been mentioned. Perhaps the most important one is the ethical issue of withholding treatment or giving a placebo to a control group or withholding treatment during the A phases of a single-case design. Sequential design comparing the conventional treatment to a new protocol is one way of dealing with this issue, as is the multiple-baseline design.

Another factor to be considered in research involving human beings is the Hawthorne effect. The Hawthorne effect derives its name from a study done by Elton Mayo and a group of researchers from Harvard University at the Hawthorne factory of the Western Electric Company between 1927 and 1932.[49] They originally started out to study the effect of lighting on fatigue and efficiency in factory workers. However, as the study progressed they soon discovered that no matter what they did to the lighting, production went up and the workers reported being less tired. As research in factory lighting it may have been a failure, but Mayo and his coworkers recognized an important ramification. In a series of subsequent experiments they were able to demonstrate that the workers' *knowledge* that they were participating in an experiment significantly changed their perceptions of the job situation and improved their productivity. The experiment became one of the classic studies in motivation, demonstrating the beneficial effects of being made to feel important and different as a result of attention being given to the individual or group.

Clearly, the Hawthorne effect could operate in a clinical research study. If the patients know that they are participating in a research study, they may be motivated to perform better, so their improvements may be due in part to the study itself and not necessarily to the treatment. With the emphasis today on human rights and informed consent, it is almost impossible to have a population of patients who do not know that they are participating in a study; a release form is usually required by law. Therefore, the clinical researcher must be aware of the Hawthorne effect, which, like the placebo, may be a powerful tool for therapeutic improvement. Perhaps the best one can do is to try to make the Hawthorne effect equally effective on all patients involved in the study.

Placebo effect has been mentioned several times in this chapter and the reader is probably already familiar with the concept, which is similar in many ways to the Hawthorne effect. In fact, Shepherd and Sartorius[50] have convincingly argued that even in animal studies therapeutic outcomes may be influenced by overcrowding, nutrition, physical activity, and similar environmental factors. "With the human subject, such psychosocial factors may assume still greater significance, especially in the therapeutic situation, when the assumption of the status of patient may be associated with unfamiliar attitudes and expectations, anxiety, fears, and the impact of the hospital milieu." In traditional pharmaceutical research the placebo is a chemically and biologically inactive substance that is usually shaped and colored to look like the active drug being studied. It is given to a control group to test the therapeutic effects of the active drug. The patients never know which drug they are getting—the active or the inactive one. Frequently the researchers use a double-blind procedure in which only one person knows who is getting the placebo and who is getting the drug. Ideally, that person has no connection with the study other than to dispense the two medications. If the active drug is no more effective than the placebo, it is generally discarded as a therapeutic tool.

However, Benson and Epstein[51] have written a fascinating article on how the placebo alone can be used for therapeutic purposes. Some investigators have been amazed at the benefits some patients derive from placebo treatment.

> The improvement actually results from the meaning of the pill as a symbol of the therapist's interest and concern as well as expertise, thereby combatting patients' feelings of isolation and improving their expectation of relief.... The placebo effect contributes substantially to the effectiveness of all medical and even some surgical procedures.[52]

Therapists have sometimes rigged modality machines, for example, ultrasound, so that they light up but deliver no energy. See Taylor and colleagues.[53] Another interesting discussion of the effects of placebos may be found in Spilker.[54] Klerman[55] has addressed the need for more research on the therapeutic effects of the placebo, including the Hawthorne effect.

Review Questions

1 Turn to the review questions in Chapter 1. Question 9 asks, ``Does goniometric biofeedback training increase functional ability?'' Develop several time-series experiments that will address this question; use both A-B-A-B and multiple-baseline designs.

2 Design an experiment using A-B-C design. How much of Appendix A was useful in designing your experiment?

3 How do the placebo and Hawthorne effects influence the studies that you designed in questions 1 and 2 above?

Additional Readings

Barlow, DH, Hayes, SC, and Nelson, RD: The Scientist Practitioner: Research and Accountability in Clinical and Educational Settings. Pergamon, New York, 1984.

Glass, GV, Willson, VL, and Gottman, JM: Design and Analysis of Time-Series Experiments. Colorado Associated University Press, Boulder, 1975.

Krishef, CF: Fundamental Approaches to Single-Subject Design and Analysis. Krieger, Melbourne, FL, 1991.

Ottenbacher, KJ: Evaluating Clinical Change: Strategies for Occupational and Physical Therapists. Williams & Wilkins, Baltimore, 1986.

References

1. Goldstein, G: A Clinician's Guide to Research Design. Chicago, Nelson-Hall, 1980.
2. Ibid., p 233.
3. Barlow, DH and Hersen, M (eds): Single-Case Experimental Designs, ed 2. New York: Pergamon Press, 1984.
4. Ottenbacher, K and York, J: Strategies for measuring clinical change: Implications for practice and research. AJOT 38:647, 1984.
5. Riddoch, J and Lennon, S: Evaluation of practice: The single-case study approach. Physiotherapy Theory and Practice 7:3, 1991.
6. Ibid., p 5.
7. Ibid., p 6.
8. Barlow and Hersen, op cit, p 49.
9. Parente, R and Parente, JA: Alternative research strategies for occupational therapy, Part 2: Ideographic and quality assurance research. AJOT 40:428, 1986.
10. Twemlow, SW and Warnock, JK: Single-subject methodology: Case history and time-series design. In Goldstein, G: A Clinician's Guide to Research Design. Nelson-Hall, Chicago, 1980, Chapter 9.
11. Riddoch and Lennon, op cit, p 8.
12. Dunbar, SB, Jarvis, AH, and Breyer, M: The transition from nonoral to oral feeding in children. AJOT 45:402, 1991.
13. Goodman, G and Bazyk, S: The effects of a short thumb opponens splint on hand function in cerebral palsy: A single-subject study. AJOT 45:726, 1991.
14. Laskas, CA, et al: Enhancement of two motor functions of the lower extremity in a child with spastic quadriplegia. Phys Ther 65:11, 1985.
15. Ostendorf, CG and Wolf, SL: Effect of forced use of the upper extremity of a hemiplegic patient on changes in function. Phys Ther 61:1022, 1981.
16. Ross, FL: The use of computers in occupational therapy for visual-scanning training. AJOT 46:314, 1992.
17. Riddoch and Lennon, op cit, p 8.
18. Goldstein, op cit.
19. Ibid.
20. Goodisman, LD: A manipulation-free design for single-subject cerebral palsy research. Phys Ther: 62:284, 1982.
21. Barlow and Hersen, op cit, pp 252–284.
22. Riddoch and Lennon, op cit, p 8.
23. Neeman, RL, Neeman, HJ, and Neeman, M: A Single-Subject Study of Clinical Utility and Social Validity of Orthokinetics Treatment for Upper Extremity Dyskinesia in a Subject with Spastic Quadriplegia. Presented in part at the 9th International Congress of Physical Medicine and Rehabilitation of the International Federation of Physical Medicine and Rehabilitation, Jerusalem, Israel, May 1984, Abstract No. 204.
24. Barlow and Hersen, op cit, p 294.
25. Sharpe, PA: Comparative effects of bilateral hand splints and an elbow orthosis on stereotypic hand movements and toy play in two children with Rett syndrome. AJOT 46:134, 1992.
26. Cermak, SA, et al: Effects of lateralized tasks on unilateral neglect after right cerebral vascular accident. OTJR 11:271, 1991.

27. Martin, JE and Epstein, LH: Evaluating treatment effectiveness in cerebral palsy: Single-subject designs. Phys Ther 56:285, 1976.
28. Barnes, KJ: Improving prehension skills of children with cerebral palsy: A clinical study. OTJ of Res 6:227, 1986.
29. Kazdin, AE: Statistical analysis for single-case experimental designs. In Barlow, DH, and Hersen, M (eds), op cit.
30. Engel, JM: Relaxation training: A self-help approach for children with headaches. AJOT 46:591, 1992.
31. Parsonson, BS and Baer DM: The analysis and presentation of graphic data. In Kratochwill, TR (ed): Single-Subject Research. New York: Academic Press, 1978, Chapter 2.
32. Wolery, M and Harris SR: Interpreting results of single-subject research designs. Phys Ther 62:445, 1982.
33. Gibson, G and Ottenbacher, K: Characteristics influencing the visual analysis of single subject data: An empirical analysis. J Applied Behav Sci 24:298, 1988.
34. Riddoch and Lennen, op cit, p 9.
35. Ottenbacher, KJ: An analysis of serial dependency in occupational therapy research. OTJ of Res 6:211, 1986.
36. Ibid.
37. Bloom, M and Fischer, J: Evaluating Practice: Guidelines for the Accountable Professional. Prentice-Hall, Englewood Cliffs, NJ 1982, p 408.
38. Ottenbacher, KJ: Reliability and accuracy of visually analyzing graphed data from single-subject designs. AJOT 40:464, 1986.
39. Hojem, MA and Ottenbacher, KJ: Empirical investigation of visual-inspection versus trend-line analysis of single-subject data. Phys Ther 68:983, 1988.
40. Woolery and Harris, op cit.
41. Payton, OD: Single-subject, behavioral and sequential medical trials research. In Bork, CE (ed): Research in Physical Therapy. Philadelphia: JB Lippincott, 1993, Chapter 7.
42. Farrell, JC: Transfer ability in a patient with spinal cord compression: A multiple baseline design. Physiotherapy Theory and Practice 7:39, 1991.
43. Riddoch and Lennon, op cit, p 9.
44. Goldstein, op cit.
45. Barlow and Hersen, op cit, pp 252–284.
46. Kazdin, op cit.
47. Kratochwill, TR: Single Subject Research. New York: Academic Press, 1978.
48. Aufdemkampe, G: Some comments on single case studies. Physiotherapy Theory and Practice 7:63, 1991, p 68.
49. Todes, JL, et al: Management and Motivation: An Introduction to Supervision. New York: Harper & Row, 1977.
50. Shepherd, M and Sartorius, N (eds): Non-Specific Aspects of Treatment. Hans Huber, Toronto, 1989, p 1.
51. Benson, H and Epstein, MD: The placebo effect: A neglected asset in the care of patients. JAMA 232:1225, 1975.
52. Frank, JD: Non-specific aspects of treatment: The view of a psychotherapist. In Shepherd and Sartorius (eds); op cit, p 97.
53. Taylor, K: Effects of interferential current stimulation for treatment of subjects with recurrent jaw pain. Phys Ther 67:346, 1987.
54. Spilker, B: Guide to Clinical Interpretation of Data. Raven Press, New York, 1986.
55. Klerman, GL: Non-specific factors in treatment: A clinician's perspective. In Shepherd and Sartorius (eds); op cit.

Group Experimental Designs: Two Data Sets

OBJECTIVES

1 Discuss the criteria by which experience becomes experimentation.
2 Define and illustrate inductive and deductive logic.
3 Discuss probability; define and illustrate type 1 and type 2 errors and power of tests.
4 Interpret given probability statements and relate null and alternate hypotheses to probability statements and levels of significance.
5 Define experimental controls, independent variable, dependent variable, error variables, experimental design, and quasi-experimental design.
6 Define and illustrate one-group and two-group experimental designs having two data sets.
7 Give examples of experimental and quasi-experimental design studies.
8 State the essential components of sequential clinical trials design.

  9 Apply sequential clinical trials design to given research
     questions.
  10 Identify statistical tools appropriate to each basic research
     design for each level of measurement.
  11 Analyze selected literature for statistical models and
     designs.

Foundations of Scientific Method

EXPERIENCE

The scientific method of research is built on three foundations: experience, logic, and probability. Physicists, psychologists, humanists, and theologians would probably all agree with the renowned experimental physiologist, Claude Bernard, who observed that experience is the one source of human knowledge. Every moment of our lives is experience: dreaming, driving to work, teaching, listening, reading, and thinking. Under what circumstances can any of these experiences be properly titled research or experimentation? Hamilton[1] quoted Bernard as saying that the experimental method is "experience [that] is . . . gained by virtue of precise reasoning based on an idea born of observation and controlled experiment." Hamilton also quoted the father of modern statistics, R.A. Fisher: "Experimental observations are only experience carefully planned in advance and designed to form a secure basis for new knowledge." From these comments and from observation of working scientists we can see that the qualities that change ordinary experience into experimentation are the qualities of control, objectivity, and replicability.

In Chapter 2 the general characteristics of experimental control were discussed; as this chapter progresses, more specificity will be brought to this concept of control. *Control* is imposed on experience in several ways: advanced planning of the research design, operational definitions of terms, precise formulation of research questions and hypotheses, careful identification of a population, randomized selection of samples, mathematical controls of statistical tests, and intellectual controls of logic.

In research, experience is made *objective* by all of the controls listed above, with an emphasis on the recording of measured observations as discussed in Chapter 3. The valid and reliable measurement tool used in a controlled way is what makes scientific experience objective. Precise and objective measurements permit replication of the study by others; thus, replication is a characteristic of an experience that can be called experimentation. **Replicability** means that other people should be able to repeat your experiment using the same controls and measurements and come out with the same results that you obtained.

LOGIC

Earlier in this text the point was made that no effort deserves the name "research" unless the researcher has obtained a logical interpretation of the data in relation to the research question. One of the major intellectual tools for interpreting data is logic. According to the dictionary, **logic** is the science that deals with the criteria for valid inferences; logic instructs us in the methodology for making inferences based on reason. Logic can be divided into two basic types: deductive and inductive. **Deductive logic** applies a general rule *to* particular instances. **Inductive logic** draws a general rule *from* particular instances.

These two processes are often interwoven in scientific thinking. One might begin inductively by thinking: If what I see in the patients in this clinic is generally true, then I can form a hypothesis of what ought to happen in all similar cases. (The thinker has gone from particular instances to a general statement. The general statement is a hypothesis to be tested.) The next step is deductive logic. If the general hypothesis is true, then it will be demonstrated in a particular experimental arrangement. (The thinker has gone from the general statement to anticipated particular instances.) Then the thinker looks at the data collected in the experimental arrangement and proceeds from those particulars to a general conclusion that the hypothesis is either supported or not supported. This last inductive reasoning from particular data to general conclusion must be based on the data alone. In the past, inductive logic was considered by many as *the* major tool of science; this is not really true. The scientific method is a synthesis of deductive and inductive reasoning as illustrated above. Let us look at a more specific example of inductive (I) and deductive (D) reasoning.

I: I have observed many patients whose skin turned bright red under hot packs. If that always happens, it might be because of the increase in arterial blood flow. (A given postulate is: arterial blood is red.)

D: Arterial blood flow will increase by a measurable amount in areas of skin subjected to a source of superficial heat above 100°F.

I: Set up an objective and controlled test situation in which observational measurements can be made on the rate of blood flow in an area under the influence of superficial heat. In a series of controlled observations each patient exposed to superficial heat demonstrates a measurable increase in blood flow as measured by plethysmography. Blood flow has thus been demonstrated to increase in a area to which superficial heat has been applied and this increase in significantly greater in the area heated than it was in the comparable unheated area on the contralateral side of the body. It is assumed that this demonstrated increase in flow involves primarily arterial blood at the surface because arterial blood is red. If the superficial increase were primarily venous, the skin color would be darker, it is reasoned.

Thus, we can see the alternate patterns of thinking from general to particular and from particular to general as being essential to several aspects of the research process. These forms of logic are important for defining the research hypothesis, for defining what observations are to be made, and for interpreting the data in the light of the question asked. In the illustration above, the data progressed from qualitative to quantitative.

PROBABILITY

Unless you observe every possible change of blood flow under hot packs that has ever occurred or that will ever occur (an obvious impossibility), you will take a chance of being wrong when you extrapolate from your sample to your population. Likewise, you cannot examine every grain of sand in the river; there is always a possibility that some of them are not really sand but gold nuggets. If you examine a thousand grains of sand on a river bank and each one of them turns out to be a grain of sand, you could be wrong if you inferred from that sample that the entire beach was composed only of similar sand. A sample of 500,000 grains from the beach might produce 10 grains of high-quality gold. In the first sample of sand the proportion of gold to sand was 0/1000; in the second sample the proportion was 10/500,000. The larger the sample, the more likely it is that the proportion in the sample represents the proportion in the population. Probability is concerned with approximating the real proportion in the population based on the observed proportion in the sample. Shott[2] defined probability as "the long-run proportion of times some event of interest will occur."

The most basic formula for probability is:

$$\frac{\text{Number of observations of an event}}{\text{Number of observations}}$$

For example, when you examine 100 people with rheumatoid arthritis and make an observation that 75 of them have pain, you would like to know how representative that is of all people with rheumatoid arthritis in the entire world. The proportion is 75/100 = 0.75. The larger your sample, the more likely it will represent the true incidence of pain in rheumatoid patients, but there is always a chance of being wrong when you extrapolate from sample to population. More will be said on this matter of extrapolation soon.

You never *prove* a hypothesis when your data are based on a sample taken from a population. The best you do is state the chances—that is, the probability—of being right and the chances or probability of being wrong when you accept or reject the hypothesis. The science of probability is concerned with allowing you to know exactly how large a risk you are taking. Most of the interesting questions in our world are related to the question of the composition of all of the grains of sand on the beach. In most instances we cannot observe every particular instance of an occurrence. Therefore, we are almost always forced to make a probability statement based on a sample taken from a population not completely accessible to us.

Type 1 and Type 2 Errors

Review the definitions of null and alternate hypotheses in Chapter 1. A null hypothesis says that there is no statistically significant difference between two methods or treatments being tested. Pursuing our example above, let us write a null hypothesis that states that there is no statistically significant difference in blood flow between a forearm that has been wrapped in a hot pack for 20 minutes and a forearm that has not been wrapped in a hot pack. In accepting or rejecting that null hypothesis, we take two risks. In the **type 1 error** we take the chance of rejecting a null hypothesis and saying that, indeed, there is a difference when in fact there is not. In other words, we run the risk of backing a loser. The risk of committing a type 1 error is symbolized by the Greek letter alpha (α). In a **type 2 error** we take the chance of not rejecting a null hypothesis and saying that there is no difference when in fact there is; we run the risk of missing a winner. The risk of a type 2 error is symbolized by the Greek letter beta (β). Nonsignificant results in a study with a small sample may represent a type 2 error. With those two risks, what chance are you willing to take of being wrong when you either reject or fail to reject a hypothesis?

One other term needs to be defined briefly in this area and that concerns the power of a test. A type 1 error was defined as the probability of rejecting the null hypothesis when it was in fact true. Conceptually, the *power* of a statistical test is defined as the probability of rejecting the null hypothesis when it is in fact false, a desirable outcome. Thus, a large type 1 error is undesirable, since you would want to reject the null hypothesis when it is in fact false; type 1 errors are generally considered more serious than type 2 errors. Therefore, the greater the power of the test the better. The power of a statistical test is the probability of reaching a correct decision and rejecting the null when it should be rejected, symbolized as $1 - \alpha$. Correctly accepting the null is symbolized as $1 - \beta$.

There is an inverse relationship between the two types of error, in that a decrease in the probability of a type 1 error will increase the probability of a type 2 error for a given sample size. Therefore, if a researcher wants to reduce the possibility of both types of errors, she must increase the size of the sample.[3,4] Type 2 errors are seldom discussed in research articles; this may lead to some mistaken conclusions. Two clear, readable secondary sources for important information on this topic may be found in Ottenbacher.[5,6] Ottenbacher demonstrated inadequate statistical power and a high rate of type 2 error in much published literature, error "which translated into a reduced sensitivity in experimental manipulations."[7] Both the power of a test and its statistical significance are influenced, in a nonlinear fashion, by sample size and effect size. The three factors—significance, power, and size—are interrelated and influence one another. Ottenbacher defined effect size as the extent to which a variable under study is truly present in a population or the extent to which the null hypothesis is false. The power of a test and its effect size should be examined when samples are small.

Level of Significance

The science of probability is concerned with helping you to define in very specific terms what kind of chance you are taking when you accept or reject a null hypothesis. Are you willing to accept a 5 percent risk—that is, are you willing to take a chance of being wrong 5 percent of the time—or are you only willing to accept a hypothesis if your chances of being wrong are at the 1 percent level? In statistics this chance of being wrong is called the **level of significance**. For example, look at paragraph 25 in the article by Beattie in Appendix C. He is saying that there is only 1 chance in 10,000 of being wrong when he says that there was a difference among the four conditions in Figure 1. More will be said on these results in the next chapter. Now look at Table 5 in the Giannini article in Appendix C. Two of the three paired, one-tailed t-tests were significant at the .05 level of significance. Why do you think they used a one-tailed test? Use paragraphs 5 and 18 to explain why the t-test uses a paired design. Interpret the statistics in Table 6 in Giannini. Goldstein[8] has stated, "The significance level is best regarded as a measure of the conflict between the evidence and the null hypothesis."

There is a long-standing tradition in research that one does not reject a null hypothesis unless the probability is .05 or less. However, that is strictly a convention; in some cases the difference between 5 chances ($P = .05$) and 6 chances ($P = .06$) in 100 of being wrong is not really a big deal. On the other hand, if it were a study of a treatment where life or death could be the outcome, one probably would not want to reject the null unless the probability statement was .01, or even .001. Statistical significance of .05 or less should never be confused with real-life significance. Statistics can give you a statement of probabilities; to interpret it you must employ human reason. As Browner and Newman[9] state, "Just as a positive diagnostic test does not mean that a patient has the disease, especially if the clinical picture suggests otherwise, a significant p value does not mean that a research hypothesis is correct, especially if it is inconsistent with current knowledge."

Each time an alternate hypothesis is tested and supported under controlled conditions, its credibility is strengthened; that is, you can put more confidence in it. Just as you never prove the alternate hypothesis, you cannot disprove the null hypothesis either, although you can demonstrate that it is highly improbable. Null hypotheses are either rejected, or they fail to be rejected. Alternate hypotheses are either supported or are inconclusive. The fewer rival alternate hypotheses, the stronger the degree of confirmation of an accepted hypothesis.

Definitions

Experimental controls were defined in Chapter 2; however, that definition is worth repeating here. **Experimental controls** are those mechanisms that so regulate or guide every aspect of the experimental situation that changes in the observed measurement can be attributed only to the uncontrolled or independent variables in the study. Because the examples of control are so varied and because there are so many aspects of an experiment that need to be controlled, it is difficult to provide a one-sentence definition of control. Students should come back repeatedly to the basic concept of control and expand their perception and understanding of this concept as they read about and experience the scientific method.

In the classic (i.e., perfect exemplar) experiment the researcher identifies a structure, function, or event to be studied and the ways in which its actions can be measured; then the researcher controls every other conceivable variable that can be controlled except the one to be studied. For example, if you wanted to study the effect of a drug on blood pressure, you would control every conceivable factor that might influence blood pressure, administer the drug, and then measure its effect on blood pressure. In this example the drug is called the *independent* or research variable; blood pressure is the *dependent* variable measured. All other factors in the environment that might influence blood pressure are potential error or *confounding* variables unless they are controlled. In a true *experimental design* one or more independent variables are identified, one or more dependent variables are identified, and all potential error variables are subject to control. The controls are those discussed in Chapters 2 and 4. At this point in your study you should emphasize the controls discussed in Chapter 2, which are concerned with making sure that your sample is truly representative of your population.

When some of the essential controls are missing, the design is more properly termed a quasi-experimental design. According to the dictionary, "quasi" means having some resemblance to or possessing certain attributes of. Therefore, a **quasi-experimental design** has some resemblance to and possesses some of the attributes of true experimental design. Campbell and Stanley[10] implied that the "when" and "to whom" of measurement are usually present in quasi-experimental designs; what is lacking is the "when" and "to whom" of treatment and the ability to randomize treatments. In this chapter and the next we will look at some classic designs, both experimental and quasi-experimental. We looked at some more innovative designs in Chapter 7.

Research Protocol

A research protocol is a detailed plan that guides the execution and reporting of a research project. The words to emphasize in this definition are "detailed plan" and "guide." It is written primarily to assist the researcher; it is also sometimes used to inform administrators and to solicit funds from financial resources. A general outline for writing a research protocol may be found in Appendix A. You have already had several occasions to examine and use parts of that protocol; now you can use it all. The protocol is a list of steps in experimental design. When this general format is applied to specific circumstances, some of the steps may drop out and others may be greatly elaborated. For example, under step 18, "procedure," the researcher may list a detailed sequence, such as

1   Turn on the electromyograph.

2   Calibrate the pen recorders.

3   Calibrate the strain gauge.

4   Invite the subject in and have her sign the release form.

(And so on)

Appendix B is an attempt by the author to reconstruct the protocol for the Giannini article.

Basic Experimental Design

To illustrate a basic research design, let us say that we are interested in studying a population of people, objects, or events. From that population we are going to draw a sample of 90 and study that sample in such a way that we can describe some of the characteristics of the population. How we draw that sample of 90 and what we do with it will ultimately determine our description of the research design used. There are several legitimate ways to draw the sample and to divide the sample into groups. There are also several ways in which we can apply treatments to the sample and measure the dependent variable. Refer to Figure 8–1. As we look at our sample and the data collection, we need to ask four critical questions.

1   Into how many groups of individuals is the sample divided?

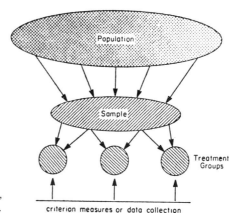

FIGURE 8–1   Diagram of population, sample, treatment groups, and data sets.

2   How did the individual get assigned to these groups?

3   How many different types of treatment were applied?

4   What data were compared; that is, how many data sets were analyzed together?

To answer question 1, the sample of 90 individuals from our population of 5000 can be treated as one undivided group; it can be divided into two groups of 45 each; or it can be divided into more than two groups, for example, three groups of 30 each or nine groups of 10 each. Mathematical convention designates any number more than two as k, therefore, we can have research designs involving one group, two groups, or k groups. Table 8–1 is a summary of these basic designs. The names in parentheses in Table 8–1 are more common in the literature than the names preferred in this text. The "block design" names go back to Fisher's agricultural experiments and are often used in statistical texts. I have two problems with

TABLE 8–1   A SUMMARY OF BASIC EXPERIMENTAL DESIGNS (ALTERNATE NAMES GIVEN IN PARENTHESES)

One-Group Designs

   1   One sample
   2   Two related samples, own control (randomized block design, repeated measures)
   3 k related samples, own control (randomized block design, repeated measures)

Two-Group Designs

   4   Two independent samples (completely randomized block design)
   5   Two related samples, matched pairs (randomized block design)

k-*Group Designs*

   6 k independent samples (completely randomized block design)
   7 k matched sets (randomized block design)

these names: they refer to agricultural research plots, with which most therapists are unfamiliar; and the same name is used for more than one design. The names preferred by the author are taken from Siegel.[11]

Questions 2 to 4 will be answered in relation to each of the possible answers to question 1. In Chapter 9 k-group designs will be discussed in more detail.

ONE-GROUP DESIGNS

In one-group designs question 2 does not apply because there is only one group, which we assume was randomly selected from the population. The answer to question 3 is that each individual in the group received the same treatment. There are three possible answers to question 4.

1   Data can be collected once (the dependent variable measured) and compared to some hypothetical standard or published norm (this will be illustrated shortly).

2   Data can be collected twice. Typically, the data are collected at the beginning of the experiment; then the group is treated and measurements are made a second time. Thus, each subject serves as his or her own control. Each individual's performance before the treatment is compared to his or her own performance after the treatment. Each data collection is often called a sample (which is a somewhat confusing convention); in this text each collection of data has been called a *data set*. This design is here called two related samples, own control.

3   Data can be collected from the group three or more times. Test results before the experiment begins are compared with other (two or more) test results, which may be measured in the middle of the experiment (during treatment), at the end (after treatment), or much later (months, years). Remember that k can stand for any whole number greater than 2. This design is here called k related samples, own control. Because this design includes three or more data sets, examples and statistical analyses will be given in Chapter 9. Table 8–2 outlines the various answers to the four questions above and expresses the designs in symbolic *formulae*.

TWO-GROUP DESIGNS

Going back to the original sample of 90 individuals, these may be divided into two groups, and this division may occur three ways. We may randomly select a group of 45 from the 5000 and then randomly select a second group of 45. A variation of this would be to take the original sample of 90 and randomly assign them to two groups.

TABLE 8–2 **SYMBOLIC OUTLINES OF CLASSIC RESEARCH DESIGNS ORGANIZED BY THE FOUR QUESTIONS POSED IN THE TEXT**

1,2 *One-Group*

    3 Same treatment for all (no control group)

    4 Two data sets compared: one to outside norm; two or *k* to each other:

One sample		T	M	N
Two related samples, own control	M	T	M	
k related samples, own control	M	T	M	M

1 *Two Groups*

    2 By randomization, matching or no control

    3 Two treatments *or* treatment and control

    4 Two data sets compared:

Two independent samples

```
                        Δ
                       / \
        R   M   T   M ─┐
                        ├─> Δ
        R   M  T/C  M ─┘
              ‾Δ‾

        R       T   M ─┐
                        ├─> Δ
        R      T/C  M ─┘
```

Two related samples, matched

```
        P   M   T   M
        P   M  T/C  M

        P       T   M
        P      T/C  M
```

Two uncontrolled samples

```
        M   T   M
        M  T/C  M

            T   M
           T/C  M
```

1 *k Groups*

    2 By randomization, matching or no control

    3 Three treatments *or* two treatments and control

    4 Three or more data sets compared:

k independent samples

```
        R   M   T   M
        R   M   T   M
        R   M  T/C  M

        R       T   M
        R       T   M
        R      T/C  M
```

k related samples, matched

```
        P   M   T   M
        P   M   T   M
        P   M  T/C  M

        P       T   M
        P       T   M
        P      T/C  M
```

**TABLE 8–2 SYMBOLIC OUTLINES OF CLASSIC RESEARCH
DESIGNS ORGANIZED BY THE FOUR QUESTIONS
POSED IN THE TEXT** *Continued*

k uncontrolled samples	M	T	M
	M	T	M
	M	T/C	M
		T	M
		T	M
		T/C	M

N =	Outside norms	R =	Randomization
M =	Dependent variable (the response to be assessed)	P =	Pairing (i.e., matching)
		C =	Control
T =	Independent variable (the treatment to be evaluated)		

A second possible way to get two groups of 45 is by matching. The process of matching was discussed at length in Chapter 2. Let us say that we want to match our individuals on only one variable, that of weight. We dip into our population and randomly select an individual who weighs 50 kilograms and assign him or her to the first group. We must then look through the population until we find another person who weighs 50 kilograms and assign that person to the second group. We continue this until we have two groups of 45 matched on the variable of weight. Some parallels to this system in clinical practice have already been discussed.

A third way of establishing two groups is by establishing nonequivalent groups; this is a quasi-experimental design. For example, Payton and colleagues[12] used this design in a curriculum validation study demonstrating change as a result of instruction. In a pre-post (M-T-M) analysis the experimental group of allied health students changed as a result of instruction; a control group of volunteer graduate students who did not receive the instruction did not change on the dependent variable.

By either of these three approaches—drawing two independent groups of 45 or establishing two groups by matching or studying two nonequivalent groups who have some characteristics in common—we have answered the second question.

With two-group designs treatment is generally given to one group and not to the other; or two different treatments form the independent variables. This answers question 3. Question 4 can be answered in either of two ways that have minimal influence on research design. As diagrammed in Table 8–2 the researcher can first calculate the difference (Δ) between pretest and posttest scores for *each* group and then statistically analyze those two differences. Or the researcher can analyze the difference between the two posttests. Either way the design is the same, and the data are treated the same way statistically.

k-GROUP DESIGNS

The *k*-group designs are discussed here from a conceptual point of view so that the student can follow the concepts throughout Tables 8–1 and 8–2. Examples and statistical analysis of three data sets will be reserved to Chapter 9.

The third way to answer question 1 is to divide the sample of 90 into more than two groups. In order to deal in whole numbers, let us say that our original sample of 90 is divided into three groups of 30 each, where each individual has an equal opportunity to be in any one of the three groups (random assignment). Or we can match the individuals in each of the *k* groups; as indicated in Chapter 2, matching several groups can become difficult and is therefore seldom used. A third alternative is to form three nonequivalent groups.

The student can avoid a great deal of confusion if the time is taken now to conceptualize the seven different designs in Tables 8–1 and 8–2 and how each of the four key questions are answered in each of these seven designs. Most of the designs found in the literature are based on these seven or are variations on them.

It should be remembered that pretreatment measures are not usually used if there is a chance that the pretreatment measure will somehow alert and bias the subject for or against the treatment, or train the subject in the taking of the measurement. These objections are particularly crucial in psychological and sociological measures such as measures of attitude, interest, or motivation.

Any of these seven designs could be made quasi-experimental by removing randomization; this is the most common omission in quasi-experimental designs. This problem of randomization is crucial in clinical research, as was discussed in Chapter 2. Another problem is that of uniform application of the treatment to each individual in each group; lack of control in this phase can also reduce the design to a quasi-experimental one. These problems are discussed in more detail in Chapter 4.

EXAMPLES OF GROUP DESIGNS

In Chapter 1 we looked at the example of two therapists in St. Hopeless Outpatient Clinic who were interested in improving joint mobility in patients with physical disabilities. They designed a series of experiments, and nine of their research questions were listed in that chapter. We have already identified some of those questions as descriptive and correlational in Chapters 5 and 6. Let us now look at their experimental questions and classify them according to our basic designs as they are numbered in Table 8–1.

	Qualitative	Semiquantitative	Quantitative	
O	1 27	2 121	3 52	200
E	20	20	160	200
	47	141	212	400

FIGURE 8–2   Hypothetical data in one sample, one-group design.

Example 1

From Chapter 1, question 4 was, "Do the medical records of St. Hopeless Clinic demonstrate the expected level of use of quantitative goniometry?" To answer this question, one sample could be drawn from the medical records. The data extracted from each record could be a nominal level measure of the type or class of goniometry recorded in that medical record. We would have a frequency count of the kinds of goniometry demonstrated in the record. To do this we might devise three categories. The first could include qualitative statements of range of motion (ROM), for examples, "The patient shows improved shoulder range of motion as demonstrated by increased ease of hair combing." The second category could be semiquantitative. "The patient has gained approximately 10° ROM in the left elbow." The third level could be strictly quantitative goniometry: "Over a 5-day period the patient's left elbow flexion increased from 28° to 42°. The figures could also be recorded on an appropriate form.

Let us say that 200 observations were taken from 76 charts. The observed (O) frequency count could be recorded in the top row of Figure 8–2. Once we have gathered these data, we can compare them to an expected level of use based on experience and/or a review of the relevant literature. The second row of Figure 8–2 could represent our expected (E) observations if the therapists had used mostly quantitative goniometry as recommended in professional standards. Let us say that we expect 80 percent of the recorded goniometry to be quantitative and the other 20 percent to be distributed over the other two categories. Those percentages can be transformed into expected frequency counts, as in Figure 8–2. Here we have an example of the first design, one sample in a one-group design, one data set compared to outside norms (Table 8–1, design number 1).

Examples 2 and 3

From Chapter 1, question 9 was, "Does goniometric biofeedback training increase functional ability?" One approach to this question would be to identify the criteria by which patients would be admitted to the study. This, in effect, would define a population. We would then admit to the sample all patients who entered the clinic and met the criteria. We would give all patients in the sample a test of functional ability, train them with goniometric biofeedback for 2 weeks, and then repeat the test of functional ability. By comparing the two sets of functional ability scores in this one group, we could draw some conclusion about the effect of goniometric biofeedback on functional ability. This would meet our criteria for the design using two related samples, own control (Table 8–1, design 2). This is a quasi-experimental design because there is no control group and we cannot, therefore, demonstrate that the patients would not have gotten the same increase (or decrease) without the treatment of biofeedback. We could have turned the same study into k related samples, own control (Table 8–1, number 3) by giving a test of functional ability before treatment, after 2 weeks of biofeedback training, and a third time 2 weeks after training ceased. This would have been quasi-experimental design also because of a lack of controls.

Example 4

Question 9 from Chapter 1 could be made into a truly experimental study by defining the criteria for admission into the study and randomly assigning individuals who meet this criteria to one of two groups. Treat one group and do not treat the other group, or give both groups some standard treatment and add goniometric biofeedback training to the experimental group. We would then have an experimental group and a control group, two independent samples (Table 8–1, number 4).

Example 5

Let us look yet again at question 9 from Chapter 1. Let us say that the first patient who enters our clinic is a potential candidate for biofeedback training because of decreased ROM. The patient is assigned randomly to one group. He is a 40-year-old man with rheumatoid arthritis, and we are going to work with his shoulder on the dominant arm. We would then look for another 40-year-old man with rheumatoid arthritis and decreased ROM in his dominant shoulder for the second group. To increase the randomness of the experiment, we could flip a coin to see which goes into the experimental group and which into the control group. We could continue this procedure over a long period of time until eventually we have both groups with a large enough n to do adequate statistical testing. In this particular example, matching was done on three characteristics—age, sex, and disease category. This arrangement would meet the criteria for two-related samples, matched pairs (Table 8–1, number 5). Many researchers would call this quasi-experimental research because they believe that matching is not an adequate control.

Practice   Now see if you can apply designs 6 and 7 for k independent samples and k related samples, matched sets to question 9 from Chapter 1. Write each example above, including your own creations, with the symbols used in Table 8–2.

NULL HYPOTHESES FOR DESIGN EXAMPLES

Each of the variations in design given above has a small but appreciable effect on the exact statement of the hypothesis and the possible interpretation of results, although all are addressed to the same general research question. The five null hypotheses for the five approaches to question 9 in the paragraphs above are as follows:

1   There will be no statistically significant difference between observed and expected scores for level of goniometric quantification in the records of St. Hopeless's therapy departments.

2   There will be no statistically significant difference *between* patient scores on a functional ability test before goniometric biofeedback training and their scores on the same test after biofeedback training.

3   There will be no statistically significant differences *among* patient scores on a functional ability test before the application of goniometric biofeedback training and their scores at the end of a 2-week training period and their scores on the same test 1 month after training ceased.

4   There will be no statistically significant differences in scores on a functional-ability test between patients treated with routine care plus goniometric biofeedback training and patients treated only with routine care.

5   There will be no statistically significant differences in measured functional ability between patients receiving routine care plus goniometric biofeedback training and patients who receive the same general training, but without the biofeedback training, when the two groups of patients are matched for age, sex, and disease category.

Variations and Limitations of Predictive Designs

From the questions presented in Chapter 1, question 7 could be written so that it would be two related samples, own control; two related samples, matched pairs; or two independent samples. Question 8 could be approached as k related, matched pairs, or k independent samples. Designs that involve measurements before and after treatment are sometimes preferable to those that make measurements only after treatment, when the first testing does not bias the second testing. This double check is particularly useful when the size of the sample is small; when the subjects vary more widely with respect to the dependent variable than they do with respect to the expected effect of the independent variable; and when the correlation within groups is extremely high, that is, when there is a high correlation between measurements made before and after treatment *within* each group. When these conditions are not present it is unwise to take two measurements;[13] it is also unwise if there is a chance that the measurement taken before treatment will sensitize the subjects to the treatments or produce a practice effect. When psychosocial factors are involved, measurements are made most often only after treatment.

QUASI-EXPERIMENTAL DESIGNS

As indicated earlier, a quasi-experimental design is one in which any potentially important confounding variables cannot be controlled. One of the most prevalent uses of quasi-experimental design is the situation in which it would be unethical or impractical to randomly divide subjects into treatment and control groups.

Quasi-experimental designs are also used when two groups are pre-existing rather than randomly chosen, as in the case of the occupational therapy class and the physical therapy class in a given university (Chapter 2). In this instance we have two intact groups, and it is assumed that the groups are approximately comparable. One is then given the treatment and the other is used as a control group (see the example by Payton[12]). On the other hand, depending on the experimental question, it could be that the experimenter has deliberately *contrasted* these two groups because it is believed that they are significantly different on some important characteristic. Some statisticians would say that it is impossible to do good research by making comparisons between such groups; however, as Nunnally has pointed out, problems do not go away simply because they create research difficulties. Researchers who are interested in such intact or comparison groups must simply impose whatever controls they can and be alert to the possible confounding variables when they make their interpretations. The basic question that is often asked when two such groups are compared is, "Do these two groups truly come from the same population?" Under these circumstances the best quasi-experimental designs provide as a control group either an intact group or a carefully chosen contrasting group and measurements before and after treatment.

Conine[14] had this to say about the choice of a research design:

> But the most significant problems in human sciences defy study by a true experimental method. Thus, in selecting a design, the researcher is besieged by the sentiment for respectability and the opposing desire for practicality; one choice may restrict him to study only simple and insignificant problems, and another may put him in an inferior position with respect to the ideal design.

In Chapter 7 we examined another solution to this problem.

As a final example of research design, let me quote a report published by Pruden:[15]

> A seventh-grader had been assigned to do some research. When he submitted his paper to the teacher, the subject of his research was "Where do babies come from?" The paper read as follows:
>
> Where babies come from is very important. I got a book from the library and read it, and I got my aunt's doctor book and read it. Then I interviewed some of my relatives. My great grandmother said she found Grandpa in the cabbage patch. Grandma said the doctor brought my Dad in his little black bag. And Mom told me she and Dad picked me out at the hospital. My research convinces me that conventional reproduction has not occurred in my family for three generations.
>
> That youngster may have shocked his teacher, but he did a lot of things right. First, he did some background reading, then some field work. Next he drew a conclusion, which his references and data seemed to justify, and he wrote up his research and turned in a paper.

Sequential Clinical Trials Design

In Chapter 7 mention was made of sequential clinical trials as a special tool for the clinician, along with the experimental study of single cases. Sequential clinical trials design has considerable potential for clinical questions that can meet the requirements of the design.[16,17] A question that would be appropriate for a sequential clinical trial is of this type: "All other things being equal (control), which of two treatments is better for this type of patient?" Thus, it is a two-data set experimental design.

Six things must be defined clearly when using this technique:

1   The criteria for admission to the study
2   The specific nature of treatment A
3   The specific nature of treatment B
4   The target behavior or characteristic to be changed, that is, the dependent variable
5   The measurement tool for the dependent variable
6   The criterion for improvement

Usually treatment A is the new, innovative, and relatively untried treatment that is to be compared to treatment B, the conventional standard of practice for this type of clinical problem. In that arrangement, A is the experimental group that receives the independent variable and B is the control group. To illustrate the technique let us look again at question 9 in Chapter 1: "Does goniometric biofeedback training increase functional ability?"

1 **Criteria for admission** Patients admitted to therapy during the experimental period must have less than 50 percent of normal ROM in one shoulder. This tightness is the result of a mastectomy and has been present for 3 months or less. The patient should have no other physical disabilities and should not be on any medication that might influence the results of the study.

2 **Treatment A** In the conventional protocol, the patients will be seen daily 5 days a week in both physical and occupational therapy. The physical therapy program will consist of hot packs to the affected shoulder followed by gentle, active stretching in all limited ranges of the shoulder using proprioceptive neuromuscular facilitation (PNF) techniques. The occupational therapy program will consist of meaningful activities designed to use the affected joint in active exercise. Length and type of treatment will be uniform for all patients in the study.

3 **Treatment B** In the experimental protocol, the same treatment will be given as in A except that during the occupational therapy program an electrogoniometer will be attached to the patient's shoulder and the patient will be taught how to read and interpret both visual and auditory feedback from the device. In this way the patient will know when he or she is using the shoulder to its full active range. The length of time for the feedback training will be uniform for all patients in this group.

4 **Target behavior** The target is ROM in the affected shoulder in all three planes of motion.

5 **Measurement tool** A standard goniometer will be used to measure the dependent variable.

6 **Criterion for improvement** More than 15° of increased ROM will be considered improvement after all ranges are totaled. (This will become more clear when we look at the rest of the design.)

Once the guidelines have been established, the therapist flips a coin, enters a table of random numbers, or otherwise decides randomly which treatment will be given to each of the first two patients who qualify for the study. Each group of two patients who qualify for the study form one "little pair."[18] For each little pair, one person is randomly assigned to receive treatment A and the other to receive treatment B. It must also be determined exactly how many treatments each pair is to receive before an evaluation is made regarding the criterion measure. For this project 10 treatments over a 2-week period will be administered to each little pair.

Let us say that the first little pair received its treatment and the patient who received treatment A gained 10° flexion, 10° internal rotation, 5° external rotation, and 10° abduction, for a total gain over the 2-week period of 35°. The patient who received treatment B gained 20° flexion, 15° internal rotation, 5° external rotation, and 15° abduction for a total gain of 55° in all ranges during the treatment period. The difference in total gains of the first little pair is 20°, and the criterion of improvement is 15° or more. Therefore, the decision for the first pair favors treatment B. For this first pair we wish to record the decision that treatment B is better than treatment A according to our previously selected criterion of improvement.

We now reach one of the beautiful aspects of the sequential clinical trials design. Figure 8–3 is a *statistical* summary, based on the binomial distribution, of our decision on each little pair that may lead to a significance level of 0.05 for the total experiment.[19] Movement along the horizontal line is a decision in favor of treatment B. Movement along the vertical line is a decision in favor of treatment A. The starting point is the X in the lower left-hand corner. The figure is like a road map that leads from the starting point to a statistical decision.

If the sample path (the graphic record of the decisions on each little pair) crosses the heavy black line, the decision line, on the treatment B side of the chart, we will decide in favor of treatment B at the 0.05 level of significance. If we cross the decision line in the upper left-hand side of the form in the direction of treatment A, we would decide in favor of treatment A at the 0.05 significance level. This is true no matter where we cross that line. You will notice that in the upper right-hand quarter of the

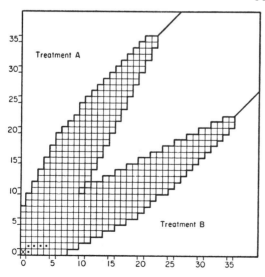

FIGURE 8–3 Sequential clinical trials with a significance level of 0.05. A hypothetical study is recorded for six little pairs (see text).

form the lines from the little squares are extended to the margin. If we cross the heavy black line, the no-decision line, anywhere on the inside of the form, we cannot reject the null hypothesis that there is no statistically significant difference between treatments.

Let us go back to our decision on the first little pair. We decided in favor of treatment B; therefore, from the starting point in the lower left-hand corner of Figure 8–3 we move one space in the direction of treatment B and make a dot. We have moved one step toward the decision line in favor of treatment B. Let us assume that our next little pair is decided in favor of treatment A. We would move one space *from our last decision point* in the direction of treatment A and make another dot. Let us assume that our third little pair did not reach a criterion of significant difference, that there was only a 7° difference between the gain of the two patients in that pair. That pair is not recorded at all. According to Figure 8–3 the next three decisions were in favor of treatment B, so our dots move in a straight line toward the B decision line. The reader can see that if we continued with our pairs and decisions long enough we would eventually cross one of the heavy black lines. This could happen after we have recorded eight pairs if the sample path moved in one straight line. On the other hand, it could take as many as 58 pairs in order to reach a decision in favor of either treatment, or to exit into the no-significance space in the middle. We could reach the no-significance area in as little as 20 moves. Bross[20] has presented two forms, at the 0.10 and 0.05 levels of significance with power set at 0.7. Armitage[21] presents formulas for drawing forms at any level of significance and power. Whitehead[22] provides similar instructions, which create slightly different forms having the same function.

Advantages of Sequential Designs

The major advantage of the Bross forms is that all the mathematical and statistical formulas have been worked into the form. A second major advantage is that it allows us to take the patients as they appear in the clinic, one at a time, and work with them so that one does not need to identify the subject sample ahead of time. This is an important consideration for clinical research because very rarely can the clinician identify a sample of 30 or more patients and randomly divide them into two groups to fit a more traditional research design. However, with sequential trials you can—over a period of years if necessary—identify a sample of 100 patients, one at a time, and randomly divide them into two groups without stressing the assumptions of the design. Another major advantage of sequential trials that is particularly appropriate to clinical studies is that as soon as you reach the level of significance, you can stop the experiment. You do not have to collect data on 50 patients and then do your statistical tests and discover that you might have been able to reach a significant outcome with half that many subjects. If our hypothetical case in Figure 8–3 turned out to favor treatment B after 11 pairs (22 subjects), you could then stop the experiment and begin to give all of your patients the preferred treatment. This potential for knowing as soon as your data have reached significance has some ethical merit in terms of providing the best known care for patients.

There are many important questions in occupational and physical therapy which are as yet unanswered. So much of what we do is based on the conventional wisdom of the profession—word of mouth and empirical case reports. As noted in Chapter 1, no one is in a better position to demonstrate the validity of clinical practice than the practicing clinicians. Given a certain modality (very broadly defined as anything done for the purpose of altering patient behavior), what are its physiological or psychological effects on normals? What are its physiological effects on patients; that is, how does pathology change the physiological effects of the modality? If pathology does change the physiological effects, under what circumstances and with what dosages, and with what pathology does it change them? What are the effects of changing the dosage, the frequency, the duration, and the intensity of any given modality of treatment? What is the therapeutic goal of using this modality in this particular case, and what normative data base does this case contribute to? What are the side effects of this modality at this dosage, frequency, duration, or intensity? Given the above information on any two modalities, how do the answers change when the two are applied concurrently? How do they interact and influence one another? If someone walked into a clinic where you were working and asked these questions about a certain modality that you were applying to any patient, what valid information could you supply as answers? The point of this long paragraph is that there are a great number of clinical questions that need to be answered in a clinical setting. Designs using sequential clinical trials make it ethical and reasonable to answer these questions clinically.

For all its intuitive appeal, clinical trials design has been little used in the published physical and occupational literature. Read Light and colleagues in Appendix C and identify all the components of the design discussed in the text. For another example, see Gault.[23]

Statistical Tools

Siegel[24] states that

When we have asserted the nature of the population and the manner of sampling, we have established a statistical model. Associated with every statistical test is a model and a measurement requirement; the test is valid under certain conditions, and the model and the measurement requirement specify these conditions.

What Siegel has said is that each statistical *test* has an associated measurement requirement (nominal, ordinal, or metric) and a statistical "model" based on sampling. If in doubt about these important factors, review Chapter 3 on levels of measurement and Chapter 2 and the earlier sections on this chapter concerning the processes of sampling related to design. Tables 8–1 and 8–2 are particularly relevant here.

Now let us bring these factors together with appropriate statistical tests.[25] Table 8–3 outlines a select number of classic statistical models as defined above. A frequently used statistical test is listed for each measurement level and for each sampling model given in Table 8–1. As discussed in Chapter 3, parametric statistics refer to those tests appropriate for metric data. Most parametric tests, especially the t-test and F test, make some important assumptions, for example, that the variances in the populations are equal and that the variables measured are normally distributed as on the familiar bell curve. Nonparametric tests make fewer assumptions and so are more widely applicable.[26] Nonparametric tests may be applied to metric data if the assumptions of the parametric tests are in question, but it is not appropriate to apply metric tests to nominal or ordinal data. More complex designs for k data sets, factorial designs, and multivariate designs will be illustrated in Chapter 9.

TABLE 8–3 **STATISTICAL TOOLS APPROPRIATE TO EACH BASIC RESEARCH DESIGN AND LEVEL OF MEASUREMENT**

Type of Design	Level of Measurement		
	Nominal	Ordinal	Metric
1. One sample	Chi-square (χ^2)	One-sample runs	t-test, related
2. Two related, own control	McNemar	Sign test Wilcoxon	t-test, related
3. k related, own control	Cochran Q	Friedman	F test, two-way AOV
4. Two independent	χ^2	Median test Mann-Whitney	t-test, independent
5. Two related, matched	McNemar	Sign test Wilcoxon	t-test, related
6. k independent	χ^2	Kruskal-Wallis	F test, one-way AOV
7. k related, matched	Cochran Q	Friedman	F test, two-way AOV

AOV = analysis of variance.

Sources: Data from Campbell, DT and Stanley, JC: Experimental and Quasi-Experimental Designs for Research, Rand-McNally, Chicago, 1973; and Daniel, WW: Applied Nonparametric Statistics. Houghton Mifflin, Boston, 1978.

Let us now begin to examine and exemplify common statistical models for two data sets. This book is intended as an introduction to basic concepts in research and research design; it is not in any sense a book on statistics. One simple example of three statistical models will be presented here. For a fuller treatment of any of the statistical models, the reader is referred to the list of statistical textbooks listed in Appendix D at the end of this book.

Table 8–4 uses the hypothetical data from Figure 8–2 to illustrate calculation of the chi-square (χ^2) statistic for nominal (frequency count) data in three categories. Among its several uses, chi-square permits the analysis of any number of categories or samples of nominal-scale data to determine statistical significance. Figure 8–2 may be called a 2-by-3 contingency table. Our null hypothesis will be that there will be no statistically significant difference between observed and expected frequency counts (2) across the categories (3). The derivation of the expected counts for this particular study was explained in connection with Figure 8–2. There are mathematical ways to calculate expected values in general, and these may be found in statistical texts such as those listed in Appendix D. The basic formula for chi-square is

$$\chi^2 = \frac{(O - E)^2}{E}$$

This formula can be simplified for calculations as in Table 8–4.

Tables of significance for chi-square can be found in the back of most statistics books. With 2 degrees of freedom (df) a calculated chi-square

TABLE 8–4   **CALCULATION OF χ^2 FOR ONE SAMPLE, ONE DATA SET COMPARED TO AN OUTSIDE NORM***

Cell	f_o	f_e	f^2_o	f^2_o/f_e
1	27	20	729	36.45
2	121	20	14641	732.05
3	52	160	2704	16.90
	200	200		785.40

$$\chi^2 = 785.40 - 200 = 585.40$$
$$df = (r - 1)(c - 1) = (2 - 1)(3 - 1) = 2$$

$^*f_o$ = Observed frequency count in each cat- r = Rows in contingency table
egory
f_e = Expected frequency count in each cat- c = Columns in contingency table
egory

Source: Data from Stahl, SM and Hennes, JD: Reading and Understanding Applied Statistics. CV Mosby, St. Louis, 1980; Witt, PL and McGrain, P: Nonparametric testing using the chi-square distribution. Phys Ther 66:264, 1986.

above the tabled value of 13.815 is significant at the <.001 level. Our calculated statistic (585.40) is far above the value in the statistical table for chi-square, so the null hypothesis can be rejected; the therapists in St. Hopeless have not met the expected standard. There is a statistically significant (as well as an obvious visual) difference between what they were observed to do and what was expected of them.

Stahl and Hennes[27] list several precautions concerning chi-square. For one, it does not indicate direction. The null hypothesis was rejected, but whether the therapists at St. Hopeless were more or less quantitative than expected must be determined logically by inspection of the raw data. Chi-square is influenced by sample size: the larger the n, the more likely you are to obtain significance. Also you should have an *expected* frequency of at least five observations in each cell, or the resulting chi-square may be distorted. Finally, chi-square assumes that the columns and rows are independent; a subject cannot appear in more than one column or more than one row. Chi-square requires independent observations, so it is not appropriate in a repeated-measures design. The categories must be mutually exclusive and account for all data. Shott[28] says that random sampling is not crucial "if the sample is not biased; the purpose of randomization, of course, is to protect against bias." Nevertheless, all of the statistics discussed in this book are used routinely in health care literature for samples of convenience.

A word about degrees of freedom: In the three categories in Figure 8–2, with a marginal total of 200, when the frequency count is known in two cells (df $= 2$), the count in cell 3 is fixed.

It can be noted in Table 8–3 that chi-square may also be used to compare two independent or k independent samples. The procedures for doing this are very similar to those illustrated in Table 8–4. According to Wang,[29] "Chi-square tests the existence of association between the variables in question; it does not estimate the degree of the association."

It is sometimes helpful to express the null hypothesis for a chi-square test as follows: There is no association between the row variable and the column variable.[30] When chi-square is used in this way it is really a test of association similar to the correlation Spearman discussed in Chapter 6. Spearman is more practical with large data sets; chi-square is more practical when the data can be summarized into a few cells, as in Figure 8–2.

Practice Using the formula in Table 8–4, calculate the chi-square statistic if the observed frequency counts in the three cells are 22, 37, and 141.

Table 8–5 provides an example of the calculation of the significance of the difference between two independent means. Example 4 on page 161 outlines an appropriate design. The criteria for admission to the study are patients referred to therapy to increase function in osteoarthritic shoulders

TABLE 8–5 CALCULATION OF t-TEST FOR TWO INDEPENDENT SAMPLES, 20 SUBJECTS IN EACH GROUP

Subject		Group E	Group C
1		10	8
2		12	5
3		8	10
.			
.			
20		15	2
		240	140
	$\bar{x}$	12	7
	s	4.2	3.1

$$t = \frac{x_1 - x_2}{\sqrt{\dfrac{n_1 \, s^2_1 + n_2 \, s^2_2}{n_1 + n_2 - 2}} \sqrt{\dfrac{n_1 + n_2}{n_1 \, n_2}}}$$

$$= \frac{12 - 7}{\sqrt{\dfrac{20(4.2)^2 + 20(3.1)^2}{20 + 20 - 2}} \sqrt{\dfrac{20 + 20}{(20)(20)}}}$$

$$= 3.571$$

$$df = (n_1 - 1) + (n_2 - 1) = 19 + 19 = 38$$

$\bar{x}$ =	Mean for the data set	s^2_1 =	Variance in group 1
s =	Standard deviation	s^2_2 =	Variance in group 2
n_1 =	Number of subjects in group 1	df =	Degrees of freedom
n_2 =	Number of subjects in group 2		

Source: Data from Stahl, SM and Hennes, JD: Reading and Understanding Applied Statistics. CV Mosby, St. Louis, 1980.

who are on no medication other than aspirin (all take aspirin). Using a table of random numbers, patients will be assigned to either an experimental or a control group. Both groups will receive an active exercise program; the experimental group will also receive goniometric (Elgon) biofeedback.

Take time to write a detailed protocol for this study using Appendix A as a guide. The independent variable is Elgon biofeedback; the dependent variable will be changes in active ROM of one shoulder after 2 weeks of therapy. The null hypothesis is, "There will be no statistically significant difference in measured active ROM of the shoulder between patients treated with active exercise and Elgon as compared to patients treated with active exercise alone."

As indicated in Table 8–3, the appropriate statistical tool for two independent samples and metric data is the t-test. The data entered in

Table 8–5 under experimental and control groups are the differences before and after treatment in active range, in degrees.

Since we expect the extra therapy to have a positive effect, based on a review of the literature, we can use a one-tailed test of significance. (If we had no idea whether the treatment would make the patients better or worse, we would have to use a more conservative two-tailed test.) Going to the statistical tables in a statistic book, we find a tabled t value of 3.570 for a significance of <.0005 with 38 degrees of freedom and a one-tailed test. Our calculated t exceeds the tabled t-test value, so our null hypothesis is rejected; there are only 5 chances in 10,000 of being wrong when we say that the Elgon made a difference. How would you state the alternate hypothesis that is supported? Calculate the t statistic if the means had been 11 and 10 with standard deviations of 3.8 and 3.6, using the formula in Table 8–5. For other easy-to-read examples of t-tests, see Witt and McGrain[31] and Lyons.[32]

As indicated in Table 8–3, there are several formulas for t depending on the method of sampling (independent, matched, or related). A slightly different formula for the t-test is used for two related samples, "own control" or "matched pairs." An interesting variation of the own-control design, which is more powerful than the one diagrammed in Table 8–2, is the *cross-over* design.[33] In the cross-over model, each patient gets both treatments and is evaluated under both treatments but at different times. This design is most useful for assessing short-term effects of treatment. The experimenter must randomly determine for each patient which treatment comes first so that no systematic bias is introduced into the data. The data for each treatment is merged, and the t-test is performed. The cross-over design may be diagrammed thus:

$$R \quad T_1 \quad T_2 \quad M$$
$$R \quad T_2 \quad T_1 \quad M$$

The t-test is intended to compare the means of two sets of data. Many statistics books warn that repeated use of the t-test in the same study may create false significance levels; this is true especially if the data sets are not independent, that is, if the score on one set may influence the score on the other set.[34] There are mathematical ways of dealing with this phenomenon. For example, Taylor and colleagues[35] stated that "Because nine [paired t-tests] were performed, we required a more stringent level of significance (P = <.0056). This level of significance was determined by applying the Bonferroni correction, which involved dividing 0.05 (the initial level of significance) by 9 (the number of repeated measures)."

Proportions were discussed earlier in this chapter. It is possible to write a null hypothesis stating that the proportion in the population (P) is equal to the observed proportion in a sample (p). Hence, P = p. For example, if you observe that 39 percent of the hemiplegic patients admitted to your hospital last year were left hemiplegics, you could ask, "What is the probability that my sample proportion represents the population proportion?" The statistical test for this question is the Z-test. Since proportion questions do not often appear in therapy literature, this test will not be further illustrated.

Now let us look at a nonparametric test for repeated measures on the same individuals (two related samples, own control) using an ordinal level of measurement for the dependent variable. As indicated in Table 8–3, one appropriate statistical tool would be the Wilcoxon Matched-Pairs, Signed-Ranks Test. The dependent variable will be pain; let us say we want to use the analog scale for pain as the measurement tool. In that scale, 1 represents "no pain" and 10, "worst pain ever experienced."

Ask each subject to rate their pain at the time of admission. Treat them for 2 weeks, then give them another analog pain test. The measurement scale is ordinal, 1 to 10. See if you can flesh out this design into a full research protocol.

Table 8–6 illustrates the steps in calculating the Wilcoxon with hypothetical data. The steps are:[36]

1 Calculate the difference between each score.

2 Assign the appropriate sign to that difference.

3 Rank the differences *without regard to sign*, giving the lowest difference a rank of 1.

4 Subjects with 0 difference are dropped from further analysis.

5 Sum the ranks with the least frequently appearing sign.

Since we expected the pain to go down, a one-tailed test is used. The tabled significance level for a T of 7, where $n = 9$, is P <.027, so we can say that our chances are about 3 in 100 of being wrong in rejecting the

TABLE 8–6 **CALCULATION OF T FOR THE WILCOXON MATCHED-PAIRS, SIGNED-RANKS TEST**

Subject	Prescore	Postscore	d	Rank	Rank of Least Freq. Sign
1	7	5	+2	5.5	
2	6	5	+1	2	
3	9	8	+1	2	
4	8	9	−1	2	2
5	4	6	−2	5.5	5.5
6	9	7	+2	5.5	
7	10	8	+2	5.5	
8	6	6	0		
9	5	1	+4	8	
10	8	3	+5	9	
	$n = 9$				7.5

null hypothesis in favor of the alternate that the treatment decreased the perceived level of pain.

Practice   The article by Gianinni in Appendix C has been referred to several times in this text. It is outlined in Appendix B. It demonstrates the use of the Spearman rank-order correlation for ordinal data and the Pearson and ICC for metric data; it demonstrates the use of the t-test for paired means, and it demonstrates the use of the Wilcoxon Matched-Pairs, Signed-Rank Test for paired samples where measurement of the dependent variable is at the ordinal level. You should be able to read the entire article now with understanding.

Computer-Assisted Statistics   Many hand-held computers are programmed to do the t-test. The directions manual that comes with each computer will tell you how to enter the data for that particular model. For larger operations the most commonly used statistical software packages are SPSS and SAS. Both SPSS and SAS are widely available in college and university statistical labs and in larger hospitals. For home use most statistical tests are available in the statistical software package SPSS/PC.[37] The computer-literate student should have little difficulty using these computer tools. For the uninitiated, a good beginning reference is Francis.[38] Computer use will be discussed further in Chapter 9.

Examples from the Literature   Dudgeon and Cunningham[39] sent a questionnaire to 176 applicants to three occupational therapy schools in the Pacific northwest. They used the SPSS computer statistical package to analyze their data by percentages, chi-square, and independent t-tests. "Location of high school graduation was different between schools, with Pacific University having a greater number of applicants from rural communities and the University of Washington having a greater number of applicants from urban settings ($\chi^2 = 13.81$, df $= 4$, P $= .007$)."[40] Here they did not have "observed" and "expected" data but rather two sets of nominal (frequency counts) data that were compared by chi-square and found to be very significantly different. In a similar fashion, they used chi-square to demonstrate an absence of statistically significant differences between the applicants to the different schools in terms of sex, marital status, ethnic origin, or residential background; they used independent t-tests to demonstrate an absence of statistically significant differences in terms of age or prerequisite grade-point averages (metric data).
Kleinam and Stalcup[41] used

a nonequivalent control group design ... to compare two noncurrent groups, the treatment group and an earlier group of patients who had not received the treatment. Assignment to groups was random to the extent that all patients who were admitted to the hospital during the two consecutive periods of the study and who met predetermined criteria were included in the study.

They further noted that

The primary hypothesis for this study was that child psychiatry patients who participate in a specific graded sequence of craft activities will be more likely to show improved posttest scores on the Developmental Test of Visual-Motor Integration than will patients who have not participated in the treatment. . . . An analysis of the data revealed that significantly more subjects in the treatment group improved their test scores by 6 months or more ($P < .05$) than did those in the control group.[42]

Kleinman and Stalcup used chi-square to test their main question. They used a t-test to demonstrate an absence of statistically significant differences between the groups in age or IQ.

In a survey questionnaire study by Domholdt and Durchholz[43]

Chi-square analyses were used to test whether therapists who had or had not practiced through direct access had different opinions about whether direct access had benefited the profession and patients. The alpha level for each test was set at 0.05.

Results indicated that the two groups differed on the benefits to both the profession and patients ($P = <.0001$).

For another example, see Trahey[44] where independent t-tests for metric data such as age and number of treatment days and chi-square for nominal data such as sex and diagnosis, were used as tests of homogeneity, that is, to prove that the groups did not differ significantly on these variables.

For an example of two related samples, own control, see Witt and MacKinnon,[45] who used the nonparametric Wilcoxon Matched-Pairs, Signed-Ranks Test and the Spearman coefficient of rank correlation with metric data because their sampling design did not meet the assumptions of the parametric tests. In a similar vein Ruth and Kegerreis[46] used a Mann-Whitney test "to determine if there was a significant difference between the control and experimental groups in the VAS measurement of perceived effort level. . . . This nonparametric method was used because equal units could not be assumed in the measurement."

Brown and her colleagues[47] studied the improvement in attitudes toward the elderly following traditional and geriatric mock clinics for physical therapy students.

A student's two-tailed t test for independent means was performed to determine any differences in the overall attitude scores of the two groups and any changes in (Kogan Old Person Scale) pretest and posttest administration. No significant difference was found between the two groups' overall attitude scores on the pretest or posttest results. Positive attitude scores increased significantly for both the experimental group ($P < .001$) and the control group ($P < .02$). Negative attitude scores decreased significantly for the experimental group (P <.05) but did not change for the control group.

In a double-blind study, Downing and Weinstein[48] randomly assigned patients to true or sham ultrasound in addition to routine treatment for 4 weeks. Physician, therapist, and patient were "blind" as to who received which treatment. Independent t-tests were used to analyze changes in ROM, the Sign test was used to study improvement in pain, and chi-square was used to evaluate pain in comparison to functional ability. Can you justify the use of each of these tests in this situation?

Howard[49] matched 12 abused and 12 nonabused children by age and family income (Table 8–1, design 5). She reported the validity and reliability data for her measurement tool. An independent t-test of homogeneity demonstrated that the matching had accomplished its purpose, the children were not significantly different on the variables of age or family income. A dependent t-test was used to determine differences between play age and chronological age *within* each group (two related samples, own control); the abused children were discrepant, the nonabused were not. Another t-test demonstrated that the two groups differed in the amount that the play age deviated from the chronological age.

Franklin[50] matched eight adolescents for age, sex, and diagnosis. Values clarification was taught to one group by computer and to the other group through group discussion. Dependent variables analyzed separately were the Tennessee Self-Concept Scale, a locus of control scale, and a questionnaire concerning perceived effectiveness. The Wilcoxon demonstrated no significance on the two scales but did show a preference (P <.05) for the computer program. How do you think the investigator could have increased the chances of finding significant differences between the two groups?

References

1. Hamilton, M: Lectures on the Methodology of Clinical Research, ed 2. Churchill Livingstone, London, 1974, pp 34–35.
2. Shott, S: Statistics for Health Professionals. WB Saunders, Philadelphia, 1990, p 24.
3. Pocock, SJ: Clinical Trials. John Wiley, New York, 1983, Chapter 9.
4. Bulpitt, CJ: Randomized Controlled Clinical Trials. Martinus Nijhoff, Boston, 1983, Chapter 10.
5. Ottenbacher, K: The significance of power and the power of significance: Recommendations for occupational therapy research. OTJ of Res 4:37, 1984.
6. Ottenbacher, K: Measures of relationship strength in occupational therapy research. OTJ of Res 4:271, 1984.
7. Ottenbacher, The significance of power and the power of significance. p 39.
8. Goldstein, G: A Clinician's Guide to Research Design. Nelson-Hall, Chicago, 1980, p 111.
9. Browner, WS and Newman, TB: The analogy between diagnostic tests and clinical research.

JAMA 257:2459, 1987. Reprinted in Hulley, SB and Cummings, SR (eds): Designing Clinical Research. Williams & Wilkins, Baltimore, 1988, p 232.

10. Campbell, DT and Stanley, JC: Experimental and Quasi-Experimental Designs for Research. Rand-McNally, Chicago, 1973.

11. Siegel, S: Nonparametric Statistics for the Behavioral Sciences. McGraw-Hill, New York, 1956.

12. Payton, OD, et al: Student-produced empathic responses: The second step in teaching communication skills to allied health supervisors. J Allied Health 7:302, 1978.

13. Nunnally, JC: The study of change in evaluation research: Principles concerning measurement, experimental design, and analysis. In Struening, EL and Guttentag, M (eds): Handbook of Evaluation Research. Sage Publications, Beverly Hills, 1975.

14. Conine, TA: Dilemmas of research in occupational therapy. AJOT 26:81, 1972.

15. Pruden, E, et al: Ins and outs of research: Problem to publication. AJ Med Technol 36:209, 1970.

16. Armitage, P: Sequential Medical Trials, ed 2. New York: John Wiley & Sons, 1975.

17. Whitehead, J: The Design and Analysis of Sequential Clinical Trials. New York: John Wiley & Sons, 1983.

18. Armitage, op cit.

19. Bross, I: Sequential medical plans. Biometrics 8:189, 1952.

20. Ibid.

21. Armitage, op cit.

22. Whitehead, op cit.

23. Gault, SJ and Spyker, JM: Beneficial effect of immobilization of joints in rheumatoid and related arthritides: A splint study using sequential analysis. Arthr Rheum 12:34, 1969.

24. Siegel, op cit, p 18.

25. Mann, WC: The choice of an appropriate statistic: A nonmathematical approach. AJOT 40:696, 1986.

26. Royeen, CB and Seaver, WL: Promise in nonparametrics. AJOT 40:191, 1986.

27. Stahl, SM and Hennes, JD: Reading and Understanding Applied Statistics. CV Mosby, St. Louis, 1980.

28. Shott, S: Statistics for Health Professionals. WB Saunders, Philadelphia, 1990, p 208.

29. Wang, M, et al, op cit, p 211.

30. Shott, op cit, p 211.

31. Witt, PL and McGrain, P: Comparing two sample means: t tests. Phys Ther 65:1730, 1985.

32. Lyons, M: Enabling or disabling? Students' attitudes toward persons with disabilities. AJOT 45:311, 1991.

33. Pocock, op cit, Chapter 8.

34. Ottenbacher, KJ: Multiplicity in rehabilitation research: A quantitative assessment. Arch Phys Med Rehabil 69:170, 1988.

35. Taylor, K, Fish, DR, Mendell, FC, et al: Effect of a single 30-minute treatment of high-voltage pulsed current on edema formation in frog hind limbs. Phys Ther 72:63, 1992, p 66.

36. Stahl and Hennes, op cit.

37. Norusis, MJ: SPSS/PC+ V3.0 Base Manual for the IBM PC/XT/AT and PS/2. SPSS, Chicago, 1989.

38. Francis, K: Computer Essentials in Physical Therapy. Slack, Thorofare, NJ, 1987.

39. Dudgeon, BJ and Cunningham, S: Occupational therapy entry-level program applicants: A survey of northwest schools. AJOT 46:583, 1992.

40. Ibid, p 586.

41. Kleinman, BL and Stalcup, A: The effect of graded craft activities on visuomotor integration in an inpatient child psychiatry population. AJOT 45:324, 1991, p 336.

42. Ibid. p 325–327.

43. Domholdt, E and Durchholz, AG: Direct access use by experienced therapists in states with direct access. Phys Ther 72:569, 1992.
44. Trahey, PJ: A comparison of the cost-effectiveness of two types of occupational therapy services. AJOT 45:397, 1991.
45. Witt, PL and MacKinnon, J: Trager psychophysical integration: A method to improve chest mobility of patients with chronic lung disease. Phys Ther 66:214, 1986.
46. Ruth, S and Kegerreis, S: Facilitating cervical flexion using a Feldenkrais method: Awareness through movement. JOSPT 16:25, 1992.
47. Brown, DS, Gardner, DL, Perritt, L, et al: Improvement in attitudes toward the elderly following traditional and geriatric mock clinics for physical therapy students. Phys Ther 72:251, 1992.
48. Downing, DS and Weinstein, A: Ultrasound therapy for subacromial bursitis: A double-blind trial. Phys Ther 66:194, 1986.
49. Howard, AC: Developmental play ages of physically abused and nonabused children. AJOT 40:691, 1986.
50. Franklin, D: A comparison of the effectiveness of values clarification presented as a personal computer program versus a traditional therapy group: A pilot study. OT in Mental Health 6:39, 1986.

Additional Readings

Bulpitt, CJ: Randomized Controlled Clinical Trials. Martinus Nijhoff, Boston, 1983, Chapter 11.
Dempsey, PA and Dempsey, AD: The Research Process in Nursing, ed 2. Jones & Bartlett, Boston, 1986, Chapter 10.
Drew, CJ and Hardman, ML: Designing and Conducting Behavioral Research. Pergamon Press, New York, 1985, Part III.
Leedy, PD: Practical Research: Planning and Design, ed 2. Macmillan, New York, 1980.
Polit, DF and Hungler, BP: Essentials of Nursing Research: Methods and Applications. Lippincott, Philadelphia, 1985, Chapters 15, 16, and 18.
Goldstein, G: A Clinician's Guide to Research Design. Nelson-Hall, Chicago, 1980, Chapter 2.

Group Experimental Designs: Three Data Sets and Related Designs

OBJECTIVES

1   Define and illustrate one-group and k-group designs having k data sets, and identify appropriate statistical tests according to level of measurement.

2   Define and illustrate factorial, covariate, and multivariate designs and associated statistical tools.

3   Analyze literature containing k data sets and factorial and multivariate designs.

4   Discuss the role of computers in the management of research data.

5   Discuss design applications to research in supervision, administration, and professional education.

k Data Sets

In the previous chapter we considered group experimental designs for two data sets. In this chapter we will examine group experimental designs

181

for three or more data sets and related designs. Review Tables 8–1, 8–2, and 8–3, which deal with research designs and statistical models for *k* related samples, own control, *k* independent samples, and *k* related samples, matched.

Let us begin by examining what is perhaps the most important and most basic statistical tool in this chapter's area of interest: one-way analysis of variance for *k* independent groups (Table 8–1, design 6). In Chapter 1, the therapists in the St. Hopeless Outpatient Clinic asked: "Which is better for maintaining joint mobility in rheumatoid arthritic patients: heat and active exercise twice daily (HA), heat and passive exercises twice daily (HP), or a functional activity program (F) twice daily?" For this study we will consider these three treatment plans as independent variables HA, HP, and F; heat, active exercise, or passive exercise will not be considered separately but only as part of the "treatment packages." Thus we have a single factor, exercise, given at three levels. (We will address factors and levels again later in this chapter.)

By now you should be able to write a research protocol for this question with a sampling model of random assignment to each of three groups. State the null hypothesis for yourself. The alternate hypothesis is that one of the treatments will be better than the other two; we will not choose which one. At this point you should have written most of the protocol for this study. Define the dependent variable as change—the difference from pretest to posttest—in measured range of motion (ROM) in the elbow of the dominant arm. We have three independent samples; therefore our design is *k* independent samples.

As indicated by Table 8–3, this design calls for the F test, one-way analysis of variance (ANOVA). According to Shott,[1] random sampling is not essential for ANOVA if the samples are not biased. That is very helpful in the health care field, where truly random samples are difficult to select. But since randomization is a powerful tool against unconscious bias, it should be used wherever possible. Shott further states that for one-way ANOVA to be valid, both the samples themselves and the observations within each sample must be independent. If the samples are not independent, as in repeated measures on the same sample or in samples that are related through matching, then two-way ANOVA must be used. For ANOVA to be used properly, the populations need to closely match normal distribution and the variances in the samples need to be similar.[2] The beginning researcher is well advised to consult a statistician before trying ANOVA to make sure that your data meet the assumptions of the statistical test.

ANOVA is a more complex statistical procedure than any presented in this text so far. It will be important to understand each mathematical expression that goes into the final formula. Table 9–1 is a general outline of the mathematical expressions that enter into ANOVA in the form of an

TABLE 9-1   **GENERAL OUTLINE OF AN ANOVA TABLE**

Source of Variation	df	Sum of Squares	Mean Squares	F ratio	p
Between means	$k - 1$	BSS	BMS		
Within groups	$n - k$	WSS	WMS		
Totals	$n - 1$	TSS			

Source: Data from Goldstein, G: A Clinician's Guide to Research Design. Nelson-Hall, Chicago, 1980, Chapter 3.

ANOVA table. ANOVA is often reported in just such a table in the literature. We will examine each expression in turn.

Let us start with one set of hypothetical data in Table 9-2. Key expressions derived from the data in Table 9-2 are sum of squares, variance, and standard deviation. The words "mean" and "square" appear frequently in what follows. They are associated with different mathematical expressions, so the beginner may need to read slowly and carefully. Table 9-3 gives some of the corresponding data for all three data sets for the question stated above plus the sum and mean of all three data sets together; this latter is called the grand or total sum and mean ($\Sigma G, \bar{x}G$).

The calculation of the group sum of (x^2) has not been demonstrated, but the method can be deduced from Table 9-2. In ANOVA the null hypothesis is as follows: there is no statistically significant difference among the

TABLE 9-2   **CALCULATION OF SUM OF SQUARES,
VARIANCE, AND STANDARD DEVIATION FOR ONE DATA SET**

Subject	Scores	$x - \bar{x}$	$(x - \bar{x})^2$	x^2
1	12	2	4	144
2	8	-2	4	64
3	15	5	25	225
4	6	-4	16	36
5	10	0		100
•				
•				
•				
20	9	-1	1	81
	Σ 200		196	2276
	$\bar{x}$ 10			

$$\text{Sum of squares} = (x - \bar{x})^2 = 196 \tag{9a}$$

$$\text{Variance} = s^2 = \frac{(x - \bar{x})^2}{n} = \frac{196}{20} = 9.8 \tag{9b}$$

$$\text{Standard deviation} = s = \sqrt{s^2} = \sqrt{9.8} = 3.13 \tag{9c}$$

TABLE 9–3   CALCULATION OF GROUP SUM, GROUP MEAN,
AND GROUP SUM OF SQUARES FOR k INDEPENDENT
SAMPLES

Subject	HA	HP	F		
1	12	9	4		
2	8	2	0		
3	15	8	2		
4	6	6	8		
5	10	4	5		
•					
•					
20	9	6	4		
Σ	200	140	100	G = 440	(9d)
$\bar{x}$	10	7	5	G = 7.3	(9e)

Group sum of squares (GSS) $= (\Sigma G)^2 / kn$ (9f)
$\qquad\qquad\qquad\qquad\quad = (440)^2 / (3)(20)$
$\qquad\qquad\qquad\qquad\quad = 193600 / 60$
$\qquad\qquad\qquad\qquad\quad = 3226.66$

Group sum of $(x^2) = 5054$ (9g)

means of several data sets. (ANOVA can be performed on two data sets; in that case it is equivalent to the t-test; t^2 for a two-tailed test $=$ F. The concept of a one- or two-tailed test does not apply in ANOVA.)

If the null hypothesis concerning the sample is not rejected, the researcher would like to infer that the means of the populations concerned are also equal; each data set is considered to be drawn from a distinct population. This is accomplished by asking whether the *sample* means and two estimates of *population* variance taken from the sample could have occurred if the null hypothesis concerning population means is true. It is a comparison of observed values in the sample with expected values in the population. Stahl and Hennes[3] observe that "the analysis of variance is a comparison of two estimates of the population variance."

So the next step in understanding ANOVA is to understand those two estimates of the population variance. We have already examined the source of the first one; it is based on the variation *within* each sample, as exemplified in Table 9–2, formula (9a). It examines variability among individuals within the data set and is called *within-group sum of squares* (WSS), or unexplained variance. The second estimate of population variance that enters into the calculation of ANOVA is based on the variation across data sets or variability among the means of the data sets; it is called *between-*

group sum of squares (BSS), or explained variance. For *k* data sets the BSS and the WSS may be calculated as follows:

$$BSS = 1/n \text{ (sum of the square of each group mean)} - GSS$$

$$= 1/20 \ [(200)^2 + (140)^2 + (100)^2] - 3226.66 \qquad (9h)$$

$$= 3480 - 3226.66$$

$$= 253.34$$

$$\begin{array}{llll} WSS = & \Sigma(x^2) - & GSS - & BSS \\ & (9g) & (9f) & (9h) \\ = & 5040 - & 3226.66 - & 253.34 \\ = & 1560 \end{array} \qquad (9i)$$

$$\begin{array}{lll} TSS = & \Sigma x^2 - & GSS \\ & (9g) & (9f) \\ = & 5040 - & 3226.66 \\ = & 1813.34 \end{array} \qquad (9j)$$

Verify the calculation as follows:

$$TSS = BSS + WSS$$

$$(9j) \quad (9h) \quad (9i)$$

The next issue has to do with degrees of freedom (df).

$$df \ TSS = n - 1 \qquad (9k)$$

$$df \ BSS = k - 1 \qquad (9l)$$

$$df \ WSS = n - k \qquad (9m)$$

where n = total number of subjects in each group and k = number of data sets. Total degrees of freedom are equal to df between plus df within.

$$(n - 1) = (k - 1) + (n - k)$$

Mean square (also called *estimated variance* or *average sum of squares*) is the average sum of squares where that average is obtained by dividing any given sum of squares by its associated df. Therefore:

$$\text{Between mean square (BMS)} = \frac{\text{BSS}}{k - 1} \qquad \begin{matrix} (9h) \\ (9l) \end{matrix}$$

$$= \frac{253.34}{2} \qquad (9n)$$

$$= 126.67$$

$$\text{Within mean square (WMS)} = \frac{\text{WSS}}{n - k} \qquad \begin{matrix} (9i) \\ (9m) \end{matrix}$$

$$= \frac{1560}{17} \qquad (9o)$$

$$= 91.76$$

We are now ready to look at the inferential test statistic called the F test or the F ratio. There are several versions of the F test based on the sampling model, the number of dependent and independent variables, and other considerations. Here we will complete one example based on the data developed above using the one-way ANOVA.

$$F = \frac{\text{BMS}}{\text{WMS}}$$

$$= \frac{126.67}{91.76} \qquad (9p)$$

$$= 1.38$$

The F ratio is the ratio between the two mathematical expressions BMS and WMS. If the F ratio approximates 1, it suggests that the population means are equal and the null hypothesis cannot be rejected. As the F ratio gets larger, the inference grows that the population means are not equal; the null hypothesis can be rejected with increasingly high levels of significance. Consult the tabled values of F in the back of a statistics book; with 2 and 17 degrees of freedom, an F ratio of 3.59 is significant at $p < .05$. Since our observed F ratio of 1.38 is less than the tabled value, we cannot reject the null hypothesis; that is, we cannot say that there is a difference somewhere among the three means of our data sets. So we have to conclude that we have not demonstrated that one of the three treatments (HA, HP, or F) is better than the other two.

Table 9–1 uses the following mathematical expressions:

Expression	Formula
BSS	(9h)
WSS	(9i)
TSS	(9j)
BMS	(9n)
WMS	(9o)
F ratio	(9p)

plus the df specified in (9k), (9l), and (9m). Table 9–1 may now be used as a model to report the results of the k independent sample study used to answer the question of the therapists from St. Hopeless. The ANOVA table for that study is found in Table 9–4.

The F test tells you if there is an *overall* difference among the means in the study. If the null hypothesis is rejected on the basis of the F test, then one may perform a **post-hoc test** to see where the greatest difference lies within the data. Three frequently used tests are the Newman-Keuls, the Tukey, and the Scheffe tests. There are different mathematical formulas for these post-hoc tests, depending on whether the basic ANOVA model is one way, one factor repeated measures, or two way. The post-hoc test will tell you which of the three treatments contributed most to the rejection of the null hypothesis by comparing data set A to B, B to C, and A to C.

Practice   Change the sums in (9d) and (9g) to 200, 150, 420, and 8452. Now rework the problem and see what results you get.

Factorial Designs

For yet another model of ANOVA, suppose that you wanted to study the effects of drugs and exercise on pain-free ROM in the knee. The dependent variable (DV) will be ROM. Here we have a situation not seen before in this text (except briefly in Chapter 7): two independent variables (IV), which may affect *each* subject in the study. When two or more independent variables are acting on a subject, we are dealing with **factorial designs.**[4]

TABLE 9–4   **ANOVA TABLE FOR THE DATA IN TABLE 9–2**

Source of Variation	df	Sum of Squares	Mean Squares	F ratio	P
Between means	2	253.34	126.67	1.38	ns
Within groups	17	1560	91.76		
Totals	19	1813.34			

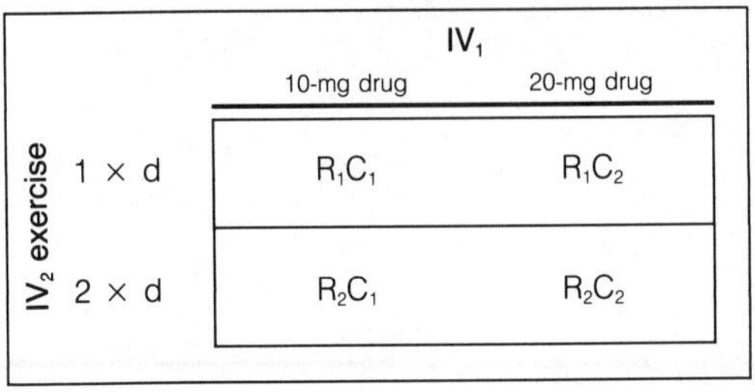

FIGURE 9–1. Diagram of a 2×2 factorial design, in which two independent variables are drugs and exercise defined at two levels.

Two-way ANOVA is used to analyze the effects of two or more independent variables on the dependent variable in *each* subject.

Please note the essential difference between this two-way ANOVA and the one-way ANOVA studied above. In the one-way model, one set of subjects received one treatment, a second set of subjects received a different treatment, and a third set of subjects received a third treatment; early in this chapter we identified that arrangement as one factor with three levels. In the two-way model being discussed here, each subject is under the influence of *both* drugs and exercise. Figure 9–1 diagrams this study in a 2×2 factorial design. In factorial designs, the *factors* referred to are the number of independent variables. Each variable may have two or more *levels*. In Figure 9–1 there are two factors, each having two levels, hence a 2×2 factorial design. Figure 9–2 illustrates the same question as a 2×3 factorial design wherein one factor, drugs, has two levels and the other factor, exercise, has three levels. In each instance the DV remains the same. A **mixed factorial design** is one in which one factor is not randomized and the other is. For example, sex is predetermined but exercise level is randomly assigned by the researcher. If Figure 9–1 were revised so that one factor was sex (male/female), and the other factor was two levels of exercise, it would be a mixed factorial design.

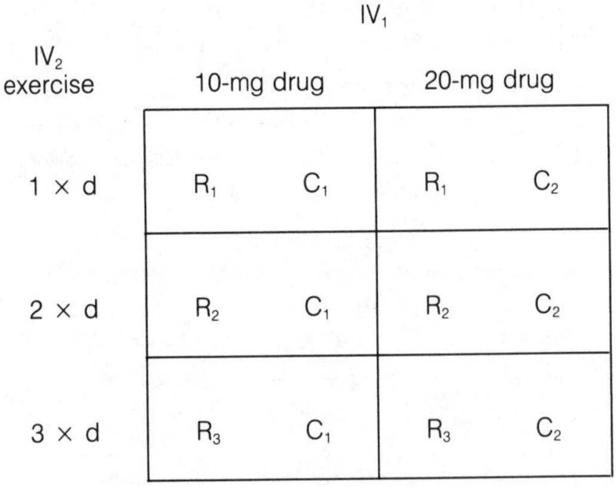

FIGURE 9–2. Diagram of 2×3 factorial design, in which the two independent variables are drug level and exercise level.

Another use of factorial designs is to study the interactive effects of treatments. If your treatment plan includes three treatment modalities and the patients get better, did one of the treatments do it while the rest were useless, did each one contribute, or was the *interaction* of the treatments more powerful than any treatment given separately? You could randomly assign patients to each of seven groups to study the effects of treatment A, B, C, A + B, A + C, B + C, A + B + C. Any one of these treatments could prove to be the most powerful.

Practice   Using Figure 9–2 as a model, design a study looking at the effects of three treatment modalities (3) and their interactive effects on fresh and mature scars (2): a 3 × 2 factorial design. (*Hint*: Each cell represents a different combination of treatments, so you will have six experimental groups. Plan to have the same number of subjects in each cell. It makes the statistics a lot simpler.)

Now carefully read the article by Stern in Appendix C. Try to identify as many elements of a research protocol (Appendix A), as you can. If it makes sense, supply what is missing. What kind of statistics are proposed in paragraph 16? Does "repeated measures" suggest one-way or two-way ANOVA? What is the research design in this study? How do you read Table 1? What kind of data are contained in Table 2?

Two-way ANOVA performs a test for each independent variable—called main effects—plus a test for the *interaction* effect between the independent variables. As the number of independent variables goes up, the number of interactions possible goes up rapidly. For example, three independent variables produce four possible interactions. Table 9–5 illustrates a two-way ANOVA table.

Factorial analysis not only allows the experimenter to study the effects of several modalities at the same time, thus mimicking the typical clinical situation, it also permits the study of interactive effects and tells the researcher how much each variable contributes numerically to the overall outcome— how much variation in the DV is due to each IV.

TABLE 9–5   **TWO-WAY ANOVA OF THE EFFECTS OF SEX AND YEARS OF EXPERIENCE ON ATTITUDES TOWARD THE DISABLED**

Source	SS	df	MS	F*	p
Main effects					
Sex		1			
Years		1			
Interaction effects					
Sex × years		1			
Error		$n - 4$			

*Three F ratios would be derived: 0, 1, 2, or all three could be significant.

Related Designs

In Table 8–2, k related samples, own control was diagrammed

M   T   M   M

k related samples require a formula called one-factor repeated-measures ANOVA. This model has its own associated formula for the Bonferroni post-hoc test. For details of this design see Shott.[5]

k independent samples was diagrammed several ways, including:

R   M   T   M
R   M   T   M
R   M   C   M

Another possibility is the split-plot ANOVA for two independent samples with repeated measures. Split-plot ANOVA may be diagrammed thus:

R   M   T   M   M
R   M   C   M   M

The split-plot ANOVA is just another in a wide variety of possibilities for the very versatile ANOVA statistical model.

You will note in Table 8–3 that two-way ANOVA is also the model used to analyze nonindependent k samples in matching or own-control sampling models. The well-known Latin square design is a member of this group in ANOVA. Advanced statistics books will give you the formulae for these applications. Unfortunately, different statistical texts use different notations and ways of presenting the various formulas, so "finding the appropriate formula for your data may be the hardest part of the analysis, especially if you are doing an experiment with a complex design."[6] Look at paragraph 15 in the Magill-Evans and Restall article in Appendix C. Why and how is one-way ANOVA used?

Analysis of covariance (ANCOVA) is a blending of ANOVA and correlation where the effect of a potentially confounding variable is removed and the remaining variation is analyzed. Schefler[7] used an example of an experiment where the effect of three diets on blood cholesterol level was tested using one-way ANOVA; no significant differences were found among the three randomly assigned groups. Then the same data were analyzed using ANCOVA; the effect of age was removed and the remaining variation produced a significant F ratio. A version of the F test is used in ANCOVA.

The Kruskal-Wallis one-way ANOVA by ranks is probably the most widely used nonparametric statistical tool for k independent samples.[8] The Kruskal-Wallis assumes that the measurement scale is at least ordinal, that the observations are independent both within and between groups, and that group assignment is random. If the Kruskal-Wallis is statistically significant, then one appropriate post-hoc test would be Dunn's Multiple Comparisons Test.[9]

Multivariate analysis of variance (MANOVA) is one the most complex topics in statistics and was little used until the advent of the computer. It is not even mentioned in most beginning text books. In essence this technique allows one to analyze the effects of the independent variable(s) on *more than one* dependent variable. Several statistical approaches to multiple DVs are possible, but an approximation to the F statistic is often recommended and is available on computer software. "The important thing to remember here is that, in making comparisons, you are not comparing a number of means, but a number of profiles or configurations of scores, and you are asking whether or not these configurations or patterns differ significantly."[10] Keppel[11] references McCall[12] for a nontechnical introduction of MANOVA.

Zito and Bohannon[13] ask what statistics are most frequently used in physical therapy literature.

A literature search of 137 articles from four physical therapy journals produced 241 reported inferential statistics. A taxonomy was constructed that classified the statistics as parametric or nonparametric, according to their basic purpose. Based on the results of our survey of research articles and support from the literature, we recommend a core of 10 inferential statistics that would permit physical therapists statistical access to almost 80% of their scientific literature. (p 13)

Of the 241 statistical tests they found, 181 were parametric and 60 were nonparametric. In order of frequency of use, the top 10 tests were ANOVA, t-test, Pearson *r*, chi-square, ICC, Mann-Whitney test, Wilcoxon, Spearman ρ, Newman-Keuls, MANOVA.

Examples from the Literature

ONE-WAY ANOVA

Newton[14] randomly assigned 44 student volunteers to one of four groups (*k* independent samples). Each subject's hip flexors were passively stretched while the posterior thigh was sprayed either with ethyl chloride, fluori-methane, isopropyl alcohol, or no spray. A one-way ANOVA demonstrated no statistically significant differences among the four treatments. For a similar design using one-factor ANOVA see Lyons.[15] Lyons used SPSS computer software to perform an ANOVA to compare four classes of occupational therapy (OT) students, freshmen through senior, on an attitudes toward disabled persons scale; there were no statistically significant differences.

Hackel and her associates[16] did a cross-sectional study of age cohorts in their sixth, seventh, and eighth decades of life, looking at changes in hand function as measured by a specific test.

The Jebsen Test of Hand Function is used to assess a broad range of hand functions required for activities of daily living. The time needed to complete a variety of subtests is measured, with high scores indicative of abnormality. Normative values have been established for men and women in two age groups: 20 to 59 years and 60 to 94 years. The purpose of this study was to determine whether hand function, as measured by the Jebsen test, declines with age in subjects over the age of 60 years. A total of 121 men and women were given the test and grouped into the following age categories (1) 60 to 69 years, (2) 70 to 79 years, and (3) 80 to 89 years. Hand function decreased with age in both men and women. There were significant positive correlations between age and time needed to complete the various subtests, and analyses of variance revealed significant differences between subjects in their 80's and those in their 60's and 70's. In only a few tasks were there significant differences between men and women within any age group. Because of the decrease in normal function with age, measurements obtained with the Jebsen test in the elderly should be compared with normative values that are obtained from similarly aged subjects.

Can you state why one-way analysis of variance would be appropriate in the Hackel study?

Mitchell and associates[17] studied the effects of two active drugs and a placebo on pain threshold. Three independent groups were formed, pretested, medicated for 14 days, then posttested. One-way ANCOVA was used to control for the wide individual variance in pain measurements by adjusting the posttest values on the basis of the pretest values before the main test was done. No statistically significant differences were demonstrated.

For other recent examples of one-way ANOVA in the literature see Robichaud, Agostinucci, and Linden[18] (who also use two-way ANOVA), and Lang, Nelson, and Bush[19] (for repeated measures, Tukey post-hoc test). Authors often do not say which formula (one-way or two-way) they used, so one has to trust both authors and editor that the proper test was used. It may make a difference only when significance is borderline. Tse and Bailey[20] had nonequivalent groups of volunteers of elderly subjects, and only ANOVA is specified. For an example of 1×4 repeated-measures ANOVA, see Kuzala and Vargo.[21] For an example of a 2×7 repeated-measures ANOVA, see Goldberg, Sullivan, and Seaborne.[22] See also Ruth and Kegerreis.[23]

TWO-WAY ANOVA

Gliner and Davis[24] provide a good example of the use of two-way ANOVA in a 2×2 factorial design. One factor, speed of movement, was measured at two levels, fast or slow; the other factor, angle of approach, was measured as altered or original. Two dependent variables, distance from the target and angle error, were statistically treated separately. (If they had taken the DV together, what statistical technique would they have used?) Forty-eight OT students were randomly divided into four groups. A two-factor between-groups ANOVA was used with a post-hoc Newman-Keuls test to pinpoint where the greatest differences lay. Their results indicated that speed made a difference, and angle did not.

Delitto and his group[25] performed a study

> to investigate the influence of personality variables and contractile forces on magnitude estimates of pain unpleasantness and pain intensity during varying levels of neuromuscular electrical stimulation (NMES). Thirty volunteers, according to their scores on a preferred coping-style questionnaire, were assigned to one of two groups, one designated "monitors" (information seekers) and the other designated "blunters" (information avoiders). All subjects were administered varying levels of two types of NMES, one causing both afferent stimulation and muscle contraction and one causing only afferent stimulation. Subjects judged the intensity and unpleasantness of each current type using magnitude estimation. Data were analyzed using a 2 × 2 × 2 × 3 (coping style × current type × pain descriptor × current level) analysis of variance. The results indicated that the rate of increase of magnitude estimates for unpleasantness and pain intensity that corresponded to increases in current were dependent on (1) the preferred coping style of the subject, (2) whether the stimulus caused a muscle contraction, and (3) whether the subject was judging the intensity or the unpleasantness of the applied stimulus. Behavioral styles appear to affect how subjects characterize the discomfort associated with NMES, and involuntary muscle contractions contribute to the discomfort felt from NMES. These results suggest that interventions tailored to a preferred coping style may increase a subject's level of tolerance to NMES and thus provide a more beneficial treatment.

In Chapter 7 we examined a single case study by Goodisman.[26] He used two-way ANOVA to analyze repeated measures of four different treatment modalities on one 5-year-old subject. Each treatment was evaluated as a main effect, and one interaction was analyzed.

Krause and her coworkers[27] used a split-plot ANOVA because of the repeated-measures aspect of their study. Duncan's new multiple-range test was used for post-hoc analysis. Sixty healthy adults were randomly assigned to two experimental groups and a control group. Pretest and posttest (repeated) measures of pain were used. They concluded that electrical stimulation at acupuncture points about the ear raised the pain threshold in the wrist.

The use of ANOVA in k related samples, own-control design is exemplified in a study by Kukulka and associates.[28] Analysis of variance was performed; Bonferroni's post-hoc t-test was used when the main test proved significant at $p<.001$. The post-hoc test was used to evaluate interactions among five trials and three test conditions on 28 healthy subjects. The three test conditions were prepressure, intermittent pressure, and post-pressure on the tendon of the soleus muscle. The dependent variable was α motoneuron excitability as measured by the H reflex. They concluded that the amplitude of the reflex decreased only during tendon pressure with minimal carryover. For another example of two-way ANOVA, see Barr and colleagues.[29]

NONPARAMETRIC ANOVA

In Chapter 3 we looked at an article by Dickstein[30] in which the ordinal data were concerned with functional independence, muscle tone, and isolated motor control. These data were analyzed by computer using the nonparametric Kruskal-Wallis one-way ANOVA. Also in Chapter 3 we examined an article by Delitto and Rose[31] where both metric and ordinal data were collected. The metric data on a visual analog scale for comfort were subjected to several one-way within-subjects ANOVAs; the ordinal rank data were analyzed using Friedman's two-way ANOVA. In Chapter 6 we reviewed an article by Filiatrault and her colleagues[32] which used the Spearman ρ and the Kendall coefficient of concordance. They also used the nonparametric Friedman's ANOVA for k related samples (see Table 8–3).

An article by Case-Smith[33] was cited in Chapter 6 illustrating the use of the Pearson r. She also used the nonparametric Kruskal-Wallis one-way ANOVA to demonstrate that children who exhibited both defensiveness and poor discrimination consistently demonstrated less efficiency in manipulative tasks. Here the Kruskal-Wallis was chosen because of the unequal sample sizes.

ANALYSIS OF COVARIANCE

Anacker and DiFabio[34] illustrate the use of covariance.

The purpose of this study was to determine how conflicting visual and ankle somatosensory inputs influenced standing balance in elders with a history of fall. Forty-seven community-dwelling elders...between 65 and 96 years of age...participated in this project....Subjects were evaluated using a sensory organization test (SOT) for standing balance and a "Get Up and Go" test (GUGT) for general mobility.... The SOT scores were evaluated using a multifactorial analysis of covariance (ANCOVA) with three factors: group (fallers versus nonfallers), surface condition (firm versus compliant), and vision (eyes open, eyes closed, and visual stabilization). Age was selected as a covariate because there is a linear relationship between the amount of body sway and age. A one-way ANCOVA was used to determine whether the GUGT scores for fallers and non-fallers were different. Tukey's *post hoc* studentized range test was used to assess multiple pairwise comparisons at an experimentwise alpha level of .05. In addition, Spearman rank-order correlation coefficients were calculated to evaluate the degree of association between the total SCOT scores and the GUGT scores.

Results demonstrated a decreased stance duration for fallers on compliant surfaces. Fallers also had significantly higher GUGT and SOT scores. For another example of ANCOVA and the Sheffe post-hoc test, see Spadone.[35]

MANOVA

Krebs and colleagues[36] used the statistical analysis system for the IBM PC "and repeated-measures multivariate analysis of variance (MANOVA) results were calculated....Multivariate statistics for multiple dependent variables were used [with an] alpha level at <.05" (p 508). They studied upper-body motions during gait, stair climbing and descending, and rising from a chair. They concluded that "upper body kinematics relative to both pelvis and gravity during daily activities are important to locomotor control.

Morton, Barnett, and Hale[37] used MANOVA for repeated measures to demonstrate no significant difference between the performance of subjects doing a single-purpose task versus subjects doing multidimensional tasks *on a number of dependent measures.* For other examples of the use of MANOVA see Cassady and Nielsen,[38] Liu and coworkers[39] and Haskvitz and Hanten.[40]

Practice   Look at the article by Magill-Evans and Restall in Appendix C. Why and how is MANOVA used?

Computer-Assisted Statistical Analysis

There are many possible ways to apply computer-assisted statistical analysis in clinical practice, administration, education, and research. The interested reader is referred to Cromwell[41] and Francis[42] for relatively brief, readable introductions to computers and their uses in therapy. Each reference deals in different ways with computers and their applications by therapists. Many computer capabilities described in these references can be used to meet the researcher's needs. For example, spreadsheets, which are used to create departmental records and reports, can be used to create tables for data management and reporting. Desktop computers can be used to store data as it is gathered. Word processing software can be used to produce text, and graphics software can produce figures and graphs.

And finally, computers can vastly speed and simplify statistical calculations. The use of pocket or hand-held calculators for simpler statistical operations was discussed in Chapters 5 and 8. ANOVA is so complex that doing the calculations by hand is both tedious and very subject to human error. If at all possible, the task should be turned over to a computer using programs such as SPSS or SAS. One should not even attempt to do any of the designs discussed in this chapter without the aid of a computer and related software. The one possible exception to this is the one-way ANOVA illustrated at the beginning of this chapter; even here, mathematical mistakes are common. Computers cannot make decisions about what formula to use; nor can computers test your data to see if they meet the assumptions of any formula. Those decisions must be made by the researcher. But the computer can do the number crunching much more accurately than most humans.

Francis has provided a quick summary of statistical packages (software) for personal computers. Most of the better statistical packages such as SAS, SPSS, and BMDP have required mainframe computers in the past, but recently new versions of these programs have become available for personal computers with hard-disk storage capability. For those with smaller personal computers using only floppy discs, Statpro, Statpak, and Epistat are available. They have varying levels of sophistication in terms of the amount of data they can handle and the types of tests they can perform. Statpro and Statpak will do some formulas of ANOVA. The journal *Physical Therapy* has a regular feature called "Computer Communication," which presents original programs written for specific clinical, administrative, or research needs and reviews of commercially available packages for statistical analysis and problem solving. For example, Krebs[43] recently published a review of the new SPSS package for personal computers. Rozier and Hamilton[44] used SPSS to analyze their data from a number of perspectives; "Among the statistical analyses used were descriptive measures, Pearson Product-Moment Correlations, reliability coefficients, t tests, analysis of variance, multiple regression, and factor analysis" (p 51). Without a computer, such analyses would have been very time consuming—and much more subject to human mathematical error.

Nonclinical Applications of Research

The most obvious difference between research in clinical sciences and research in other aspects of professional practice is the nature of the questions asked and the methodology. In the areas of education, administration, and supervision, as in all other areas of research, the goal is to produce a body of knowledge—concepts, principles, generalizations, and laws to predict behavior, develop procedures and practices, and effectively control events in a given situation.

Only a few relevant questions will be listed here in order to give the reader an introduction to these areas. What are the major supervisory problems that arise between professional and technical therapists or assistants? Do aides and orderlies respond differently to assistants as supervisors than they do to staff therapists as supervisors? Is there a measurable difference between clinical educators perceived by students as good teachers and clinical educators perceived by students as not good teachers? On what characteristics? Will the introduction of the management by objectives (MBO) form of administration reduce the number of supervisory problems in a given department? What characteristics of the typical clinical environment facilitate student learning, and what characteristics impede student learning?

Research in education, administration, and supervision share with other behavioral sciences some methodological problems that are less bothersome in the natural sciences and almost never a problem in the physical sciences. As with clinical studies, it is often difficult to identify an appropriate population for behavioral research and even more difficult to select an appropriate sample for study. Randomization is frequently difficult to achieve, and the researcher in education and administration is often forced by circumstances to use quasi-experimental designs. The complexity of human behavior can create severe problems, particularly where one cannot count heavily on the randomization procedure for the equalization of groups. Thus, it is often difficult to arrive at a cohesive educational, administrative, or supervisory theory on which sound research can be based. In many instances, these areas of study may be good places for intensive case studies and single-case designs.

For example, Coren and her coworkers[45] sent questionnaires to students in 14 schools ($n = 326$) to obtain biographical, experiential, socioeconomic, and attitudinal data, and to correlate this material with intent to work with the elderly. Chi-square analysis was used to demonstrate a statistically significant relationship between intent to work with the elderly and 15 items in the questionnaire.

References

1. Shott, S: Statistics for Health Professionals. WB Saunders, Philadelphia, 1990, p 149.
2. Ibid.
3. Stahl, SM and Hennes, JD: Reading and Understanding Applied Statistics. CV Mosby, St. Louis, 1980, p 285.
4. Robinson, PW: Fundamentals of Experimental Psychology, ed 2. Prentice-Hall, Englewood Cliffs, NJ, 1981, Chapter 11.
5. Shott, op cit, Chapter 9.
6. Goldstein, G: A Clinician's Guide to Research Design. Nelson-Hall, Chicago, 1980, p 74.
7. Schefler, WC: Statistics for Health Professionals. Addison-Wesley, Reading, MA, 1984, Chapter 16.
8. Daniel, WW: Applied Nonparametric Statistics. Houghton-Mifflin, Boston, 1978, p 200.
9. Daniel, op cit, p 211.
10. Goldstein, op cit, p 112.

11. Keppel, G: Design and Analysis: A Researcher's Handbook, ed 2. Prentice-Hall, Englewood Cliffs, NJ, 1982, p 539.
12. McCall, RB: Addendum. The use of multivariate procedures in developmental psychology. In Mussen, PH (ed): Carmichael's Manual of Child Psychology, Vol 1, ed 3. Wiley, New York, 1970, pp 1366–1377.
13. Zito, M and Bohannon, RW: Inferential statistics in physical therapy research: A recommended core. JPTEd. 4:13, 1990.
14. Newton, RA: Effects of vapocoolants on passive hip flexion in healthy subjects. Phys Ther 65:1034, 1985.
15. Lyons, M: Enabling or disabling? Students' attitudes toward persons with disabilities. AJOT 45:311, 1991.
16. Hackel, ME, et al: Changes in hand function in the aging adult as determined by the Jebsen Test of Hand Function. Phys Ther 72:373, 1992.
17. Mitchell, MJ, Daines, GE, and Thomas, BL: Effect of L-tryptophan and phenylalanine on buring pain threshold. Phys Ther 67:203, 1987.
18. Robichaud, JA, Agostinucci, J, and Linden, DWV: Effect of air-splint application on soleus muscle motoneuron reflex excitability in nondisabled subjects and subjects with cerebrovascular accidents. Phys Ther 72:176, 1992.
19. Lang EM, Nelson, DL, and Bush, MA: Comparison of performance in materials-based occupation, imagery-based occupation, and rote exercise in nursing home residents. AJOT 46:607, 1992.
20. Tse, SK and Bailey DM: T'ai Chi and postural control in the well elderly. AJOT 46:295, 1992.
21. Kuzala, EA and Vargo, MC: The relationship between elbow position and grip strength. AJOT 46:509, 1992.
22. Goldberg, J, Sullivan, SJ, and Seaborne DE: The effect of two intensities of massage on H-Reflex amplitude. Phys Ther 72:449, 1992.
23. Ruth, S and Kegerreis, S: Facilitating cervical flexion using a Feldenkrais method: Awareness through movement. JOSPT 16:25, 1992.
24. Gliner, JA and Davis, CG: The effects of movement speed and initial position on movement reproduction accuracy. OTJ of Res 4:181, 1984.
25. Delitto, A, et al: A study of discomfort with electrical stimulation. Phys Ther 72:410, 1992.
26. Goodisman, LD: A Manipulation-free design for single-subject cerebral palsy research. Phys Ther 62:284, 1982.
27. Krause, AW, et al: Effects of unilateral and bilateral auricular transcutaneous electrical nerve stimulation on cutaneous pain threshold. Phys Ther 67:507, 1987.
28. Kukulka, CG, et al: Effects of intermittent tendon pressure on alpha motoneuron excitability. Phys Ther 66:1091, 1986.
29. Barr, AE, et al: Biomechanical comparison of the energy-storing capabilities of SACH and carbon copy II prosthetic feet during the stance phase of gait in a person with below-knee amputation. Phys Ther 72:344, 1992.
30. Dickstein, R, et al: Stroke rehabilitation: Three exercise therapy approaches. Phys Ther 66:1233, 1986.
31. Delitto, A and Rose, SJ: Comparative comfort of three waveforms used in electrically eliciting quadriceps femoris muscle contractions. Phys Ther 66:1704, 1986.
32. Filiatrault, J, et al: Motor function and activities of daily living assessments: A study of three tests for persons with hemiplegia. AJOT 45:806, 1991.
33. Case-Smith, J: The effects of tactile defensiveness and tactile discriminiation on in-hand manipulation. AJOT 45:811, 1991.
34. Anacker, SL and DiFabio RP: Influence of sensory inputs on standing balance in community-dwelling elders with a recent history of falling. Phys Ther 72:575, 1992.

35. Spadone, RA: Internal-external control and temporal orientation among Southeast Asians and white Americans. AJOT 46:713, 1992.
36. Krebs, DE, et al: Trunk kinematics during locomotor activities. Phys Ther 72:505, 1992.
37. Morton, GG, Barnett, DW, and Hale, LS: A comparison of performance measures of an added-purpose task versus a single-purpose task for upper extremities. AJOT 46:128, 1992.
38. Cassady, SL and Nielsen, DH: Cardiorespiratory responses of healthy subjects to calisthenics performed on land versus in water. Phys Ther 72:532, 1992.
39. Liu, HI, Currier, DP, and Threlkeld AJ: Circulatory response of digital arteries associated with electrical stimulation of calf muscle in healthy subjects. Phys Ther 67:340, 1987.
40. Haskvitz, EM and Hanten, WP: Blood pressure response to inversion traction. Phys Ther 66:1361, 1986.
41. Cromwell, FS (ed): Computer Applications in Occupational Therapy. Haworth Press, New York, 1986.
42. Francis, K: Computer essentials in physical therapy. Slack, Thorofare, NJ, 1987.
43. Krebs, D: A review: SPSS PC+ (A statistical package). Phys Ther 66:1434, 1986.
44. Rozier, CK and Hamilton, B: Why students choose physical therapy as a career. JPTEd. 5:51, 1991.
45. Coren, A, et al: Factors related to physical therapy students' decisions to work with elderly patients. Phys Ther 67:60, 1987.

Additional Readings

Goldstein, G: A Clinician's Guide to Research Design. Nelson-Hall, Chicago, 1980, Chapter 7.
Norton, BJ and Strube, MJ: Guide for the Interpretation of One-Way Analysis of Variance. Phys Ther 65:1888, 1985.
Norton, BJ and Strube, MJ: Guide for the Interpretation of Two-Way Analysis of Variance. Phys Ther 66:402, 1986.
Polit, DF and Hungler, BP: Essentials of Nursing Research. JB Lippincott, Philadelphia, 1985, Chapter 17.

The Library as a Tool

The Library Search

The library serves several functions in the basic and continuing education of any professional. This chapter concerns the library as a research tool.

The purpose of reviewing the literature in a given field was mentioned in Chapter 1. The difference between primary and secondary sources was also discussed. Once you have identified your goal or established a research hypothesis, the review of related literature should answer two main questions: Has my research question already been answered? What have other people learned that will help me to answer my question? The latter may include research strategies and designs, procedures, and measurement tools and their results and conclusions. We can learn from the mistakes of others as well as from their successes.

Researchers should have at least a general goal in mind before beginning library search. A researcher who enters the library with only a general goal can read to get an overview of the entire area of interest. The library search will require three basic supplies: paper, pencils, and patience. It takes a long time to find, read, understand, and integrate information contained in the literature. Dempsey[1] has suggested that one should plan to spend 2 weeks in the library for a term paper in a semester course. Say, as an example, that you begin with the topic of human movement, or kinesiology. With an interest this large you would probably go to general textbooks on the subject in order to get a wide sampling of what is known in the area. Table 10–1 is an outline for reading in the subject of kinesiology; it gives an idea of the various directions that your research could explore. The student could spend considerable time getting just a superficial knowledge of what is known in each of the five major areas listed there. Usually the researcher has already completed this initial mastery of the subject matter long before approaching a specific research project. Such broad areas of interest are generally encompassed in an introductory course.

What about the two therapists from St. Hopeless Outpatient Clinic who were introduced in Chapter 1? Their original goal was improving joint mobility in patients with physical disabilities. They eventually decided to conduct a series of experiments with two specific goals in mind: to evaluate the accuracy of various tools for measuring joint mobility and to evaluate several therapeutic procedures for increasing joint mobility. They developed a series of questions that we have examined throughout this textbook.

Before they could carry out any of those research projects, they had to review the related literature. If these therapists started with the outline in Table 10–1, their first goal would come under item III, Biomechanics. They could then outline their reading in this area as shown in Table 10–2.

TABLE 10–1   **OUTLINE FOR READING IN THE BROAD AREA OF KINESIOLOGY**

Goal: to understand how people achieve purposeful movement
I. Structural and functional kinesiology
A. Gross anatomy
B. Functional anatomy
II. Exercise physiology
III. Biomechanics
IV. Developmental studies
A. Physiological
1. Motor
2. Sensory
B. Psychosocial
V. Psychological aspects of movement

TABLE 10–2 OUTLINE FOR READING IN BIOMECHANICS*

Biomechanics
A. Statistics
B. Dynamics
  1. Kinetics
  2. Kinematics
    a. Planes of movement
    b. Levers and axes
      1. Types
      2. Measurement
    c. Displacement
    d. Normal ranges

*Heading III from Table 10–1.

Much of this reading would still be at the secondary source (textbook) level of reading. Eventually, in order to address their first purpose of evaluating tools for measuring joint mobility, they will do some very specific reading about measurement. They would then be ready to read seriously in the primary sources to get an in-depth understanding of what has been done and what is known about the measurement of joint mobility. They have completed the first three steps in writing a research protocol.

As the researchers approach their task they should always keep their specific research questions in mind so that they do not get distracted by interesting, but irrelevant reading. What methodology and procedures did other workers in the same area use? The reading may suggest new ideas and techniques that had not originally occurred to them. What results did they obtain? How do those results relate to my topic and to my question? Findley[2] has suggested doing a *conceptual* review of literature. (Concepts were discussed briefly in Chapter 1 and will be discussed again in the next chapter.)

As researchers read, they take careful notes. Many use index cards for this purpose. At the top of the card the main topic covered by the card—from an outline such as those found in Tables 10–1 and 10–2—would be identified. Full bibliographic references should be written down clearly with attention to spelling and page numbers so that the researcher does not have to go back to the literature later when compiling the references. A full bibliographic reference includes the author's full name, the title of the article, the journal or book title, volume, page numbers, and year of publication. For books, the publisher, city of publication, and edition are necessary. Include the library call number in case you need to go back to the reference again later.

The researcher should then take careful notes of all information that is relevant to the research question, as well as anything that is related to the broader topic of joint mobility. At the bottom or on the back of the card it is helpful to make a few brief notes about how the article relates to your question and how you think you might be able to use the information in developing your research protocol.

Look over the hypotheses in Chapter 1. It is obvious that the therapists from St. Hopeless are going to need information about standard goniometry and electrogoniometry, since both measuring devices are involved in several of their hypotheses. The next question they must answer, then, is this: How can the relevant primary literature be located in that mass of material in the medical library?

Entry Points into the Literature

You step through the front door of the library and there they are: several floors, jam-packed with thousands of books and bound journals. Where do you begin? Perhaps with a guided tour of the facility to find out where major types of materials and services are located. After that, there are a number of reference resources, which are organized for the express purpose of assisting you in your review of the literature. But even with all of these aids, the beginning researcher should be reminded that one of the major requirements of effective library searching is patience. Be organized and take good notes to avoid the frustration of having to repeat the same search more than once.

The major entry points into a medical library are as follows:

Card catalogs, or their computerized equivalent

Index Medicus

Computer-assisted searches

Reference books

    Books in Print

    Annual reviews

    Journal indexes

    Excerpta Medica and other abstract compilations

Citation Index

    Current Contents

The librarian

Let us take a brief look at each one of these.

CARD CATALOGS

The card catalogs are the heart of the library and the most important single entry point into everything in the library's holdings. There is at least one card for every piece of literature in the library, including books, journals (but not individual journal articles), filmstrips, microfilm, microfiche, audio tapes, and videotapes. In most libraries there are three separate sets of cards, one for authors, one for subjects, and one for titles. In many libraries, the "card catalog" is now on computer, but the same three headings are usually found. Many hospital libraries still use cards. In the card catalog, each set of cards is arranged in alphabetical order; in the computer other arrangements may prevail. It is assumed that the reader is already familiar with the general layout of libraries and the card catalogs, so a great deal of time will not be spent on this. If readers are not familiar with the card catalogs and the call numbers [either the National Library of Medicine (NLM) System in a medical library, or the Library of Congress System or Dewey decimal system, found in most general libraries], they should ask for assistance from one of the librarians.

The subject heading catalogue is most useful in the early stages of a literature search. When you have identified an interesting title in the card catalog, go to the shelves to find that book. Look also at other books on the same shelf, and other books with the same general number. For example, *Brunnstrom's Clinical Kinesiology* has the NLM number QP301. Other books with the same number will be in the same general subject area and can often provide you with a whole shelf full of references. The references and bibliographies in the books you have located will alert you to other secondary sources and many primary sources upon which the textbook material is based. When you write down a reference which you find in a textbook such as Brunnstrom, it is helpful also to note where you found the reference (e.g., page number) in case you make some mistake in transcribing and need to go back to your source. If Brunnstrom refers to a textbook by Wells, you can go back to the author headings in the card catalog to find that book, assuming you have not already discovered it on the same shelf with Brunnstrom.

In order to illustrate some of the complexities of the card catalogs, the author searched for *Brunnstrom* in the subject card catalog. It was not under "kinesiology." In fact, there was no subject heading for kinesiology in the cards. It was not found under "anatomy" or "functional anatomy" either. *Brunnstrom* was finally found under the subject heading "movement." The computerized card catalog, however, was much more helpful. The Automated Library Information System (ALIS) in use in the author's medical library listed 33 books under the subject heading "kinesiology," including *Brunnstrom*. When searching in card catalogs, with the computer, or in references such as *Index Medicus,* you will find synonyms most helpful.

The MESH (Medical Subject Headings) list of *Index Medicus* provides a useful list of key words. The beginning researcher in a medical library will probably find that it would pay off in the long run to spend some time looking through the MESH book to see how information is categorized by the National Library of Medicine.

INDEX MEDICUS

Before the advent of MEDLARS, MEDLINE, and related electronic information retrieval systems, the *Index Medicus* was the major entry point into periodical medical literature (i.e., articles in journals). It has been estimated that 6000 to 7000 scientific articles are written each day, increasing the scientific and technical literature by over 13 percent each year.[3] It is still useful to start with the paper copy called *Index Medicus* because it is the source of the more sophisticated electronic sources. The *Index Medicus* is published on a monthly basis and bound into a multivolume set by years. The yearly edition lists all journals that are indexed in the *Index Medicus;* both *Physical Therapy* and the *American Journal of Occupational Therapy* are among the journals indexed. The January issue includes a list entitled Medical Subject Headings (MESH), which is published in a separate volume as well. These are the key phrases used in the electronic databases as well as the topic headings under which journal articles appear in the *Index Medicus.* In the early part of a search the reader may find it helpful to go to the list of medical subject headings to find the keys under which the topic may be found. There is an author index and a subject index in each yearly accumulation.

In looking for the literature on goniometry while preparing some of the examples and illustrations used in this text, the author discovered that the word "goniometry" is not in the list of medical subject headings. The words "test" and "measurements" are also not usable keys. After some searching around in the list of headings, the author found "physical examination." There were no subheadings under this title in MESH, but in the cumulative index for 1986 there were five subheadings: Economics, Methods, Psychology, Standards, and Veterinary. A sixth subheading, Instrumentation, was found in 1984 and 1985. Under each subheading articles are listed in alphabetical order according to the title of the journal in which they are published. "Goniometry" did not appear under any subheading of Physical Examination in *Index Medicus* for 1984, 1985, or 1986, although several titles, such as "Examination of the Knee," might have dealt with goniometry in the text. By way of contrast, in the cumulated index for 1976 under the topic heading Physical Examination, subheading Instrumentation, three articles are listed. (One of those articles was published in 1974, another in 1975, and the third in 1976; this points to the fact that articles don't always get into the *Index Medicus* the year they are published.) Two of these three articles are concerned with goniometry. One was published in the *Medical Journal of Zambia* and the other in *Plastic and Reconstructive Surgery.* Also in 1976, under Methods, 17 articles are listed. Five of those are in foreign languages (the language is specified). Of those 17 articles, one is clearly related to goniometry because the word "hydrogoniometer" appears in the title. Another article, "Measurement of Spinal Mobility: A Comparison of Three Methods," may deal with goniometry but you would have to check the original article to be sure. It seems probable that the people who do the indexing at NLM changed the way they do it between 1976 and 1987. The point is, a search pattern that works for you in a given year in *Index Medicus* may not work in other years. Also different journals come and go in the list of those indexed in *Index Medicus.*

Since "movement" was a minor key in the Townsend article cited in the section below under "Computer Searches," the author went to that listing in the *Index Medicus* for 1985; seven articles of potential interest were found. Those included a study about range of motion in the lower extremities published in the *Archives of P M & R,* an article on a method for measuring arm movements in *Ergonomics,* one on measurement of ankle movements in *Injury,* a study on increasing angle of passive straight leg raising in *Physical Therapy,* another in *Physical Therapy* on range of motion, and one on measurement of finger mobility written in Danish with an English abstract, published in 1984. The only listing under "movement" in the 1985 *Index* with the word "goniometry" in it was entitled, "Goniometric Reliability for a Child with Spastic Quadriplegia" published in *J Pediatr Orthop* in 1985. Four articles of potential interest were found under the Movement subheading in the 1986 *Index,* and three of possible interest under that heading in 1976. As the reader can see, articles of possible interest are published in a very wide variety of journals.

With the information found in *Index Medicus* serious searchers now have two choices. They can go through every year of the *Index Medicus,* beginning with the latest and working backward, and check under several headings. Or they can make a computer printout of everything listed under the headings Physical Examination: Instrumentation and Methods and Movement. Before initiating such a computer search, researchers would probably find a conference with the reference librarian very helpful.

COMPUTER-ASSISTED SEARCHES

The computer, like *Index Medicus* but unlike the card catalog, provides an entry point into recent literature that is not confined to a single library. It can often reduce the amount of time spent in library search by as much as one half. In order to use the computer in your search, you need two things: (1) a key word or a set of key words that will be recognized by the computer and (2) a reference librarian.

The major computer systems of most interest to readers of this book are MEDLARS or MEDLINE. MEDLARS is the older of the two systems and requires the assistance of a medical librarian. MEDLARS stands for Medical Literature Analysis and Retrieval System; this is maintained by the National Library of Medicine (NLM) and contains over 6 million references to journal articles and books published since 1965. All of the references in MEDLARS are filed under the key words used by the MESH system of *Index Medicus.* Therefore, in order to get into the computer database in MEDLARS you must know certain key phrases. MEDLARS is the electronic version of the *Index Medicus.* It is on-line, meaning that the computer is directly connected by telephone to the database in the source computer in the NLM in Bethesda, Maryland. The reference librarian can be of great assistance to you in learning to understand computer language and how to use the system.

There are several other computerized databases that might be of interest to some readers. The Education Resources Information Center (ERIC) is a database maintained by the U.S. Office of Education. *Psychological Abstracts* is maintained by the American Psychological Association, and SOCABS is the code name for the Sociological Abstract Service of the American Sociological Association. Each of these services has lists of key words needed to access the system.

In 1986 the NLM provided a new service, which you can access on your own personal computer at home or in the clinic. The new service is a software package called *GRATEFUL MED.*[4] With GRATEFUL MED, a modem (computer to telephone connector), and membership in your local telecommunications network (TELENET, TYMNET, or APTA-NET), you can do your own search just like MEDLINE, at less cost. Other databases are available through similar connections. For more information on these systems, see Chapter 7 in Francis and Chapter 8 in Lane and Chisholm.[5] Shearer, Wall, and Burnham[6] have provided an interesting example of how many databases may be used to search the literature on gait very broadly.

One of the latest advances in computer searching is called CD-ROM (compact disk, read only memory).[7] The MEDLINE database back to 1966 is on a compact disk (CD) and can be searched in a fashion similar to the computerized card catalog.[8,9] Several companies sell the sofware for MEDLINE on CD. Other CD databases include Excerpta Medica, Science Citation Index, Cumulative Index in Nursing and Allied Health Literature (CINAHL), PSYC literature, and ERIC. Each database has its own separate disk. In the author's library the MEDLINE disk is part of the Compact Cambridge package. This MEDLINE disk includes citations from *Index Medicus, the International Nursing Index,* and the *Index to Dental Literature.*

For example, the author used the CINAHL disk to search for references for Chapter 11 of this book. The searcher is allowed to search using MESH headings or by topic or author. A thesaurus, provided on the CD, will help in the search for key words. Key words can be linked with "and," "or," "and not," or "within": for example, "theory and process." After some searching I typed "theory construction" and was given 90 references. Each reference gave title, source, year of publication, major subject headings, minor subject headings, and—in most instances—an abstract. A copy of each interesting reference could be printed with the press of a button.

If you are interested in a topic such as goniometry, which does not appear in the MESH indexing key, you can "ask" the MEDLAR or MEDLINE computer to give you a printout of all articles that have that word in their title. This approach is ordinarily used when you do not know any other way of gaining access to the material. With the assistance of a reference librarian, the author asked MEDLINE to search on-line for articles with the word "goniometry" in the title. In 1978 that request, covering four years, resulted in a printout of four articles. In 1987 the same request, covering five years, resulted in 22 documents containing the word "goniometry" in their title and 49 documents containing "goniometry," "goniometric," or related words in the title. The computer printout looks something like this:

AU   Townsend, M.A., Izak, M. and Jackson, R.W.
TI   Total Motion Knee Goniometry
SO   J Biomech. 10:3:183–193, 1977
MJ   Knee
MN   Adult, Aged, Arthritis, Biomechanics, Gait, Human, Male, Movement

In 1992 the CD-ROM for 1987 through September 1992 showed the word "goniometry" in only four titles—two in 1987 and two in 1992.

The computer printout above may be translated as follows: the authors of the article are Townsend, Isak, and Jackson. The title of the article is *Total Motion Knee Goniometry.* It appeared in the *Journal of Biomechanics,* volume 10, number 3, pages 183–193, in 1977. MJ stands for major keys; this article's major MEDLAR listing is under "knee." The last line lists minor keys under which it is also listed; note that this particular article can be found by the computer under any of eight minor key words, but not under "goniometry," since that key word is not in MESH. This list of key words might give the researcher some cues as to other ways to approach the computer's database. Note the similarity to the "major subject headings, minor subject headings" information on the CD-ROM.

REFERENCE BOOKS

Other entry points into the literature, when you have only a general topic to search, are reference books. There are many useful reference books, and not all of them can be listed here. There are, however, a few important ones that are likely to be of interest to readers of this book.

Books in Print

Books in Print comprises three huge volumes; one for authors, one for subjects, one for titles. These list all of the books currently available from publishers in the United States. There is also a *British Books in Print.* These are most useful when you have a broad topic to search, if you only have the name of an author or the title of a book, or if you have discovered an author whose books you like and you want to know what else he or she has written. The subject guide of *Books in Print* has a section on kinesiology.

Annual Reviews

There is also a series of books published under the general title of *Annual Review of _____.* " Two examples are *Annual Review of Physiology* and *Annual Review of Psychology.* Typically each chapter in these reviews is written by a different expert, who reviews the latest information and thinking on a given topic and writes an integrated summary and update. Not every topic is covered every year. These review articles are also listed separately in the *Index Medicus.*

Journal Indexes

Many journals print an index in the December issue of the journal. Articles are usually indexed by both author and title, and sometimes also by general subject heading. Also, some journals—*Physical Therapy* and *American Journal of Occupational Therapy* among them—publish cumulative indexes every 5, 25, or 50 years. These indexes are helpful in obtaining the entire history of developments in a particular area. The *Cumulative Index to Nursing and Allied Health Literature,* published since 1956, is a resource for many topics (and is now available on CD-ROM, as well as in book format). The *Hospital Literature Index* is concerned with the literature in health care planning and administration.

Abstract Compilations

There are a number of journals or books that print nothing but abstracts of articles that appear in journals. An abstract includes a bibliographic reference and a brief summary of what the article had to say. Some important publications in this area are *Psychological Abstracts, Sociological Abstracts, Biological Abstracts, Dissertation Abstracts,* and *Excerpta Medica.* *Excerpta Medica* is especially useful since its several yearly volumes cover a variety of disciplines, including anatomy, pediatrics, neurology, geriatrics, internal medicine, and rehabilitation. Abstracts in *Excerpta Medica* are taken from journals published all over the world; they are not necessarily the same journals in *Index Medicus,* although there is a large overlap. *Excerpta Medica* publishes over 40 sections a year. Section 19 is "Rehabilitation and Physical Medicine." Each recent volume on rehabilitation is divided into 20 topics, and many topics have subsections of their own. These include sections on functional tests, physical therapy, occupational therapy, kinesiology, and activities of daily living. *Excerpta Medica* is now also on CD-ROM.

In looking for literature on goniometry the author went to *Excerpta Medica,* section 19, volume 20, 1977. Under subsection 6.0, "Functional Tests," there were three abstracts of articles dealing with goniometry by three different authors: Low, Bojd, and Owen. Abstract 1248 gave the following bibliographic reference.

AU Low, JL (Auckland)
TI The Reliability of Joint Measurement
SO Physiotherapy. 62:7:227–229, 1976

That article was then abstracted in two short paragraphs so that the reader would know whether or not he wanted to read the entire article. In the same volume there is also an author index and a cumulative subject index. Under the cumulative subject index there is a subject heading Goniometry. Listed here were the abstracts of Low and Bojd, found earlier in the main body of the volume, as well as two others. Both of the two new ones dealt primarily with knee evaluation and therefore had not been listed under functional tests. The author then found the subject heading Electrogoniometry, which included the article by Owen, found earlier under "Functional Tests," as well as three other articles that did not deal primarily with functional tests but made some mention of electrogoniometry. One of these latter three was an article that appeared in volume 30 of the *American Journal of Occupational Therapy.* In volumes 28 and 29 (1985 and 1986) of section 19, no references to goniometry were found under "Functional Tests"; however, four references were found by using the subject indexes in the back of the volumes. What is important here is that even with all the help of key words, topic headings, and subheadings, you still have to search. Also, the format may change from year to year. For example, in volume 34, 1991, of *Excerpta Medica*—now in section 3, "Diagnosis, Functional Tests & Evaluation"—four abstracts were given, none dealing with goniometry. However, in the subject index of the same volume there were six abstracts concerning goniometry, two of the knee and two concerning gait. *Excertpa Medica* has both a subject and an author index.

In *Excerpta Medica,* section 19, volume 13, 1970, the author found the subject heading index "Electrogoniometry," under which abstract 967 was listed. This article is old enough to be traced forward as well as backward and will be used to illustrate several points.

In the main body of the volume, abstract 967 gave the following reference:

AU Johnston, RC and GL Smidt
TI Measurement of Hip Joint Motion during Walking:
     Evaluation of an Electrogoniometric Method
SO   J Bone and Jt Surg (Boston) 51A:6:1083–1094, 1969

This is one of the references that will be used in Table 11–3 in the next chapter and also below to illustrate the uses of the *Citation Index*.

CITATION INDEX

The fifth resource listed earlier is the *Citation Index*. There are two branches of the *Citation Index:* the *Science Citation Index* and the *Social Science Citation Index*. The *Science Citation Index* is now also available on CD-ROM.

In book form, the *Science Citation Index* is published quarterly; cumulations are published yearly and every 5 years. It has four sections: the *Citation Index,* the *Source Index,* the *Permuterm Subject Index,* and the *Corporate Index* (the latter will not be dealt with in this text). These are most useful after you have found an article that is in some way important to your research question. Unfortunately, the *American Journal of Occupational Therapy* is not indexed by *Citation Index; Physical Therapy* has been added since 1978. However, it is still useful for articles found in other journals. Having found the reference in *Excerpta Medica* to the article by Johnston and Smidt, the author went to the 5-year cumulative index of *Science Citation Index* for the years 1970 through 1974. The original article has been published in 1969. In the *Citation Index* section the author found the article by Johnston and Smidt listed. Under it were 19 articles that *referred to* the Johnston article in their reviews of related literature or otherwise in their articles. So here are 19 authors who thought Johnston and Smidt were important enough to cite in their work, and these are 19 potentially important studies related to our study using the Elgon.

In the *Citation Index,* the seventh article that referred to the Johnston and Smidt study was:

J Bone Jt Surg A52:775, 1970, Kettelka

Following the citation to the article by Kettelka in the *Journal of Bone and Joint Surgery (JBJS),* the author went to the *Source Index* section of the *Science Citation Index* and looked up Kettelka in the cumulative 5-year index for 1970–1974. There was a long list of articles published by him during that 5-year period, including the 1970 article in the JBJS. In the 1970 article, Kettelka was senior author; the other authors were Johnson, et al. The full title of the article is "An Electrogoniometric Study of Knee Motion in Normal Gait." It was not until the author went to the bound volumes of the JBJS and found the article itself that he discovered that Kettelka is an abbreviated form for Kettelkamp.

The Johnston and Smidt article has 9 citations in the *Citation Index* cumulative section for 1975 to 1979, and 20 citations in the cumulation for 1980–1984. So that article continues to hold the interest of researchers in its area. Between 1970 and 1984 48 articles cited Johnston and Smidt. In 1990 there were four citations, and in 1991 only one. Many of those articles may be of interest to anyone who finds the work of Johnston and Smidt pertinent to their own study.

The third section of the *Science Citation Index* of interest to us is the *Permuterm Subject Index*. Looking in the 5-year cumulation from 1970 to 1974 under the subject heading "Electrogoniometric," there was only one article listed—the one by Kettelka. Continuing in the *Permuterm Subject Index,* under "goniometer," there were approximately 300 articles listed. Each one is identified with a key term; hence, for each article you have a pair of terms, such as goniometer-account, goniometer-device, goniometer-electronic, goniometer–x-ray, etc. There were also approximately 50 articles under the term "goniometers," another 100 under "goniometric" and 9 under "goniometry." There were about 12 articles listed under "goniophotography." In the 1980–1984 cumulation of the *Permuterm Subject Index* there were over 270 articles connecting some other word to "goniometer," 2 to "goniometers," 40 to "goniometric," and 44 to "goniometry."

Current Contents is published by the same company that issues *Science Citation Index*. It consists of three series: *Clinical Medicine, Life Sciences,* and *Physical, Chemical and Earth Sciences.* Each series is published weekly and consists of three major parts. The first section is a copy of the table of contents pages from almost 850 journals and multiauthored books. The second section is the word index, which lists in alphabetical order all of the key words contained in the titles of the articles listed in the table of contents section. The final major section of *Current Contents* is the author index for all articles appearing in the table of contents section. *Current Contents* is intended to be a quick means of access to the current literature; perhaps the most useful approaches are through journals of particular interest to you or through the word index. *Physical Therapy* is covered in the *Clinical Medicine* series. *Current Contents* is available in both paper and computer disk formats. *Reference Update* is a similar service provided on disk only.

THE LIBRARIAN

The last—but not least—general entry point into the literature is the librarian. The librarian is listed last only to suggest that researchers should make some attempt to solve their own problems before going to the librarian.

Guide to Library Search

Table 10–3 is a generalized guide to a library search for purposes of research. If you have only a general topic, there are a number of places to go to get into the literature: subject headings in the card catalog or MESH for the *Index Medicus* or MEDLARS; any one of several computer databases; various reference books; and the *Permuterm Subject Index* of the *Citation Index*. If you have the name of an author who has written in your area of interest, you can look under the various author listings. Finally, if you have a good primary source that is relevant to your research question, you can follow it in two directions: backward, by looking at the references cited by the author in his or her review of literature; and forward, through the *Citation Index* list of articles that mention it in *their* studies.

TABLE 10–3 **GUIDE TO A LIBRARY SEARCH**

If you have a topic:
    Card catalog, subject index
    Computer
        MEDLINE: CD-ROM or other source
        MEDLARS
        ERIC
        Psychological Abstracts
    Index Medicus
        Medical Subject Headings
    Reference books
        Books in Print, subject index
        Annual Reviews
        Journal indexes
        Abstracts, especially *Excerpta Medica,* subject index
    Citation Index
        Permuterm Subject Index
If you have a name (author):
    Card catalog, author index
    Computer, author entry
    Index Medicus, author index
    Reference books, author indexes
    Citation Index
        Citation index
        Source index
If you have a reference:
    Bibliography
    Citation Index

Review Questions

1 Return to review question 2 in Chapter 4 and answer it again using the new information you have acquired in this chapter.

2 Start with a general research goal in an area of interest. Use the library to do a superficial review, and make note of particularly helpful resources. Narrow the area down to a more specific research purpose, and read in that area. Finally, write a research hypothesis and do a thorough review of the relevant literature using the guide provided in Table 10-3.

References

1. Dempsey, PA and Dempsey, AD: The Research Process in Nursing. Jones and Bartlett, Boston, 1986, p 39.
2. Findley, TW: Research in physical medicine and rehabilitation II. The conceptual review of the literature or how to read more articles than you ever wanted to see in your entire life. Am J Phys Med Rehabil 68:97, 1989.
3. Fitzsimmons, J: Foreword, In Lane, ND and Chisholm, ME (eds): Information Technology. GK Hall, Boston, 1991.
4. Francis, K: Computer Essentials in Physical Therapy. Slack, Thorofare, NJ, 1987, pp 89–91.
5. Main, L: Personal computer software, In Lane, ND and Chisholm, ME (eds): Information Technology. GK Hall, Boston, 1991.
6. Shearer, BS, Wall, JC, and Burnham, JF: Anatomy of a literature search. Clin Manage 12:23, 1992.
7. Lane, ND: CD-ROM and multimedia publishing. In Lane, ND and Chisholm, ME (eds): Information Technology. GK Hall, Boston, 1991.
8. Lee, JM: Telecommunications applications. In Lane, ND and Chisholm, ME (eds): Information Technology. GK Hall, Boston, 1991, p 77.
9. Lane, ND, op cit, p 164.

Additional Readings

Beatty, WK: Searching the literature and computerized services in medicine: Guides and methods for the clinician. Ann of Internal Med 91:326, 1979.
Hauer, M: Books, Libraries and Research, ed 3. Kendall-Hunt, Dubuque, 1990.
Lane, ND and Chisholm, ME (eds): Information Technology. Design and Applications. GK Hall, Boston, 1991.
Lehmkuhl, D: Techniques for locating, filing and retrieving scientific information. Phys Ther 58:579, 1978.
Watters, C: Dictionary of Information Science and Technology. Academic Press, Boston, 1992.

White House Conference on Library and Information Services. Information 2000: Library and Information Services for the 21st Century. Government Printing Office, Washington, DC, 1991.

Williams, RM, Baker, LM, and Marshall, JG: Information Searching in Health Care. Slack, Thorofare, NJ, 1992.

The Role of Theory in Research

Theory

The central theme of this chapter is the concept of a theory. A **theory** is a set of interrelated principles (in this context often called "postulates" or "propositions") that are based on solid evidence. A theory organizes what is known about the subject and acts as a stimulus to research. Let us look at some of the essential characteristics of this definition of a theory.

First of all, it is a set of interrelated principles. You will recall from Chapter 1 that a principle is a statement of relationship between two or more concepts. If necessary, it might serve the reader to go back to Chapter 1 and review the definitions of concepts and principles, for they are the building stones of a theory.

The next essential ingredient in our definition is that its principles are based on solid evidence. This evidence has usually been reported in research studies and summarized in textbooks. This solid evidence is the body of facts possessed by a discipline or a profession, and it almost always includes the generally accepted interpretation of what those facts mean. Evidence is not hearsay. It is not opinion. It is the body of substantiated facts that are generally held to be true by respected professionals in a particular subject area.

The next critical ingredient in our definition is that it organizes what is known. Here the word "organizes" places an emphasis on the relationships and interrelationships among the facts, concepts, and principles of a subject.[1] A good theory should organize and encompass everything that is known about that particular subject. A good example of the organization of a theory is the periodic table of elements, which people generally study in chemistry. The periodic table organizes and summarizes the theory of chemical elements in tabular form and graphically illustrates the relationships between the various elements (concepts) in the theory. Other examples of theory are the atomic theory of matter, the wave theory of light, quantum theory, and social learning theory.

Most theories can be classified along at least two continuums. A theory may be anywhere along a continuum that is at one end partial, specific, or limited and at the other end global and general. The same theory may also be classified as qualitative or quantitative, depending on whether it is expressed mostly in words (e.g., social learning theory), or in mathematical symbols, (e.g., wave theory of light). An example of a large global theory is the germ theory of disease. The germ theory attempts to explain everything that is known about pathology in living organisms that is caused by other living organisms. However, it is not so global or all-encompassing that it attempts to explain everything that is known about all disease and dysfunction; it is applicable only to those disorders caused by living organisms. So aneurysmatic strokes, for example, are not covered by the germ theory of disease.

The last element in our definition of a theory is that it acts as a stimulus to research, which generates new principles. This element in the definition specifies that most important and most meaningful purpose of a theory. On the basis of the theory, predictive statements are made and then tested for accuracy. Ultimately, "the function of a theory, then, is to describe, explain or predict limited properties of reality."[2] In the language of Chapter 1, we might say that *if* the theory is correct, *then* certain things will happen. The if-then statement becomes a hypothesis (which, within the context of theory, is often called a deduction). We can then set up an experiment to test the hypothesis to see if we can produce the results that we predicted on the basis of the theory. Research either generates or tests theory. Fawcett and Downs[3] even contend that there are three types of theory—descriptive, explanatory (correlational), and predictive—corresponding to the three types of research. A progression can often be found through these three types of research as a theory grows, as mentioned in Chapter 1.

ESSENTIAL COMPONENTS OF A THEORY

There are three essential components to a theory when it is formally stated. Table 11–1 is an example of a very limited theory; it explains a very specific and restricted set of phenomena. Such limited theories are sometimes called "conceptual frameworks." The three components shown are definitions, postulates, and deductions. You have already met all three of these under other names.

Definitions

Within a formal statement of a theory, definitions represent concepts. Each concept is defined very precisely in language so concrete and technical that there is no question as to when and where it applies. The definition should use terms that are so clear, concrete, and precise that one could divide everything in the world into those things that are included in the definition and those that are not. A term often used for this kind of definition is *operational definition,* which was discussed in Chapter 2. Fawcett and Downs[36] distinguish between *constitutive definitions, operational definitions,* and *empirical indicators.* Pursuing the example given in Chapter 2, the dictionary definition of intelligence is the constitutive definition; it defines the concept with other concepts. The research definition is the operational definition, which defines intelligence in terms of observable, manipulatable data. The Stanford-Binet Test of Intelligence is the empirical indicator or measurement tool.

Postulates

The second essential element in a theory is a postulate (principle, proposition, generalization). Postulates state *demonstrated* relationships between the concepts defined. In order to qualify as even a partial theory, a statement must have some principles based on valid, generally accepted evidence. Table 11–1 is deficient in this area. It has improved, however,

TABLE 11-1 **LIMITED AND PARTIAL THEORY OF GONIOMETRY**

---

*Definitions**

1. *Goniometry:* Art, process, or science of measuring angles.[4] (A constitutive definition.)
2. *Goniometer:* An instrument for measuring angles.[5] (A constitutive definition.)
3. *Measurement:* Assignment of numerals to objects or events according to rules.[6]
4. *Protractor arthrometer:* Two rigid shafts intersecting at a union allowing movement at right angles to their longitudinal axis; a protractor is fixed to one of these shafts so that its center corresponds with this union; the other shaft can move independently of the protractor and acts as an indicator.[7] (An operational definition.)
5. *Axis of rotation:* An imaginary line, itself at rest, about which a rotating limb turns in a plane at right angles to the axis.[8,9]
6. *Joint center or fulcrum:* The axis about which a bony lever pivots.[10,11]
7. *Bony lever or limb segment:* A rigid bar (bone) that pivots about a fixed point.[12]
8. *Range of motion* (ROM): Quantitative measure of motion of bony levers at joint axis of rotation; measured in terms of that portion of an arc of motion which the moving limb segment describes on a hypothetical 360° circle.[13]
9. *Active ROM:* Measurement of joint range achieved by active contraction of the governing muscles.[14]
10. *Passive ROM:* Measurement of joint range achieved by the examiner when the governing muscles are relaxed.[15]
11. *Normal ROM:* A composite of normal ranges of joint mobility reported in the literature.[16,17]
12. *Planes of motion:* Sagittal, frontal, or transverse directions of movement from the anatomical position.[18,19]
13. *Joint mobility:* The ability to produce or allow a range of motion in diarthroidial articulations.[20]
14. *Accurate measurement:* Requires placing the shafts of the arthrometer over or parallel to the bony lever and in the same plane of motion, with the union of the shafts over the axis of motion, when the mesaurement is read.[21,22] (Based on experience.)
15. *Use of goniometry:* To measure and record active and passive ranges of motion in patients with actual or potential loss of joint mobility, in the evaluation of physical disability, in planning therapeutic interventions, and in evaluation therapy.[23,24] (Based on experience.)

Postulates†

1. Compensatory motion at joints may interfere with accurate recordings, particularly at shoulder, forearm, back, hip, and ankle.[25] (Based on experience.)
2. Repeated measurements under controlled conditions will fall within 4 angular degrees of each other 95 percent of the time, intrarater reliabilities being higher than interrater.[26] (Based on experimental data.)
3. Goniometric measurements of the knee are reliable and valid.[27] (Based on experimental data.)
4. Intratester and intertester goniometric measurements of knee and elbow in clinical settings are reliable using three common goniometers.[28] (Based on experimental data.)
5. Sources of error in goniometry of the elbow are alignment of goniometer arms, identification of bony reference landmarks, and force used at end of passive ROM.[29] (Based on experimental data.)
6. Standardized methods make elbow goniometry reliable and valid.[30] (Based on experimental data.)

TABLE 11-1 LIMITED AND PARTIAL THEORY OF GONIOMETRY *Continued*

Postulates† **Continued**

---

7. Intratester reliabilities are higher than intertester reliabilities.[31,32] (Based on experimental data.)
8. Three common goniometers are equally reliable in measuring finger joints.[33] (Based on experimental data.)
9. Intertester reliability is moderate and validity is low using four different instruments to measure lumbar spine and pelvic positions.[34] (Based on experimental data.)
10. Intratester reliability in shoulder goniometry is greater than intertester reliability.[35] (Based on experimental data.)

Deductions

---

1. If patients with reduced joint mobility demonstrate an increase in active ROM that is equal to or greater than 25 percent of their recorded loss, then they will concurrently demonstrate a significant increase in functional ability.
2. If a patient has a painful joint that demonstrates significantly less active than passive ROM, then 20 percent reduction in pain, as measured on the visual analog scale, will significantly increase active ROM.

---

*These definitions are not fully exhaustive. For example, joint, specific joints, pain, functional ability, physical disability, and therapeutic interventions are concepts that are assumed rather than defined.

†The postulates listed here are representative only. For a more detailed review of the literature on goniometry, see Miller.[17]

since the first edition of this book 14 years ago. Chapter 5 discussed what you can do if you have not reached the point where you can define even a limited theory in the area in which you are interested, that is, exploratory descriptive research.

Fawcett and Downs[37] define nonrelational propositions, which state the existence or level of existence of a concept, and relational propositions. **Nonrelational propositions** may state the existence of a relationship: its direction, shape, strength, symmetry. **Relational postulates** may define concurrent or sequential relationships, deterministic or probabilistic relationships, and sufficient or contingent relationships. Postulates may be ordered in hierarchial sequence from concrete to abstract.

Deductions

The last essential element in the formal statement of a theory is the deduction, which, for research purposes, is our old friend hypothesis. A deduction is a logical if-then inference derived from the principles. If proven, confirmed, and accepted by a significant proportion of the professional community, it becomes a new postulate or principle. A deduction may eventually become a principle on its own, or it may be combined with a number of proven hypotheses to form a new principle. Twain[38] notes that

> Construction of adequate theory is a profoundly difficult but essential task ensuring that each research project grows out of the previous one in logical, developmental progression. To the degree that theory is effectively utilized, both human service practice and the process of research are facilitated. (p. 27)

PROPERTIES OF A THEORY

Every theory has some generality in that it can be applied to more than one instance. Theories are about kinds or classes of phenomena rather than about unique or individual phenomena. A theory should be consistent in the sense that it does not contradict itself. And it should be complete; that is, its set of postulates should explain everything that the theory intends to explain, however global or limited that may be. A theory is useless if it is not testable. It should be as simple as is commensurate with the task of being complete; this latter statement is sometimes called the law of parsimony.

No theory is ever final. It merely represents the current state of knowledge about a given topic. As more facts become available, as more refined methods of experimentation and/or analysis and more refined observational techniques are developed, as more research is done, the theory changes and improves. New concepts relative to the topic may be incorporated into the definitions and new postulates and hypotheses formulated. Theory is not an affirmation; it is only a method of analysis. A theory may prove, with new data, to be a formulation of one's ignorance; it is to be used as long as it is helpful and then discarded. Its function is to organize the available evidence in the search for better evidence.

The Uses of Theory

Kurt Lewin, the famous psychological theorist, has said that there is nothing as practical as a good theory. Theory organizes what is known, explains past and current facts or events, predicts future events, and, through prediction, introduces the possibility of controlling future events. For example, a theory that successfully explains the causes of past and present heart attacks may predict ways to control (prevent) future heart attacks. "Theory connects practice and ideas."[39] Through theory we increase knowledge; it guides hypothesis generation and research.[40]

It cannot be emphasized too strongly that the major purpose of theory is to stimulate the search for new facts, concepts, and principles that will either substantiate the theory or alter it in ways that will make it more accurate, more effective, more predictive, or more comprehensive. "Theory-testing research seeks to develop evidence about hypotheses derived from a theory. Thus, deductive reasoning forms the basis for theory testing."[41] One of the essential characteristics of a profession is that it possesses a unique body of knowledge; the greater the organization of that body of knowledge into theoretical formulations, the higher the degree of professionalization. As noted earlier, one of the basic principles of this text is that research that grows out of theory is more likely to be useful and productive than research that grows out of trial and error or happenstance. This is not to deny unexpected benefits of serendipity or the use of intuition, although fruitful intuition quite frequently comes to those who are well grounded in theory. Through the development of theory, a hypothesis becomes substantiated to the point where it can be called a principle. In time the principle may be so widely accepted that it becomes a law.

In all professions, and most especially in new and developing professions such as physical and occupational therapy, there is a continuous and urgent need to substantiate and further solidify the principles upon which clinical practice is built. There is an equally pressing need to organize those principles so that they assist the clinician in developing new principles that will improve practice. In other words, there is an urgent need for occupational and physical therapists to make explicit the theories on which they are now operating and to develop those theories so that they can act as a stimulus to further development. Of particular importance in this context is the idea that important, researchable questions will be highlighted in the process of writing out the theories on which we operate, and in the process of operationally defining terms and organizing what is known into a theory format. By this process of theory building it will become much more obvious what information is missing, so that wasted effort can be avoided and high priority questions can be identified more quickly. Fawcett and Downs[42] have discussed a method for reading a research report, and outlining and detailing the theory contained therein, that is much like parsing a sentence in English grammar. Acton, Irvin, and Hopkins[43] have made a statement for nursing that is equally applicable to physical and occupational therapy. "To establish nursing as distinct and separate from other health care professions, we nurse scientists must identify and validate that body of knowledge that is uniquely ours. Essential to this task is the establishment of a solid theoretic base upon which to develop knowledge, conduct research, and guide practice."

One of the very useful functions of organizing and writing out what we know in theory form is that it helps us to see clearly what we really know, based on solid evidence (principles), and what we think we know (hypothesis). Dykes[44] has very forcefully called our attention to the problems created when we confuse hypothesis with knowledge (substantiated postulates). Dykes attributes much poor medical practice to this confusion.

Although there can be no scientific method without the hypothesis, a clear distinction must be made between a formulative, but untested hypothesis and a tested and accepted one. . . . Unfortunately, however, a report of a group of anecdotal cases sometimes assumes the appearance of a bona fide structured, scientific investigation. . . . Thus, through lack of critical thinking, engendered by lack of time, material that should at best generate no more than a weak hypothesis, unfortunately may soon be offered as proof of a causal relationship.

Dykes recognized that when pressed by the need to treat patients, one must often proceed on hypotheses that are untested or poorly supported. However, if one recognized clearly the status of the hypothesis on which one treats the patient, then the way is laid for the scientific testing and eventual validation or rejection of that hypothesis. What Dykes said for medicine is true for the therapies, but progress is being made.

"Unfounded, charismatic verbal rationale and dogma often are recited mistakenly as 'theory' by physical therapists," says Krebs.[45] Acton, Irvin, and Hopkins[46] have suggested 15 criteria for research testing of theory. Their criteria have been culled from a review of literature on theory and theory in nursing.

1 The purpose of the study is to examine the empirical validity of the constructs, concepts, assumptions, or relationships from the identified theoretic frame of reference.

2 The theoretic frame of reference must be explicitly described and summarized.

3 The constructs and concepts to be examined are theoretically defined.

4 An overview of previous studies that are based on the theoretic framework, or that clearly show the derivation of the concepts being tested, must be included in the review of the literature.

5 The research questions or hypotheses are logically derived from the definitions, assumptions, or propositions of the theoretic frame of reference.

6 The research questions or hypotheses are specific enough to put the theoretic frame of reference at risk for falsification.

7 The operational definitions are clearly derived from the theoretic frame of reference.

8 The design is congruent with the level of theory described in the theoretic frame of reference.

9 The instruments must be theoretically valid and reliable.

10 The theoretic frame of reference guides the sample selection.

11 The statistics used are the most robust possible.

12 The analysis of data must provide evidence for supporting, refuting, or modifying the theoretic framework.

13 The research report must include an interpretive analysis of the findings in relation to the theory being tested.

14 The significance of the theory for nursing is discussed in the report.

15 Ideally, the researcher makes recommendations for further research on the basis of the theoretic findings.

Kielhofner[47] has provided a very good example of a partial, limited theory of temporal adaptation with definitions, seven propositions, and suggestions for ways to develop clinically relevant deductions. Barris et al[48] did a predictive study using a model of human occupation as a theoretical framework. The theory distinguished normal subjects from those with psychological problems and accurately classified subjects with different psychiatric problems.

Models

Sometimes a theory may grow out of a more speculative working model. A **model** represents complex phenomena in a simpler way. Examples are the globe as a model of the earth, a road map, a table of organization for a hospital, or an architect's plans for a building; these are replica models. Sometimes a model is expressed as an analogy; for example, a molecule is like the universe. Sometimes hypothetical constructs become models; these are symbolic models. "Paradigm" is a current buzz word in many circles; it seems to be used interchangably with theory, model, or worldview. According to the dictionary, it means example or archetype, which seems closer to "model" than anything else.

A *hypothetical construct* is a verbal symbol for something that cannot be seen. Examples are intelligence, motivation, facilitation, inhibition, mechanical ability, physical therapy, or occupational therapy. None of these things can be seen. We infer their existence as causes behind specific behaviors that we observe. It is possible to see an occupational therapist, and it is possible to see a patient who is receiving something called occupational therapy, but you cannot see occupational therapy per se. Its existence is inferred from what we see, and therefore it is called a hypothetical construct; it is a concept constructed from a hypothesis regarding the causation of things seen. Occupational therapy is also a symbolic model for a group of related behaviors. The interested student may find other models in the literature. See "Additional Readings" at the end of this chapter. The word "model" has also been used synonymously with protocol, a description of steps to be taken. DeRosa and Porterfield[49] have described such a model for the treatment of low back pain. In their review of literature, DeRosa and Porterfield identified a number of issues in low back care.

In an attempt to organize our thoughts about a comprehensive physical therapy strategy to deal with this complex problem, we will address the following five topics: (1) the dilemma of diagnosis, (2) the information gained from the assessment, (3) a patient classification system, (4) the objectives of the treatment process, and (5) a proposed physical therapy intervention model that matches the objectives of treatment to the classification of the patient.

DeRosa and Porterfield then continue to review the literature under these five headings. From this they create five tables: a modified physical therapy diagnosis classification, patient classification of activity-related spinal disorders, objectives of treatment, approaches used to generate controlled forces, and treatment plan. These five tables constitute a protocol, or model, that can be used to guide the total management of patients with low back pain.

Rogers and Holm[50] reviewed the literature on the factors influencing the use or disuse of assistive technology devices (ATD). They found many commentaries but few scientific studies of the topic.

A model is proposed to guide empirical research aimed at identifying non-device users from the outset of treatment so that interventions to improve ATD use may be initiated or alternative interventions implemented. The variables comprising the model pertain to the patient, the patient's living environment, the therapist prescribing the device, and the device itself.

The editorial by Rothstein[51] on the use of models in research was commented on in Chapter 5. He cited two articles[52,53] in the same issue that reported on the use of a pressure-sensitive implant in the hip of a 73-year-old woman to "model" pain, range of motion, and other rehabilitation activities. The idea was that the information for this model might be used to govern rehabilitation activities of other patients with endoprostheses.

Taxonomy

The word "taxonomy" is derived from two Greek words, which translate as "the law of arrangement." One of the earliest and most famous taxonomies was that of Linnaeus. Blakiston's medical dictionary[54] defines taxonomy as "the science of the classification of organisms." However, the word has a more generic meaning as the science of classification of any set of related phenomena. In education there are two very famous taxonomies; Bloom[55] and Krathwohl[56] have developed taxonomies of educational objectives in the cognitive and affective domain, respectively. A lesser-known companion to these two is Harrow's[57] Taxonomy of the Psychomotor Domain. One of the major advantages of a taxonomy is that it gives one a quick overview of an entire field of study or area of interest in a way that elucidates the relationships between components of that field. For example, one can find a chart of the animal kingdom based on the Linnaean taxonomy that summarizes on one large page all of the known animals and their presumed anatomical and/or physiological relationship to one another. In a sense, a taxonomy is a special form of a model; like the table of elements, a taxonomy can provide the astute observer with clues that may lead to the discovery of important information.

From Basic to Applied Research

Hilgard and Bower[58] have provided a model for research in education that has implications for research in the therapies. The Hilgard-Bower model is shown in Table 11–2; it has been modified in Table 11–3 to make it relevant to clinical practice. Table 11–3 is proposed as a model that can be used in conjunction with the model of a theory proposed earlier in this chapter, the protocol guide in Appendix A, and the guide to library research provided in Table 10–3. These four models form a combination of tools that may be used to validate and expand clinical practice. They are certainly not the only tools available and, like any other tool, they should be used only when their use is productive.

The original model outlined by Hilgard and Bower listed three steps under basic science research and three steps under technological research and development in the field of education. Table 11–2 outlines the Hilgard-Bower model and gives one example of each step. A similar model was developed by Smidt.[59] His six steps were

- Fundamental
- Design and development

TABLE 11–2 **THE HILGARD-BOWERS RESEARCH MODEL**

Basic Science Research
    Step 1.   Not directly relevant to education (e.g., animal maze learning)
    Step 2.   Topic-relevant (e.g., concept learning)
    Step 3.   School-relevant (e.g., learning math concepts)
Technological Research and Development
    Step 4.   School laboratory research (e.g., studies using special settings and special teachers)
    Step 5.   Normal classroom "try-out" (e.g., step 4 repeated in normal setting)
    Step 6.   Adoption (e.g., write textbooks and train teachers to use step 4 process or materials)

TABLE 11–3   A GENERALIZED MODEL FOR RESEARCH IN OCCUPATIONAL AND PHYSICAL THERAPY

Basic

Step 1.   Microbiological Research
  A. Elasticity of tendon *in vivo*
  B. Movement time in manual dexterity
  C. Nonphysical affective stimulation in children ages 6 to 12
Step 2.   Biological Systems Research
  A. Mechanisms of diarthroidial articulation
  B. Eye-hand coordination in manual tasks
  C. Normal affect related to body image in children ages 6 to 12
Step 3.   Pathokinesiology
  A. Typical course of rheumatoid arthirits in the knee joint—histological and mechanical
  B. Measurement of manual dexterity in spasitc victims of cerebral palsy
  C. Body image in children ages 6 to 12 with congenital spasticity in comparison to children with acquired spasticity

Applied

Step 4.   Therapeutic Kinesiology
  A. Influence of active exercise on range of motion in rheumatoid knees
  B. Influence of rhythmic stabilization exercises for shoulder, elbow, and wrist on subsequent hand dexterity in patients with spastic cerebral palsy
  C. Influence of group socialization activities on body image of spastic children ages 6 to 12
Step 5.   Therapeutic Regimens
  A. Interactive effects of drugs, exercise, and heat modalities on function of rheumatoid knees
  B. Interactive effects of drugs, exercise, and vocational training on employment of spastic adults in light industry
  C. Interactive effects of group socialization activities, rational-emotive therapy, and ADL training on spastic children ages 6 to 12

- Evaluation and standardization on normals
- Evaluation and standardization on abnormals
- Clinical application
- Clinical implementation

Smidt's system is particularly well suited to the development and evaluation of clinical and research instruments and therapeutic modalities.

Table 11–3 is a model for research relevant to occupational and physical therapy. It was developed for this text using Hilgard and Smidt as guides. In the context of this model, kinesiology is defined as a study of human movement that encompasses all aspects of and influences on movement: biological, psychological, and social. The model has five steps. The first three are classified as basic research and the last two are classified as applied research. Under each step, three examples are given. In each instance, example A is in the physical-biological area, example B is in the psychomotor area, and example C is in the psychosocial area. These examples are not intended to be specific research hypotheses or even goals or purposes. They are general areas of interest. All five A examples are loosely interconnected, as are the B examples and C examples, but no clear-cut progression is intended through the five steps at any of the levels. It is, then, only a generalized model in need of further development.

Let us first examine the five basic steps, Step 1 is microbiological research. It is "micro" because it looks at only one small part of a larger phenomenon; it is "biological" in the sense that it refers to life, and in this case, to human life. Example A is at the tissue level, example B deals with only one small component of the concept of manual dexterity, and example C is looking for a general list of nonphysical things that stimulate affective responses in children.

Step 2 is biological systems research. Example A is concerned with the general mechanisms of all kinds of dyarthroidial articulations. Example B deals with one aspect of the complex required to perform a manual task. Example C is concerned with normal children and one affective attitude, that of body image.

In a sense, step 3 is at the same level as step 2 in that it is looking at biological systems. But step 3 is looking at biological systems in which pathology is present. In another sense, there is a sequence between steps 2 and 3 since the student usually finds it helpful to understand what is normal before trying to define the pathological. The examples follow the same sequence of biological, motor, and psychosocial.

Research done in steps 1 and 2 is frequently done by anatomists, physiologists, psychologists, and sociologists. Research at these two levels may be done by occupational and physical therapists with advanced training in the basic sciences. However, it could also be done by people with no knowledge or interest in these therapeutic professions.

Step 3 deals with subject matter of particular interest to therapists, and research at step 3 can and should be done in research laboratories staffed, at least in part, by physical and occupational therapists. In working out the details of many questions in this area, and in interpreting the data generated at step 3, the therapist would frequently call upon the expertise of basic scientists and medical specialists to contribute to the development of principles in pathokinesiology.

In steps 4 and 5 we have moved into the applied sphere—clinical therapeutics. The examples in step 4 deal with therapeutic elements in a laboratory setting. The kinds of questions that would be asked in step 4 tend to isolate one independent variable at a time and study its effects on selected measurements. Step 4 relates fairly closely to Hilgard's step 4: laboratory research using special settings and specially trained clinicians. Step 4 is designated as laboratory research because active exercise usually is not the only treatment for rheumatoid knees (example A), and rhythmic stabilization is usually not the only therapeutic technique used in training spastic victims of cerebral palsy (example B). The major purpose in step 4 is to isolate independent variables and to identify their specific effects. Research at this level is almost always the exclusive domain of therapists.

As Hilgard's step 5 was normal classroom research, so step 5 in this model is normal clinical research. It represents an attempt to define the cumulative effect of a total therapeutic regimen. If the health care team gives its best to patients with rheumatoid knees, a number of therapeutic modalities will most likely be applied under the supervision of physicians, nurses, physical therapists, and occupational therapists. These various aspects of treatment interact with one another. Drug therapy may enhance or inhibit the effectiveness of exercise procedures. Conversely, the effects of exercise may support or oppose the action of certain drugs. Our ultimate concern is the total welfare of the patient, and therefore the ultimate research questions must be the total net effect of the entire therapeutic complex on the life and well-being of one human being. That one individual is often studied as a member of a group of similar human beings, but the therapist should never lose sight of the most important question of all: What good are we doing *this* individual, and how are we doing it? Step 5 of our model looks at the therapeutic environment and asks questions about the net effect of that total environment on individuals or groups. Therapists can do this kind of research singly, as primary investigators with proper input from the other health professionals involved in the care of the patients, or as members of an interdisciplinary team of researchers.

Uses of the Research Model

This generalized model may serve several useful purposes. To the reader it may serve as a reminder to evaluate each bit of newly acquired information, and determine where it can best contribute to the overall understanding of the problem. Earlier in this text we discussed the danger of taking results from animal research and applying them clinically without researching the appropriateness of that application. Many clinicians have been unnecessarily disillusioned and disheartened by failing to see the necessary progression, and by assuming that an answer to a question at step 1 is equivalent to the answer to a question that should be asked at step 4 or 5 of the model in Table 11–3.

The second use of the model is to assist the student in organizing what he or she knows about a given topic and in developing a set of definitions, postulates, and hypotheses about a given topic. If the definitions and postulates are at step 1, are the hypotheses at step 2 or do they jump to step 5? For example, Tokizane[60] published a study in which, among other things, he studied the labyrinthine reflex and its influence on flexor and extensor muscle tone. His subjects were five adults with normal hearing and one adult who was deaf. He concluded that with the head in a specific position, stimulation of the labyrinthine reflex would facilitate extensor tone and decrease flexor tone in selected muscles throughout the body. On the basis of that information, would you put a brain-damaged child or adult in a head-down, inverted position to stimulate the extensor tone in their musculature? What about the influence of that position on other reflexes or its influence on systems other than the muscular? What is its influence on the cardiovascular system? What other neurological mechanisms may be stimulated or inhibited by this method of stimulating the labyrinthine reflex? All of those questions are still in steps 1 and 2, as was Tokizane's research.

What about the myriad of questions that need to be answered in step 3? What does the presence of various kinds of pathology do to influence the labyrinthine reflex and all of its neuromuscular connections? What are the specific therapeutic effects of the inverted position in different types of patients and in individual patients, and, finally, what are the interactive effects of the inverted position with other therapeutic procedures that may be applied to patients with cerebral palsy or hemiplegia? Bits and pieces of this information are just beginning to become available. See for example the article by Haskvitz,[61] reviewed in Chapter 9.

A third potential use of the model grows out of the second one. The model may suggest specific questions that need answering and a general approach to answering them. Suppose that a clinician learns of a new therapeutic modality and wants to answer some questions about its effectiveness on her patients. The question of interest is clearly at step 4 or 5. The model suggests that there are some more basic questions underlying the question of clinical interest. A search of the literature may provide some of these answers and information from the earlier stages can assist the clinician in refining the question in ways that will make her research project as useful as possible.

What has been said so far is not intended to imply that research *must* progress from step 1 through step 5. In some instances that may be the ideal progression, and it is certainly the most efficient approach for long-term studies. However, there are times when this progression is not feasible or even fruitful. Therapeutic procedures that have grown out of clinical experience and empirical trial and error may generate defendable hypotheses at the clinical level. People with a basic science interest and expertise may then take these clinically demonstrable facts, develop hypotheses that will explain the underlying mechanisms at steps 1, 2, and 3, and thus support the clinical practice in question. In an earlier chapter the example was given of the development of smallpox vaccine that was clinically effective before the microbiological basis of the disease and of the vaccine was discovered. The essential point here is that the model is not a magic formula; it is a tool to be used creatively in the search for more reliable knowledge.

A separate step—dissemination of information—was not included, in imitation of Hilgard's step 6, in Table 11–3 because it is a component of each of the five steps. Researchers have a clear obligation to report the results of their studies so that their professional colleagues can share the information and use it. Publishing results is thus a professional and educational obligation as much as it is a specific step in the research process.

Summary

The diligent reader should now have the basic tools for reading, understanding, and using the evidence provided by the professional literature. Like any other skill, from algebraic equations to piano playing, skill in reading and interpreting research comes with practice, and one can frequently learn as much from mistakes as from successes. Once some modicum of skill is developed in reading, interpreting, and applying other people's research, and in understanding how they arrived at their results, conclusions, and interpretations, the reader is then ready to embark, at some modest and meaningful level, on the high and rewarding adventure of making an original contribution to our understanding of useful therapeutic procedures.

Review Questions

1	What is a theory, and what are the essential components of a theory?
2	What is a conceptual framework?
3	How does theory aid research?
4	What is a model? How does it relate to theory?
5	What is a hypothetical construct? How does it relate to theory?
6	What is a taxonomy? How does it relate to theory.
7	Look at the article by Beattie in Appendix C.

    a   Define the key concepts in the article. If the necessary definitions are not in the article, go to a dictionary or to the literature.

    b   Find and/or define other concepts necessary for a partial theory of the effects of mobilization on low back pain.

    c   List the postulates (principles) supported by some evidence, as presented in the article.

    d   Write several alternate hypotheses based on the definitions and postulates derived above.

Final Review

As a final self-examination the reader is invited to undertake the following procedures:

1 Select a topic which you are interested in.

2 Do a review of the literature concerning what is known about that topic. Use the guide developed in Chapter 10 and analyze each reading critically, following the outline suggested in Appendix A.

3 Organize what you have learned in the form of a formal statement of the theory underlying the therapeutic procedure that you are studying. Use the model of a theory developed earlier in this chapter and illustrated in Table 11-2.

4 Spread out the information that you gathered in steps 2 and 3 using the research model developed in Table 11-3.

5 Identify several research questions that you believe to be important and useful.

6 Select the research question that you believe you are most capable of answering and most willing to devote time and energy to. Develop that question into a research protocol using the model provided in Appendix A. Select your dependent variable, using information provided in Chapter 3.

7 Execute the study. Remember, where there's a will, there's a way—and enjoy!

References

1. Kerlinger, FN: Foundations of Behavioral Research, ed 2. Holt, Rinehart & Winston, New York, 1973, p 9.
2. Fawcett, J and Downs, FS: The Relationship of Theory and Research. Appleton-Century-Crofts, Norwalk, CN, 1986, p 3.
3. Ibid, p 4.
4. Webster's Seventh New Collegiate Dictionary. O & C Merriam Co, Springfield, MA, 1963.
5. Webster's Ninth New Collegiate Dictionary. Merriam-Webster, Springfield, MA, 1985.
6. Stevens, SS: On the theory of scales of measurement. Science 103:2684:677, 1946.

7. Salter, N: Methods of measurement of muscle and joint function. J Bone Joint Surg 378:474, 1955.
8. Dyson, G: The Mechanics of Athletics, ed 4. University of London Press, London, 1967.
9. Moore, ML: The measurement of joint motion, Part 2: The technique of goniometry. Phys Ther 29:256, 1949.
10. Moore, op cit.
11. Kelly, DL: Kinesiology: Fundamentals of Motion Description. Prentice-Hall, Englewood Cliffs, NJ, 1971.
12. Ibid.
13. Poland, JL, Hobart, DJ, and Payton, OD: The Musculoskeletal System. Medical Examination Publishing Company, Flushing, New York, 1977.
14. Hurt, SP: Joint measurement. AJOT 1:209, 1947; 1:281, 1947; and 2:13, 1948.
15. Ibid.
16. American Academy of Orthopaedic Surgeons: Measuring and Recording Joint Motion. Author, Chicago, 1965.
17. Miller, PJ: Assessment of joint motion. In Rothstein, JM (ed): Measurement in Physical Therapy. Churchill-Livingstone, New York, 1985.
18. Kelly, op cit.
19. Poland, op cit.
20. Ibid.
21. Moore, op cit.
22. Hurt, op cit.
23. Salter, op cit.
24. Hurt, op cit.
25. Ibid.
26. Mayerson, NH and Milano, RA: Goniometric measurement reliability in physical medicine. Arch Phys Med Rehabil 65:92, 1984.
27. Gogia, PP, et al: Reliability and validity of goniometric measurements at the knee. Phys Ther 67:192, 1987.
28. Rothstein, JM, Miller PJ, and Roettger, RF: Goniometric reliability in a clinical setting: Elbow and knee measurements. Phys Ther 63:1611, 1983.
29. Fish, DR and Wingate, L: Sources of goniometric error at the elbow. Phys Ther 65:1666, 1985.
30. Ibid.
31. Hamilton, GF and Lachenbruch, PA: Reliability of goniometers in assessing finger joint angles. Phys Ther 49:465, 1969.
32. Boone, DC, et al: Reliability of goniometric measurements. Phys Ther 58:1355, 1978.
33. Ibid.
34. Burdett, RL, Brown, KE, and Fall, MP: Reliability and validity of four instruments for measuring lumbar spine and pelvic positions. Phys Ther 66:677, 1986.
35. Riddle, DL, Rothstein, JM, and Lamb, RL: Goniometric reliability in a clinical setting. Phys Ther 67:668, 1987.
36. Fawcett and Downs, op cit, pp 21–24.
37. Ibid. pp 24–32.
38. Twain, D: Developing and implementing a research strategy. In Struening, EL and Guttentag, M (eds): Handbook of Evaluation Research. Sage, Beverly Hills, CA, 1975.
39. Krebs, DE, et al: Theory in physical therapy. Phys Ther 66:661, 1986.
40. Oyster, CK, Hanten, WP, and Llorens, LA: Introduction to Research: A Guide for the Health Science Professional. Lippincott, Philadelphia, 1987, p 18.
41. Acton, GJ, Irvin, BL, and Hopkins, BA: Theory-testing research: Building the science. Adv Nurs Sci 14:52, 1991.
42. Fawcett and Downs, op cit, Chapter 2.

43. Acton, Irvin, and Hopkins, op cit, p 52.
44. Dykes, MHM: Uncritical thinking in medicine: The confusion between hypothesis and knowledge. JAMA 227:1275, 1974.
45. Krebs, DE, et al, op cit, p 682.
46. Acton, Irvin, and Hopkins, op cit, pp 56–59.
47. Kielhofner, G: Temporal adaptation: A conceptual framework for occupational therapy. AJOT 31:235, 1977.
48. Barris, R, et al: Occupational function and dysfunction in three groups of adolescents. OTJ of Res 6:301, 1986.
49. DeRosa, CP and Porterfield, JA: A physical therapy model for the treatment of low back pain. Phys Ther 72:261, 1992.
50. Rogers, JC and Holm, MB: Assistive technology device use in patients with rheumatic disease: A literature review. AJOT 46:120, 1992.
51. Rothstein, JM: Making models more attractive. Phys Ther 72:689, 1992.
52. Strickland, EM, et al: In vivo acetabular contact pressures during rehabilitation, Part 1: Acute phase. Phys Ther 72:691, 1992.
53. Givens-Heiss, DL, et al: In vivo acetabular contact pressures during rehabilitation, Part 2: Postacute phase. Phys Ther 72:700, 1992.
54. Hoerr, NL and Osol, A (eds): Blakiston's New Gould Medical Dictionary. McGraw-Hill, New York, 1956.
55. Bloom, BJ, et al (eds): Taxonomy of Educational Objectives. Handbook 1: Cognitive Domain. David McKay, New York, 1956.
56. Krathwohl, DR, et al: Taxonomy of Educational Objectives. Handbook 2: Affective Domain. David McKay, New York, 1964.
57. Harrow, AJ: A Taxonomy of the Psychomotor Domain. David McKay, New York, 1972.
58. Hilgard, ER and Bower, GH: Theories of Learning, ed 3. Appleton-Century-Crofts, New York, 1966.
59. Smidt, G: Research in Musculo-skeletal Disorders. Paper presented to the Section on Research, American Physical Therapy Association, Houston, Texas, June 27, 1973.
60. Tokizane, T, et al: Electromyographic studies on tonic neck, lumbar and labyrinthine reflexes in normal persons. Jpn J Physiol 2:130, 1951.
61. Haskvitz, EM and Hanten, WP: Blood pressure response to inversion traction. Phys Ther 66:1361, 1986.

Additional Readings

GENERAL

Fawcett, J: Approaches to knowledge development in nursing. Canadian J Nurs Res 23:23, 1991.
Nolan, M and Grant, G: Mid-range theory building and the nursing theory-practice gap: A respite care case study. J Adv Nursing 17:217, 1992.
Reynolds, PD: A Primer in Theory Construction. Macmillan, New York, 1971.
Roy, C and Roberts, SL: Theory Construction in Nursing: An Adaptation Model. Prentice-Hall, Englewood Cliffs, NJ, 1981, Chapter 1.
Walker, LO and Avant, KC: Strategies for Theory Construction in Nursing. Appleton-Century-Crofts, Norwalk, CN, 1983, Chapter 2.

PHILOSOPHY OF SCIENCE

Aronson, JL: A Realist Philosophy of Science. Macmillan, London, 1984.
Causey, RL: Unity of Science. D. Reidell, Boston, 1977.
Suppe, F (ed): The Structure of Scientific Theories, ed 2. University of Illinois Press, Chicago, 1977.

EXAMPLES

Adams, JA: A closed-loop theory of motor learning. J Motor Behav. 3:111, 1971.
Harris, FA: Inapproprioception: A possible sensory basis for athetoid movements. Phys Ther 51:761, 1971.
Heard, C: Occupational role acquisition: A perspective on the chronically disabled. AJOT 31:243, 1977.
Mosey, AC: An alternative: The biopsychosocial model. AJOT 28:137, 1974.

Outline for Writing a Research Protocol*

1 Long-range goal
2 Immediate purpose
3 Specific question(s) to be answered by this study
4 Research hypothesis (H_A)
5 Null hypothesis (H_0)
6 Operational definitions of critical terms
7 Assumptions and limitations of this study
8 Type of study
9 Population
10 Sample
    a   Pertinent selection criteria
    b   Methods of selection and assignment
11 Independent variable(s)
    a   Treatment schedule or control
12 Dependent variable(s)
13 Potential error variables and their controls
14 Research design (as applicable)
15 Level of measurement
16 Measurement tool
    a   What will the data consist of or look like?
17 Statistical tool(s)
18 Procedure (Where is data? How will it be obtained? How will it be used? etc.)
19 Results
20 Clinical value (interpretation)
21 Anticipated problems
22 Informed consent
23 Time table
24 Budget
25 References

*Also called a prospectus proposal.

Reconstructed Protocol for Article by Giannini and Protas in Appendix C*

1 Long-range goal: To improve the quality of life for children with juvenile rheumatoid arthritis (JRA).

2 Immediate purpose: To obtain quantitative information on cardiovascular response to exercise for children with JRA. (2)

3 Specific questions to be answered by this study:

- Is there a difference in heart rate (resting, submaximal, and peak); peak Vo_2; highest workload completed; and exercise duration between subjects with JRA and normal subjects matched for age, sex, and body surface area (BSA)? (3)

- Is there a relationship between peak Vo_2 and articular disease severity? (Abstract)

4 Research or alternate hypotheses (H_A):

- There will be a statistically significant difference between the JRA patients and their matched controls in that the JRA patients' heart rate would be of greater magnitude (resting, submaximal, and peak).

- There will be a statistically significant difference between the JRA patients and their matched controls in that the JRA patients' Vo_2 will be less.

- There will be a statistically significant difference between the JRA patients and their matched controls in that the JRA patients would demonstrate lower workload completed than the controls.

- There will be a statistically significant difference between the JRA patients and their matched controls in that the JRA patients would not be able to exercise as long as the controls.

- There will be a strong inverse correlation between peak Vo_2 and

*Numbers in parentheses refer to paragraphs in the article.

articular disease severity or number of joints with active arthritis. (derived from 3)

5   Null hypotheses (H_0):

- There will be no statistically significant difference between subjects with JRA and their controls matched for age, sex, and BSA on the variable of heart rate (resting, submaximal, and peak).
- There will be no statistically significant difference between subjects with JRA and their controls matched for age, sex, and BSA on the variable of peak Vo_2.
- There will be no statistically significant difference between subjects with JRA and their controls matched for age, sex, and BSA on the variable of highest workload completed.
- There will be no statistically significant difference between subjects with JRA and their controls matched for age, sex, and BSA on the variable of exercise duration.
- There will be no statistically significant correlation between peak Vo_2 and articular disease severity or number of joints with active arthritis in subjects with JRA and their controls matched for age, sex, and BSA. (derived from 3)

6   Operational definitions of critical terms:

JRA   Children between the ages of 7 and 17 who fulfill the 1977 revised American Rheumatism Association criteria for a diagnosis of JRA. (5)

BSA   Calculated from the Du Bois nomogram using a specified formula. (10)

Vo_2   The score obtained from using an open-circuit computerized gas analysis system according to manufacturers' instructions. (9)

Peak Vo_2   Defined as the highest rate of Vo_2 achieved in any 20-second period. (12)

Articular disease severity   Defined by the number of joints with active arthritis and the articular disease severity score obtained using the standardized methodology of the Pediatric Rheumatology Collaboration Study Group. (8)

Highest workload completed   Highest rate of work that was reached and maintained for the 2-minute duration of each stage of exercise; this score was obtained from a specified protocol using a Monark bicycle ergometer. (12, 9, 10, 11)

Exercise duration   After a brief training period, time from the beginning of the exercise test until voluntary exhaustion or until the child was no longer able to pedal at a constant rate. (10, 11)

Peak heart rate   Determined for the final minute of exercise of the highest workload, as monitored with a Narco Physiograph CMP-4A using a CM5 chest lead configuration. (12, 9)

Submaximal heart rate   Recorded at the end of the second stage of exercise. (12)

7   Assumptions and limitations of this study: Assume that each child did his or her best during ergometer testing, and that each child met the inclusive and exclusive criteria for admission to the study. (5, 6) A limitation is that the control group may not be representative of the general population. (25)

8   Type of study: Predictive. (18)

9   Population: Children between the ages of 7 and 17 with JRA. (5)

10   Sample: Thirty subjects with JRA who met inclusionary and exclusionary criteria and 30 control subjects matched for age, sex, and BSA who volunteered for the study. (5, 6)

   a   Pertinent selection criteria: Children with JRA as defined above who were not undergoing a change in their current medical therapy, had sufficient lower-extremity ROM to pedal a bicycle, had sufficient mouth-opening capability to use the mouthpiece, did not have bilateral knee pain on resisted extension, had not had lower-extremity surgery within 6 months and had no specific precautions for exercise. (5, 6)

   b   Methods of selection and assignment: Consecutive patients and their parents who were scheduled to be seen by the pediatric rheumatologist; met the criteria for diagnosis, age, and stable medical status; and volunteered for the study. Matched controls recruited through professional colleagues from the Texas Medical Center. (6)

11   Independent variable: JRA

   a   Treatment schedule or control: None; treatment was done in one sitting.

12   Dependent variables:

   a   Heart rate (resting, submaximal, and peak)
   b   Peak Vo_2
   c   Highest workload completed
   d   Exercise duration
   e   Articular disease severity (3)

13   Potential error variables and their controls:

   a   Intrasubject variability controlled by limiting measurement to a single testing day for any one subject (16)
   b   Intersubject variability controlled by matching control group for age, sex, and BSA, and by inclusionary and exclusionary criteria for JRA subjects (5, 6)
   c   Instrument variability controlled by reliability testing based both on literature and on-site testing (13 through 17)

    d   Data error controlled through calibration of data collection instruments and through a specific exercise protocol (8, 9, 10, 11)

14 Research design (as applicable): Two related samples, matched pairs. (5) Samples of convenience were assumed to be independent. Each dependent variable was analyzed separately, as if they had done six separate studies. (18, 19)

15 Level of measurement: Metric for peak Vo_2, exercise duration, heart rate, and number of joints with active arthritis; ordinal for the highest workload completed and the severity score. (18, 19)

16 Measurements tools: A count of the number of joints with active arthritis; the articular disease severity score; a Sensormedics open-circuit gas analysis system; a Monark bicycle ergometer; a Narco Physiograph; and a stop watch. (8 through 12) Data consist of a frequency count, numerical scores (ordinal and metric) on the tests, and time.

17 Statistical tools: Paired t-tests, Wilcoxon matched-pairs, signed-rank test, Pearson's Product Moment Correlation, and Spearman Rank Order Correlation Coefficient. (18, 19) ANOVA and ICC are also mentioned as part of the reliability testing. (17)

18 Procedure: Where is data? How will it be obtained? How will it be used? etc. (8, 10, 11, 12)

19 Results:

- Null hypothesis 1 was rejected for peak and submaximal heart rates but not for resting heart rate. (21)
- Null hypothesis 2 was rejected and alternate 2 was accepted. (22)
- Null hypothesis 3 was not clearly treated in the text. (24 and Figure 2); one might say that the results are equivocal with a trend in favor of the control group.
- Null hypothesis 4 was rejected and alternate 4 was accepted. (Table 6 and paragraph 22)
- Null hypothesis 5 was not rejected. (23)

20 Clinical value (interpretation): Paragraphs 26 and 35 concerning the prevention of deconditioning in JRA children.

21 Anticipated problems: None listed. Some problems noted at the end are discussed in 34.

22 Informed consent: Inferred at the end of paragraph 6.

23 Time table: Not stated. It may have taken several months to find all 60 subjects.

24 Budget: Not stated. Probably slight because their laboratory may have already contained all necessary equipment. This is supported by the statement that this was part of a larger study. (4)

25 References: Most are in paragraphs 1, 13 through 17, and the discussion.

APPENDIX C

Reprints of Seven Articles Discussed in the Text

Occupational Therapists in Private Practice

LINDA McCLAIN, JULIE McKINNEY,
and JULIE RALSTON

Key Words • career choice • motivation • risk-taking

Although increasing numbers of occupational therapists are choosing to work in private practice, little data exist describing this sector of the profession. In the present study, experienced occupational therapists were asked about their moves into private practice, including (a) their motivation, (b) their preparation, and (c) their perceptions of the move's risks and benefits before and after the move.

A survey was sent to a national random sample of 105 occupational therapists, 74 of whom responded. According to the survey, autonomy was the most important motivating factor for occupational therapists moving into private practice. However, once they were in private practice, the occupational therapists noted that increased income was a major benefit. These occupational therapists had planned for the risks of reimbursement, referral sources, and overhead but had not anticipated problems with staffing shortages.

Incomes increased for occupational therapists who moved into private practice. The survey compared the incomes of occupational therapists before and after they

Linda McClain, PhD, OTR, FAOTA, is Associate Professor and Graduate Program Director of Occupational Therapy Education, University of Kansas Medical Center, 3901 Rainbow Boulevard, Kansas City, Kansas 66160–7602.

Julie McKinney is a Staff Occupational Therapist, Dwight D. Eisenhower Department of Veterans Affairs Medical Center, Leavenworth, Kansas. At the time of this study, she was a senior occupational therapy student, University of Kansas Medical Center, Kansas City, Kansas.

Julie Ralston is a Staff Therapist, Healthtech Rehabilitation Inc., Warrensburg, Missouri. At the time of this study, she was a senior occupational therapy student, University of Kansas Medical Center, Kansas City, Kansas.

This article was accepted for publication February 27, 1992.

245

entered private practice. It also compared their income and educational levels. Other comparisons included income and work experience, income and work role, and income and geographic location.

Autonomy and financial considerations appear to be the overriding issues for occupational therapists choosing careers in private practive. Almost unanimously, the survey respondents said that private practice was a good career choice.

1 Reimbursement, referrals, overhead, quality control, parking, Medicare certification, liability insurance, medical insurance, tax structures, and small business loans are but a few of the concerns of the occupational therapist considering a move into private practice. With so many potential headaches, what can account for the mass exodus of occupational therapists from traditional work settings into private practice?

Literature Review

2 The private practitioner contracts to provide services for a fee through a small business that provides specific services. An individual practice consists of a single occupational therapist providing contracted services, whereas a partnership has two or more co-owners. An associate private practice typically has one therapist, who serves as director and employer for other professional and technical staff members of the same professional group (Punwar, 1988). The private practitioner may or may not be self-employed; a private practice may include both owners and employees. This paper presents a brief history of the private practice movement as well as current opinion and data relating to professional autonomy, ethics, and the financial implications of private practice.

3 The growth of private practice and consultation began in the 1960s, bringing with it an expansion of community services. This growth was fostered by legislation, economic issues, personnel shortages, and technology (Epstein, 1985). In 1973, 7.3% of American occupational therapists were in private practice (Hershman, 1984). That number had grown to 14.4% by 1978 and 18.3% by 1982. By 1990, 26.4% of registered occupational therapists were self-employed (I. Silvergleit, personal communication, April 3, 1991).

4 The expansion of private practice is not dominated by one practice area. Occupational therapists have written about private practice in

the areas of workers' compensation and personal injury (Shriver, 1985), pediatric programming (Hinojosa, Anderson, & Strauch, 1988; Shuer & Weinger, 1985), hand rehabilitation (Hershman, 1984), upper extremity rehabilitation (Tiernan, 1991), and skilled nursing facilities (Faust & Meaker, 1991). Usero (1991) described herself as a traveling consultant; in her unique practice, she actually moves from setting to setting assessing departmental operations, systems, and programs and making recommendations for improvement.

5 It is unlikely that the trend toward private practice will slow. Bruhn's (1991) projections for the 21st century included the prediction that more occupational therapists will become self-employed and begin to market themselves. Bruhn stated that, as this occurs, payment for services in agencies and institutional settings will become more acute, and institutions will use more and more contract service providers. Bruhn also predicted that in the future more occupational therapists will be consultants, private practitioners, and case or care managers.

6 According to Howard (1991), it is not theory or research that is driving these changes in service provision, but rather societal influences. She cited health care reimbursement as the key issue affecting the definition of occupational therapy, its practice, management, and ethics. Howard also stated that individualism and private enterprise are valued in our society, and she challenged occupational therapists to become active in health care policy.

7 Many occupational therapists want to establish their own pay schedules, make their own hours, and use their creativity and imagination in their own programs (Saltz, 1990). According to Epstein (1985), being in business for oneself can be exciting and rewarding, but it requires a major commitment of time, energy, and money.

8 Not all occupational therapists agree that the proliferation of private practice is a positive trend for the profession. Crabtree (1991) stated that referrals for profit limit free and fair competition among therapy companies and create an ethical dilemma for private practitioners. According to Crabtree, both the consumer and the occupational therapist suffer serious losses in autonomy as a result of behind-the-scenes referrals for profit. To illustrate his point, he presented the following examples of potential conflicts of interest: (a) A group of allied health professionals has a financial interest in a nursing home corporation that contracts with a private rehabilitation practice that it also owns; (b) an occupational therapist provides contract services to an acute care hospital and recommends to patients a long-term care facility where he or she also works on a contract basis; and (c) a hospital owns a skilled nursing facility where it refers patients at discharge. Crabtree noted that, in the third scenario, the possibility existed that

patients with Medicare would be referred to the hospital-owned facility, but those patients with poor insurance coverage would be referred elsewhere. According to Crabtree, the reciprocal nature of referral for profit makes fair competition among occupational therapists difficult if not impossible, because both the therapist and the physician stand to gain from the constant flow of patients that occurs in some private settings.

9 Occupational therapists in private practice are faced not only with new ethical decisions, but also with new legal ones. Steich (1991) stated that private practitioners need an attorney to advise them on applicable laws and help them avoid liability in the areas of business organization, contracts, accounts receivable and collections, employee relations, employee benefits, insurance, and taxes. An attorney can also provide needed advice on third-party reimbursement, fraud, and abuse as well as on licensure, confidentiality, and Medicare. Steich also described sole proprietorships, partnerships, and corporations, which are the three basic types of business organizations, and listed the advantages and disadvantages of each.

10 Although the literature encompasses many opinions and positions on private practice, little research has been reported on the subject. In a survey of Canadian occupational therapists, 54% said a desire for autonomy was their primary reason for going into private practice (Bridle & Hawkes, 1990). They cited the limitations of institution-based practice as their second reason for entering private practice and the potential for higher income as their third reason.

11 In the last quarter century, the movement toward private practice has spread to a number of practice areas. This movement appears to be spawned by motives of autonomy and financial reward, and it brings with it new questions of ethics and legal needs. Grady (1991) discussed professional change in terms of being prepared for it. She stated that the process of change must be considered as important as the change itself for it to be successful.

12 In the present study, we asked experienced American occupational therapists what motivated them to enter private practice and what they did to prepare themselves for the move. We also asked them for their perceptions of the risks and benefits of private practice, both before and after their move.

Method

SUBJECTS

13 A random sample of 105 occupational therapists was generated from the pool of registered occupational therapists who indicated that they

were in private practice in the American Occupational Therapy Association's (AOTA) *1986 Member Data Survey* (AOTA, 1987). The 105 surveys were coded, but the subjects were assured confidentiality. Seventy-four (70%) of the surveys were returned. Of those who responded, 70 were female and 4 were male. The ages ranged from 27 years to 72 years, with a mean of 38 years. Based on the geographic configuration in the *Statistical Abstracts of the United States, 1988* (U.S. Department of Commerce, 1987), 22 (29%) of the respondents lived in the Midwest, 19 (25%) lived in the West, 18 (24%) lived in the South, 14 (19%) lived in the Northeast, and 1 (2%) lived in Puerto Rico.

14 The highest degree held by 45 (61%) of the subjects was a bachelor's degree; the other 29 (39%) held master's degrees. Sixty percent of the occupational therapists in the present study described themselves as co-owners or owners of their practices. Not all of the respondents answered every question, so the total number responding varies slightly across questions.

INSTRUMENT

15 A two-page survey was developed, pilot-tested on a convenience sample of therapists in private practice ($N = 6$), and revised prior to its use in the present study. The survey was designed to provide demographic information as well as information on the motivating factors and preparation of private practitioners. The survey asked the occupational therapists for their pre-move perceptions of the risks and benefits of private practice and whether those perceptions changed once they became private practitioners. The data were analyzed with descriptive statistics.

Results

16 Before entering private practice, 39% of the survey respondents worked in general hospitals, 25% worked in rehabilitation hospitals, and 14% worked in school systems. The remaining 22% listed more than one setting. At the time of the study, 25% of the respondents worked in a hand clinic setting, 25% worked in a pediatric setting, and 25% worked in a home health setting. The remainder listed more than one current setting. The respondents' work experience in occupational therapy, prior to private practice, ranged from less than a year to 23 years with a mean of 7 years.

FULL-TIME VERSUS PART-TIME

17   Eighty-two percent of the respondents reported that they had worked full-time before their move to private practice, but only 54% reported working full-time after the move. Eleven percent worked more than half-time (but not full-time) before their move into private practice, compared with 36% after the move. Seven percent worked less than half-time before entering private practice; 10% did so after their move.

PREPARATION

18   When asked to rank the three most beneficial methods of preparation for a move into private practice, 67% of the respondents listed work experience as the most beneficial. The ability to obtain information from others in private practice was listed as the second most beneficial method, and the opportunity to observe others in private practice was listed as the third most beneficial method. Formal training (e.g., workshops, texts, and courses) was mentioned less often.

BENEFITS

19   Survey respondents were asked to list the three most important motivating factors or potential benefits that influenced their decisions to enter private practice. The most common answers to this question related to autonomy. In order of importance, respondents ranked flexible hours first, being their own boss second, and independence in clinical decisions third. Once in private practice, their perceptions changed little. Flexible hours and being their own boss was still ranked first and second; however, the potential of an increased income was ranked third.

RISKS

20   The subjects were also asked to rank the three potential risks they had perceived as greatest before their moves to private practice and the risks they perceived as greatest now that they were private practitioners. Respondents ranked reimbursement as the highest perceived risk and referral sources as the second highest risk both before and after the move into private practice. Respondents considered overhead (e.g., rent and equipment) to be the third highest risk before they moved to private practice; however, after the move, they considered problems with staffing shortages the third highest risk.

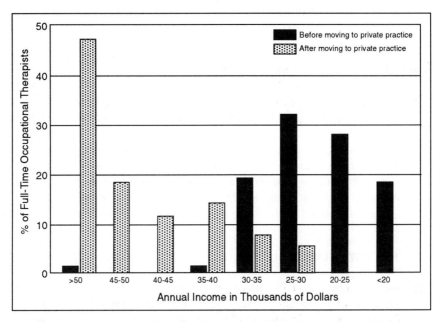

FIGURE 1   Incomes of full-time occupational therapists before and after becoming private practitioners.

INCOME

21   The present study indicates that occupational therapists who move to private practice experience dramatic salary changes (see Figure 1). For example, only 4% of the survey's respondents made $35,000 or more before they moved to private practice; 87% earned this income after they moved to private practice. Several different comparisons were made relative to income.

INCOME AND EDUCATION

22   We looked at the occupational therapist's income in relation to his or her level of education. Of the full-time private practitioners with bachelor's degrees, 50% had annual incomes above $50,000, and another 17% had incomes between $45,000 and $50,000. Of the full-time occupational therapists with master's degrees, 43% had annual incomes above $50,000, and another 4% had incomes between $45,000 to $50,000.

23   Of those occupational therapists with bachelor's degrees who worked part-time but more than half-time, 20% made more than $50,000 a year. Of those occupational therapists with master's degrees who worked part-time but greater than half-time, 11% made more than $50,000 a year. It appears a master's degree is not a financial advantage in private practice.

INCOME AND WORK EXPERIENCE

24 The number of years of work experience (combining both prior work and work within private practice) does relate to income. More than $50,000 a year was earned by 67% of those with 11 to 15 years of work experience, 62% of those with 6 to 10 years of work experience, and 35% of those with 0 to 5 years of work experience. Respondents who earned $45,000 to $50,000 a year included 17% of those with 11 to 15 years of work experience, 20% of those with 6 to 10 years of work experience, and 11% of those with 0 to 5 years of work experience.

INCOME AND WORK ROLE

25 We also compared the incomes of owners and co-owners with the incomes of occupational therapists who had employee status (see Figure 2). Sixty-one percent of the owners and co-owners who worked full-time had incomes above $50,000 a year, compared with 25% of

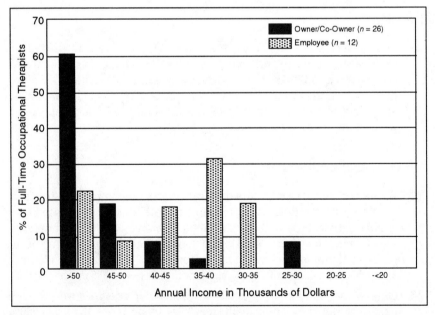

FIGURE 2   Incomes of full-time occupational therapists in private practice by owner or employee status.

the occupational therapists who worked full-time as employees. Figure 2 also shows that 19% of the owners and co-owners who worked full-time were in the $45,000 to $50,000 income category, compared with 8% of the full-time employees. More employees than owners and co-owners were at the lower ends of the income scale.

26 A similar comparison was made for those who worked part-time but more than half-time, and similar trends emerged. Of these owners and co-owners, 30% made more than $50,000 annually, compared with 15% of the employees. Another 15% of the part-time owners and co-owners were in the next income category of $45,000 to $50,000, compared with 10% of the part-time employees. Of the part-time employees, 40% earned $30,000 to $35,000.

INCOME AND GEOGRAPHIC LOCATION

27 Figure 3 shows a comparison of salaries by geographic location for full-time private practitioners. The highest incomes were reported in the Northeast, followed by the South. The Midwest and the West reported lower incomes.

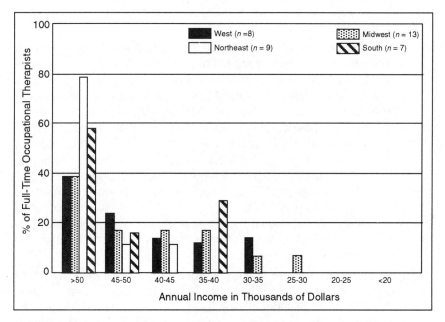

FIGURE 3   Incomes of full-time occupational therapists in private practice by geographic region.

**OPINION REGARDING THE MOVE INTO
PRIVATE PRACTICE**

28　The survey asked the occupational therapists to respond to the statement, "The move into private practice has been a good career choice
for me," using one of the following ordinal answers: (a) strongly agree,
(b) agree, (c) neutral, (d) disagree, or (e) strongly disagree. Responses
were as follows: 68% strongly agreed, 28% agreed, 3% were neutral,
0 disagreed, and 1% strongly disagreed. Survey participants were asked
in an open-ended question what the overriding variable was in their
decision to move to private practice. Among those who strongly agreed
or agreed that their decision to move to private practice was a good
one, the most common answers in order of prevalence were flexibility
of hours, personal satisfaction, independence with decisions, an
increased income, the opportunity to specialize, and more control for
quality care.

Discussion

29　The 70% response rate to the present study is good; however, the
sample size is small, given that one-quarter of the profession (10,000
members) is in private practice. Replication of this study with a large
sample size is needed.

30　A number of trends are noted. Those who moved from traditional work
settings to private practice tended to move from full-time to part-time
work. Those who responded to this survey appeared to have been
prepared for the move, they used their work history and observation
of others as preparation. However, this may not reflect the current
trend. The occupational therapists in the present study's sample were
selected from the *1986 Member Data Survey* (AOTA, 1987) and had
already been in private practice for several years. Recently developed
educational resources such as *Private Practice: Strategies for Success*
(Hertfelder & Crispen, 1990) and workshops on the local and national
level were not available in the early 1980s. It would be interesting to
learn whether occupational therapists who are currently entering private practice are using more formal avenues of training to prepare for
their moves.

31　It is interesting to note that the perceived risks and benefits before
and after the move into private practice were similar. These occupational therapists had done their homework and were ready for the
benefits of flexible hours and autonomy as well as the risks of reimbursement and referral sources. It appears the therapists were less

prepared for the salary increases and the problems with staffing shortages they experienced once in private practice. Staffing shortages have spiraled nationally in the last few years, becoming a worry not only to those in private practice but also to employers in medical, educational, and community arenas.

32   Although the salary increases may seem graphic, two basic limitations must be considered when interpreting the data. First, the pre-private practice salaries that the respondents reported were an average of 6 years old. Additionally, the study did not take into account the cost-of-living and potential merit raises the occupational therapists may have received if they had stayed in traditional work settings. It did not account for general inflation either. Therefore, it may be assumed that a portion of the gain is due to a general rise in salaries across years. Second, this survey did not address issues of management costs and benefits as a separate salary issue. Questions were simplified to consider only income. We assume the respondents reported accurate information; however, it is possible that the respondents did not calculate the loss of such benefits as health insurance and malpractice insurance into their differential incomes (before and after the move). In this regard, the survey provides a simplistic analysis.

33   Having a master's degree does not appear to be a financial benefit to the private practitioner, but having substantial work experience does. Those who worked in what might be considered the high-risk categories of owner and co-owner actually made higher salaries than employees of an associate practice. This was true for both full-time and part-time workers. Incomes did vary somewhat by geographic location. Although incomes in the Northeast were highest, when the cost of living is taken into account, those in the South may actually see the largest financial gain by moving to private practice.

34   The high degree of satisfaction reported with the move to private practice is encouraging. These results are tempered by the possibility that some of the 31 occupational therapists who chose not to return the survey may have done so because they were not happy with their career choices and had returned to their original practices. It would be interesting to see if similar findings would emerge in terms of motivating factors, preparation, and perceived risks and benefits from a survey of those who have made a more recent move into private practice.

References

American Occupational Therapy Association. (1987). *1986 member data survey.* Rockville, MD: Author.

Bridle, M, & Hawkes, B (1990). A survey of Canadian occupational therapy private practice, *Canadian Journal of Occupational Therapy 57*, 160–166.

Bruhn, JG (1991). Occupational therapy in the 21st century: An outsider's view. *American Journal of Occupational Therapy, 45*, 775–780.

Crabtree, JL (1991). The effect of referral for profit on therapists' and clients' autonomy and fair competition. *American Journal of Occupational Therapy, 45*, 464–466.

Epstein, CF (1985). Consultation: Communicating and facilitating. In J Bair & M Gray (eds), *The occupational therapy manager* (pp 299–317). Rockville, MD: American Occupational Therapy Association, Inc.

Faust, L & Meaker, MK (1991). Private practice occupational therapy in the skilled nursing facility: Creative alliance or mutual exploitation? *American Journal of Occupational Theraspy, 45*, 621–627.

Grady, AP (1991). Directions for the future: Opportunities for leadership. *American Journal of Occupational Therapy, 45*, 7–9.

Hershman, AG (1984). Reimbursement in private practice. *American Journal of Occupational Therapy, 38*, 299–306.

Hertfelder, SD & Crispen, C (eds.). (1990). *Private practice: Strategies for success.* Rockville, MD: American Occupational Therapy Association, Inc.

Hinojosa, J, Anderson, J, & Strauch, C (1988). Pediatric occupational therapy in the home. *American Journal of Occupational Therapy, 42*, 17–22.

Howard, BS (1991). How high do we jump? The effect of reimbursement on occupational therapy. *American Journal of Occupational Therapy, 45*, 875–881.

Punwar, AJ (1988). *Occupational therapy: Principles and practice.* Baltimore, Williams & Wilkins.

Saltz, DL (1990, October 11). Therapists find satisfaction on their own. *OT Week*, pp 5, 16.

Shriver, DJ (1985). A new arena for private practice in occupational therapy: Worker's compensation and personal injury. In FS Cromwell (ed.), *Private practice in occupational therapy* (pp 25–36). New York, Hawthorn.

Shuer, J & Weiner, L (1985). Developing pediatric programming in a private occupational therapy practice. In FS Cromwell (ed), *Private practice in occupational therapy* (pp 53–67). New York, Hawthorn Press.

Steich, T (1991, August 8). Focus: Private practice. Legal considerations when you're the boss. *OT Week*, pp 16–17.

Tiernan, K (1991, August 8). Focus: Private practice. A unique formula. *OT Week*, pp 12–13.

U.S. Department of Commerce, Bureau of the Census. (1987). *Statistical abstract of the United States, 1988* (108th ed.). Washington, DC: Author.

Usero, PA (1991, August 8). Focus: Private practice. Have dog, will travel. *OT Week*, pp 14–15.

Early Neuromuscular Development of the Premature Infant

RUSSELL E. CARTER, MPH
and SUZANN K. CAMPBELL, PhD

A case study is presented which documents the neuromuscular development of a premature infant (34–35 weeks gestation) during the first eight weeks of postnatal life. The development of postural tone, spontaneous activity, and responsiveness to stimulation is described and compared with that of the full-term infant. This information is of value to physical therapists involved in evaluation and therapeutic intervention programs for high risk infants.

1 The motor patterns and muscle tone of the premature infant differ from those of the full-term baby in the neonatal period and early months of infancy.[1-3] In attempting to assess the presence of central nervous system deficits in premature infants examined in the Special Infant Care Clinic at North Carolina Memorial Hospital, we found that our experience and knowledge of the appropriate responses to stimulation or test procedures were frequently inadequate. While helpful, the descriptions by Saint-Anne Dargassies of the premature infant's development are primarily subjective, making difficult the determination of *degrees* of change which are appropriate during early infancy.[2,3] We, therefore, performed a longitudinal study of the neuromuscular development of a "normal" premature infant, using objective ratings and subjective observations, to improve our ability to recognize abnormalities, as well as appropriate responses, in these infants. We described the following responses from birth to forty-two weeks postmenstrual age: muscle tone, sucking and rooting reactions and other primitive

Mr. Carter was a Pediatric Fellow in the Division of Physical Therapy, Department of Medical Allied Health Professions, School of Medicine, University of North Carolina at Chapel Hill, Chapel Hill, NC, when the study was conducted. He is currently Mental Health Administrator III, Illinois State Pediatric Institute, 1640 W. Roosevelt, Chicago, IL 60608.

Ms Campbell is Assistant Professor, Division of Physical Therapy, Department of Medical Allied Health Professions, School of Medicine, University of North Carolina at Chapel Hill, Chapel Hill, NC 27514.

This study was supported in part by Grant 149 from the Bureau of Community Health Services, U.S. Public Health Service.

reflexes, spontaneous activity, behavioral state, and head control with the child in the prone and upright positions and when pulled to sitting from the supine position.

Methods

SUBJECT

2 A white male infant, N.M., was randomly selected from the infants residing in the premature nursery of North Carolina Memorial Hospital at the time the study began. The infant's mother was twenty-four years old and had not experienced any complications during this second pregnancy. The 1,700 gram infant was the first-born of twins delivered with low forceps, occiput anterior presentation, after a four and one-half hour labor at thirty-four to thirty-five weeks gestation. Oxytocin was used as well as the epidural anesthetic, bupivicaine. Suctioning and bagging with oxygen were required to elicit respiration. The Apgar scores were 4 at one minute and 6 at five minutes.[4]

3 The infant had mild respiratory distress during the first hours of life which resolved within the first twenty-four hours. An umbilical catheter was inserted but was removed during the first twenty-four hours. A sugar-water solution was offered during the first two days and formula was begun on day 3. On day 4, the infant appeared to be jaundiced, and a diagnosis of hyperbilirubinemia was made on day 5. Phototherapy[5] was employed in the resolution of the jaundice until day 6. On day 9, breast milk was first fed, and, on day 10, breast feeding began with formula supplementing the diet. Body temperature fluctuations were reported on day 10, with stabilization on day 12. Conditioning, the process of allowing the infant to regulate his own body temperature, was instituted at seventeen days. On day 20, the infant was removed from the incubator and placed in a crib. On day 25, he was circumcised. An electrocardiogram was performed on day 27 to rule out suspected peripheral pulmonary stenosis; normal heart sounds were reported. On day 28, N.M. was discharged home weighing 2,160 grams. His subsequent medical course was reportedly unremarkable. The infant, as well as his twin, has been followed in our Special Infant Care Clinic and at thirteen months of age, both infants appear to be normal in all respects.

METHOD OF EXAMINATION

4 The neurological examination followed a format similar to that described by Prechtl and Beintema in The Neurological Examination of the Full

Term Newborn Infant[6] supplemented by the work of André-Thomas, Chesni, and Saint-Anne Dargassies.[7] Objective scores were assigned when possible. Throughout the study, consistent observation under standard conditions was attempted. These conditions were as follows:

(1) Time of examination. Prechtl and Beintema reported that the optimal time for an infant examination is two or three hours after a feeding[6]; this timing was also suggested for the examination of the premature infant since the infant would be less likely to be irritable or to fall asleep.[8] We adopted such a schedule for the testing of our subject.

(2) Place of examination. The examination was conducted in the premature nursery, under thermoneutral conditions (isolette or radiant heater). After the infant was discharged, examinations were conducted in the home in a well-lighted area of constant warm temperature.

(3) State of the baby. Since the physiological status of the infant is reflected in the quality of responses elicited during an examination,[9] the following behavioral states were scored and recorded during each test:

State I: Eyes closed, regular respiration, no movements
State II: Eyes closed, irregular respiration, no gross movements
State III: Eyes open, no gross movements
State IV: Eyes open, gross movements, no crying
State V: Eyes open or closed, crying
State II/IV: Eyes closed, gross movements[6,10]

During the examinations in the first five days of postnatal life, the infant was in State II/IV. Neither State III nor State IV was observed by the investigator before day 6. From that day until the end of the study, the infant was examined consistently during State III or IV.

(4) Personnel conducting examinations. All examinations were conduced by the first author.

(5) Item sequence. The sequence of administration of the test items was the same on each day. The items in each basic test position were conducted in a sequence proceeding from least demanding to most demanding of the infant, minimizing the actual amount of handling of the infant in an effort to maintain a constant state.

(6) Testing frequency. The subject was examined daily through the first ten days, twice during the third week, and weekly thereafter.

Because of interrupting circumstances (for example, health of the infant or investigator), testing was not possible on day 4 and during the fifth week. A total of sixteen examinations was completed between birth and forty-two weeks of postmenstrual age (a chronological age of 8 weeks).

5 Each assessment began with a three-minute observation of the spontaneous postures and motor activity of the supine infant. After this observation, reflexes and reactions were evaluated. The following rating system was used[6,7]:

Supine

(1) *Spontaneous Activity*—observation of infant for three minutes, accounting for basic postural set, state, amount of movement, type of movement, and direction and results of movement, such as autoelicitation of reflexes and tremors. The amount of time the child was active was scored:

0—none
1—spontaneous activity during less than 30 percent of the observation time
2—infant active more than 50 percent of the observation time
3—infant constantly active during observation with only brief pauses of inactivity (less the 10 seconds)

(2) *Sucking Response*—insertion of approximately three centimeters of the examiner's little finger into baby's mouth. The ease or difficulty encountered in eliciting the suck was described. The strength of the suck was graded:

0—no response
1—one or two sucking movements in ten seconds with little lip or tongue pressure on the examiner's finger
2—several sucking movements (3 to 6) in ten seconds with full stripping by tongue, and lip pressure on examiner's finger
3—long sucking (6 or more) in ten seconds with full stripping by tongue, and lip pressure on examiner's finger
4—full and uninterrupted sucking (15 seconds or more)

(3) *Rooting Responses*—elicited by lightly stroking the perioral area, the upper lip, and the lower lip with the little finger. The head was in the midline. The responses were scored:

0—no response
1—only lip movements toward stimulus
2—lip and tongue movements visible, plus incomplete turning of the head
3—full turn of the head toward stimulus

4—full turn, with lip grasping (requiring repeated stimuli)

5—easily elicited full turning and lip grasping (single stimulus)

(4) *Palmar Response*—elicited by placing the examiner's index finger in the infant's palm from the ulnar side and producing a slight stretch on the flexor muscles. The response was scored:

0—no response

1—incomplete flexion of fingers, not touching examiner's finger throughout test

2—complete flexion of fingers, but only lightly touching examiner's fingers through full test (examiner may easily remove finger from infant's grasp)

3—full flexion, but maintained for less than ten seconds (examiner may raise infant's arm off mat before infant's grasp releases)

4—full flexion maintained for longer than ten seconds (infant's arm and shoulder can be raised off mat)

5—fingers strongly flexed and have to be retracted by the examiner

(5) *Tonic Labyrinthine Reflex*—posture of shoulders, arms, and legs, and possible opisthotonos when lying supine were first noted. Then the examiner placed a hand behind the infant's head and passively flexed the head to the chest. The amount of resistance to passive motion was graded:

0—floppy, no resistance to passive neck movements

1—resistance through any part of range, but easily moved through the full range

2—resistance strong in initial part of range, some resistance throughout the range which increases in velocity of neck movement

3—head and neck firmly press into examiner's hand; difficult to initiate movement but full range possible; resistance throughout the range

4—head and neck firmly press into examiner's hand, trunk arching; difficult to passively move head and neck, and full range is not possible without strong effort by examiner

(6) *Muscle Tone*—resistance to passive movement of the arms and legs was scored:

0—floppy

1—resistance to passive emotion, but falls back to initial position

2—resistance through full range, with immediate rapid return to position

3—resists passive motion, restricted range, immediate return to initial position

(7) *Asymmetrical Tonic Neck Reflex*—first the examiner tried to elicit active head rotation to one side and then to the other by visual distraction. If active head rotation could not be obtained, the examiner passively turned the head to one side, and then to the other. After the head was rotated, a description of the infant's posture was recorded.

(8) *Pull to Sit*—the examiner gradually pulled the infant from supine to sitting while supporting the infant by the upper arms and shoulders. The movement was scored:

0—head passively hangs; no attempt to right head
1—head hangs down, but infant attempts to assist slightly with shoulders and neck
2—head hangs down through the first 60 degrees, then infant can right head
3—head hangs down through the first 45 degrees, then infant can right head
4—infant cannot initiate, but brings head up through most of the range
5—infant actively pulls to sit, using head and arms

(9) *Head Control and Posture When Sitting*—the examiner rated the sitting posture and head control after pulling the infant to sitting. Head control and posture were scored:

0—head passively hangs with no attempt to bring head upright; body slumps forward
1—head hangs down, but infant attempts to right head; spine and body slumped forward
2—head remains upright for several seconds with minimal movement
3—head remains upright with only several movements; upper spine is straightening up
4—head remains upright for three to four seconds and upper spine is straight
5—head is steady and upright; spine is straight but still needs some support

(10) *Moro Reflex*—the examiner held the infant in the supine position. The reflex was elicited by a quick extension of the neck, allowing the head to drop into the examiner's hand. The response was described, and then objectively scored:

0—no response (within 30 seconds)
1—minimal abduction (less than 45 degrees) or extension (less than 45 degrees) of arms
2—minimal arm motion involving abduction or extension, or both, of greater than 45 degrees
3—full abduction or extension, or both, of the arms
4—immediate and full response to a short head drop
5—any handling elicits a Moro reflex

Prone

(1) *Spontaneous Activity*—the infant was observed in the prone position for three minutes. Subjective observations regarding posture and movement were recorded.

(2) *Head Lifting*—the examiner described the infant's attempt to clear his head from the supporting surface when placed in the prone position. The response was scored:

0—no effort is made to clear the face

1—minimal effort involving visible contraction of neck muscles, but the face does not clear the surface

2—the face is cleared several times for a few seconds

3—sustained head lift for three to four seconds

4—the head is cleared for ten seconds with any degree of clearance

5—the head is upright with the face vertical to the supporting surface

(3) *Tonic Labyrinthine Reflex*—the examiner first described the infant's posture when lying prone. The examiner then placed a hand beneath the infant's forehead and passively extended the head. The amount of resistance to passive motion was graded using the same scale as the tonic labyrinthine reflex in the supine position.

(4) *Galant's Reflex*—with the infant in the prone position, the examiner firmly stroked the paravertebral muscles in a cephalocaudal direction from approximately midthoracic area to low lumbar area. The response was scored:

0—no response

1—slight movement of supine and wrinkling of skin after repeated stimulation

2—slight movement of spine to each stimulus

3—obvious full spine incurvation with each stimulus

4—obvious full trunk incurvation sustained for three seconds

(5) *Ventral Suspension*—the examiner picked up the infant from the prone position, supporting the baby with both hands about the thorax. The posture the infant assumed was described and graded:

0—no attempt to raise head

1—several unsuccessful efforts to raise the head and neck; body mostly flexed over examiner's hands

2—weak head raising successful but never attains the horizontal plane

3—head sustained in the horizontal plane for several seconds

4—head extended with retracted shoulders

5—head, shoulders, spine, and hips extended to horizontal

6—head, shoulders, spine, hips, and knees extended above the horizontal plane.

Vertical

(1) *Head Control When Held in Standing*—subjective description

(2) *Placing Reaction of the Feet*—the examiner held the infant upright with both hands about the thorax. The dorsum of the foot was touched against the under edge of the table. The response was described and graded:

0—no response
1—stimulated leg flexed and then extended; foot is not placed
2—placing response, but difficult to elicit (requires repeated stimulation)
3—full placing response, easily elicited but placed briefly (only one or two stimulations needed)
4—full response, easily elicited and placed for ten seconds

6 The average examination time was ten minutes. Twenty minutes was the maximal time allotted for the examination, allowing time to calm the infant if he was crying or to stimulate him if he was asleep. If not completed within twenty minutes, the examination was discontinued and attempted at another time.

Results

7 In general, alertness and reactiveness to stimuli increased with time, but fluctuations were noted in several scores on the days that hyperbilirubinemia was present, during time of body temperature instability, and when breast feeding was initiated.

8 State differentiation evolved from a state of continual somnolence during the first two weeks of life, but especially the first days of life, to precisely defined states of sleep and wakefulness when the infant was about forty weeks of postmenstrual age. Concomitantly, N. M. became more active and responsive to stimuli.

SPONTANEOUS ACTIVITY

9 Motor activity was almost totally suppressed during the first two days of life, then increased and fluctuated with changing medical conditions over the next two weeks, finally increasing steadily to attain the maximal possible score (Table). Motor patterns noted during the early weeks of life included gyrating arm movements, bilateral reciprocal leg flexion and extension rolling to one side, hand-to-mouth activity, and head turning. Tremors were common. The motions of the premature infant were wide-ranging with more elbow, hip, and knee exten-

TABLE RATINGS OF DEVELOPMENTAL REFLEXES AND MOTOR PATTERNS FROM DAY 1 TO DAY 56 (APPROXIMATELY 42 WEEKS POSTMENSTRUAL AGE) OF POSTNATAL LIFE

| | Item Rating[a] | | | | | | | | | | | | | | | |
Test Item	Day 1	2	3	5[b]	6	7	8	9	10[c]	14	16	20	35	40	50	56
Supine																
Spontaneous activity	0	0	1	1	1	1	2	1	1	1	2	3	3	3	3	3
Sucking	2	2	2	1	3	3	3	3	4	3	3	3	4	4	3	3
Rooting	1	1	1	1	3	3	3	5	4	4	4	4	4	5	5	5
Palmar response	3	3	3	3	4	4	3	3	3	4	3	4	4	4	4	4
Tonic laybrinthine reflex	1	2	2	1	1	2	2	2	2	2	2	2	2	3	2	2
Muscle tone	2	2	2	1	2	2	2	2	2	2	2	2	2	2	2	2
Pull to sitting	1	1	2	1	2	2	2	2	3	3	2	4	4	4	4	4
Head control (sitting)	1	1	1	1	1	1	1	1	1	1	1	2	1	2	2	2
Moro reflex	2	3	3	2	3	4	4	4	3	4	4	4	4	4	4	4
Prone																
Head lifting	1	1	1	1	1	1	1	1	1	1	1	1	1	2	2	2
Tonic labyrinthine reflex	2	2	2	1	1	1	2	2	2	2	2	3	2	2	2	1
Galant's reflex	1	0	1	1	1	1	1	1	1	1	1	2	2	2	0	0
Ventral suspension	0	0	0	0	1	1	1	1	1	1	1	1	1	2	2	2
Vertical																
Placing reaction	0	0	0	0	1	1	1	0	1	1	1	2	2	3	3	3

[a]See text for scoring system.
[b]Hyperbilirubinemia diagnosed.
[c]Breast feeding initiated and body temperature fluctuations noted.

265

sion than are seen in the full-term infant. During the fourth week (38 weeks postmenstrual age), bridging (elevation of the hips in supine) was observed as well as reciprocal kicking and increased facial contact by the hands; although the activity level was high, there were fewer wildly gyrating limb movements than previously.

10   In both supine and prone, flexion postures were assumed with increasing frequency, first in the legs and later in the arms as the infant matured. At no time, however, did the degree of hip, knee, or elbow flexion approach the degree of flexion seen in full-term neonates. In the prone position, a flexed posture with the arms flexed tightly against the chest was consistently observed. The hips were typically abducted and flexed, but occasionally assumed a relaxed extended posture. As N.M. became older, hip flexion increased and abduction decreased, causing the hips to elevate from the surface. They were, however, never adducted and flexed to the degree seen in full-term infants in the prone position.

ORAL REFLEXES

11   Sucking and rooting activity were present immediately and increased gradually in strength and duration during the first week and one-half. The sucking score peaked on day 10 when breast feeding was initiated (Table). Both scores dropped in succeeding days and remained constant until the expected date of delivery when maximal ratings were again obtained. At eight weeks of age, the infant refused to suck when a nonnutritive stimulus was offered. Apparently, he was able to recognize the difference between breast and pacifier and, when hungry, reacted appropriately by refusing to suck a pacifier.

MUSCLE TONE

12   The objective muscle tone ratings remained almost constant during the first eight weeks of life (Table). During the first days of life, little resistance to passive movement was encountered. Upon release of the limb, rebound occurred after a brief latency. The rebound in the early examinations was more brisk and consistent in the legs than in the arms. Resistance to displacement, especially to extension, progressed with maturation to such a degree that proximal stabilization was needed to obtain full extension of the limbs; nevertheless, full range of motion was always present in each joint, making it impossible for the infant to obtain a score above 2, despite the fact that resistance to displacement and the resulting rebound to the starting position became stronger over time.

ASYMMETRICAL TONIC NECK REFLEX

13 Postural changes were first seen in the leg toward which the face was turned. The arms became consistently responsive during the second week of postnatal life. Trunk participation began at seven weeks of age (41 weeks postmenstrual age). The most consistently obtained response was elbow flexion on the occiput side. The reflex was never noted to be obligatory.

HEAD CONTROL

14 Head control during the pull-to-sitting test improved steadily until three weeks of age when righting the head was obtained after the first 45 degrees of trunk flexion (Table). This response remained static until the end of the study when the infant was two months old. In the sitting position, by the end of the first week, the baby was able to extend his head to the vertical, a position which seemed to facilitate ease of respiration. Attempts at head righting when supported in sitting became more effective with increasing age (Table). He began to rotate his head laterally during the third week of life at thirty-seven postmenstrual weeks and maintained his head in an oscillating, erect position for several seconds at six weeks of age.

15 Head lifting in the prone position showed little change during the course of the study (Table). For the first month and a half, the infant made minimal efforts at neck extension involving visible contraction of neck muscles, but he was unable to clear his face from the supporting surface. At five weeks of age (approximately equal to term), he became able to clear his face repeatedly for a few seconds, a response which was still present at the end of the second month of life.

VENTRAL SUSPENSION

16 The ability of the infant to resist the force of gravity when supported about the thorax in ventral suspension improved gradually (Table). No response was noted during the first five days; head, trunk, and limbs conformed to the pull of gravity. From the end of the first week to the fifth week of age, the infant made several unsuccessful efforts to raise his head during each test while the body remained flexed over the examiner's hands. At an age equivalent to term, the infant was able to raise his head successfully to a level slightly less than the horizontal plane, the best response obtained during the course of this study. The rest of the body never participated overtly in the reaction which begins at two to three months of age, according to Milani-Comparetti and Gidoni.[11] The knees and elbows remained extended; however, the trunk muscles showed a gradual increase in extensor tone as evidenced by decreased trunk curvature over the examiner's hand during suspension.

MORO REFLEX

17   The Moro reflex increased from an upper extremity response of slightly more than 45 degrees of shoulder abduction or elbow extension on day 2 to an immediate and full response to a short head drop by one week of age, a behavior which then remained stable (Table). The initial low postural tone of the infant was reflected in a large displacement of the arms when the Moro reflex was elicited. As flexor tone increased, the range of arm displacement decreased and the velocity of response increased. The range, however, remained greater than noted in a full-term infant with typical flexor hypertonicity.

PLACING REACTION

18   The placing reaction of the feet could not be elicited for the first five days (Table). It then appeared as a flexion-extension response of the leg following contact of the foot, but without placing. At three weeks of age, a full placing reaction could be elicited after repeated stimulation, and at five weeks of age the foot was placed for a few seconds after one or two stimulations.

19   The tests of palmar grasp, tonic labyrinthine, and Galant's reflexes produced no reliable trends during the age period observed in this study, and the results of these tests will not be discussed further. The scores for these items are presented in the Table.

Discussion

20   Several major patterns of change emerged from the daily and weekly observations of this infant. These changes included differentiation of state, the influence of birth shock, and the quality and quantity of motor activity.

21   Birth shock was present during the first two days of life accounting for the minimal amount of spontaneous activity and a depressed sucking reflex. Beintema has reported a significant number of subjects with a depressed sucking reflex during the first four days of life,[10] and other

studies have also attributed a depression in infant activity and responsiveness during the first few days of life to birth shock.[12,13] Escardó and de Coriat have reported a significant number of cases of birth shock resulting from anesthesia employed during labor.[12] A check of the mother's labor history revealed the use of anesthesia during labor.

22 As anticipated, the infant's activity level increased with age and with changes in physiological state. The level of spontaneous motor activity progressed from an initial level of minimal or no motor activity during the first weeks of life to an almost continually active infant during the final examination eight weeks later. The initial low level of motor activity was found in the presence of physiological instability, low muscle tone, and a state of somnolence.

23 In addition to increased quantity of motor activity, the overall quality of the infant's movements became more coordinated. In the first few weeks, arm and leg movements were bizarre, writhing, and often tremulous. As the infant matured, constraint of the wildly gyrating limbs occurred. Similar observations of mobility changes in premature infants have been noted by others.[2,3,14]

24 The first apparently intentional movements were noted in the oral area when the infant was able to differentiate nutritive from nonnutritive objects he was offered to suck. This behavior is acknowledged by Piaget as one of the infant's first intelligent acts, developed by repeated contacts with objects associated with either food or nonnutritive stimulation.[15] Sucking of the hand is used in self-comforting according to Brazelton,[16] but Burpee[17] has reported that premature infants from birth to forty weeks postmenstrual age appear to exhibit hand-mouth behaviors infrequently compared to full-term neonates.

25 The subjective descriptions and the objective scores for the selected test items appeared to reflect accurately the premature infant's motor development, as subjectively described by Saint-Anne Dargassies.[2,3] More specifically, the descriptions and scores document the caudocephalic development of muscle tone and its influence on motor development. The premature infant's muscle tone during the first days and weeks of life is essentially flaccid. The more premature the infant, the more flaccid he appears.[2,3] Correspondingly, little or no spontaneous activity accompanies the global hypotonia of the premature infant of twenty-eight to thirty weeks gestation. As the infant matures, his muscle tone develops progressively in a caudocephalic direction. Flexor muscle tone initially dominates in the legs, as was seen in N.M., and is observed in handling of the infant, in the quality of spontaneous movements, and in the resting postures of the infant, such as that produced by the asymmetrical tonic neck reflex. Eventually the flexor tone influence plateaus; however, previous to this flexor plateau, the

development of extensor tone is occurring, resulting in active extension of the legs and, later, of the trunk when placed in standing, followed by decreased hip flexion in prone and intial attempts at neck extension. Eventually equilibration of these tonal influences becomes evident overtly in the attainment of a synergistic motor skill such as head control in sitting.

26 Consistent differences from the full-term infant in postures and muscle tone were observed in the premature infant from birth to an age equivalent to forty-two weeks postmenstrual age. Not only is the muscle tone of the thirty-four- to thirty-five-week premature infant initially low and asymmetrically distributed between arms and legs, but the degree of flexor hypertonicity noted in the full-term neonate is never achieved.[2,3] The full-term neonate moves less than the premature infant, his ranges of movement being restricted by flexor hypertonicity. The premature infant, in contrast, has full range of motion into extension; resting postures feature less flexion and adduction of the hips than seen in the full-term infant; and stimulation of the Moro reflex results in wide opening of the arms.

27 The apparent low flexor muscle tonicity in the premature infant may be caused by the early influence of gravity exerted on the postural, extensor musculature resulting in strong extensor muscles relative to flexor muscles. (The infant in utero, by contrast, is surrounded by amniotic fluid so that the extensor muscles are not subjected to an equivalent gravitational stretch, and he is experiencing an increasing amount of mechanical compression as parturition approaches.[18]) The flexor muscles of the premature are not *without* tone after the initial period of hypotonia. They are merely opposed by relatively stronger extensor muscles; thus, at term-equivalent age, the premature infant is able to initiate head righting when pulled to sitting from supine and successfully maintains an erect head for a few seconds in sitting, while the full-term neonate exhibits complete head lag when pulled up and makes only weak attempts at neck extension when held erect.[14] Early development of head control and of neck muscle cocontraction, therefore, appears to be facilitated by early experience.

28 Unfortunately, the rating scale chosen to assess muscle tone, response to *passive* limb displacement, was not valid for the premature infant. The scale did not reflect early asymmetry between arms and legs, failed to measure all of the muscle tone changes which occurred, and showed almost no variance despite changes in posture and movement observed during spontaneous activity and testing procedures.

29 Observations of resistance to passive stretch do not appear useful in predicting the quality of performance of functional activities involving coordination of mobility and postural stability with adequate force,

velocity, and sequence of muscle activation. Attempts to improve each recognition of central nervous system pathology must include development of a satisfactory quantitative assessment of postural tone since the authors have subjectively observed that muscle tone abnormalities, particularly in the legs, are often observed before retarded motor development or abnormal movement patterns are recognized in evaluation of the premature infant. In addition, clarification of the caudocephalic direction of muscle tone development is needed. Clearly, tonicity is present in the muscles of mastication before it becomes apparent more caudally, and sucking is a relatively mature skill even before birth. The actual timing of the appearance of tonicity in individual muscle groups remains to be described adequately.

30 The Rosenblith Neonatal Behavioral Assessment Scale contains a comprehensive measure of muscle tone in which a rating is derived from several items, including resting posture, passive limb displacement, degree of trembling, and quality of resisted movement.[19] This scale may find increasing use as the test becomes more widely known and validated. Another approach to evaluation of muscle tone in infants might be use of the tonic vibration reflex to examine motoneuron excitability indirectly,[20–23] since the quality of tonic reflexes may have more significance than the phasic reflexes in the prediction of postural control abnormalities.

31 The purpose of performing this clinical study was to enhance our understanding of neuromuscular development in the premature infant, especially in those areas in which it differs from that of the term infant. While evaluation of one infant is not sufficient for establishing developmental norms, it has assisted us in appreciating the quality of movement patterns in premature infants and comparing them with the patterns observed in full-term infants. This information is vital for physical therapists who evaluate high risk infants in the first months of life in order to avoid false identification of cerebral dysfunction. Large ranges of movement, trembling, relatively dominant extensor tone, and presence of asymmetrical tonic neck reflex effects on muscle tone in the legs are normal findings in the premature infant in the early weeks of postnatal life and, unless they persist, should not be interpreted as abnormal symptoms.

Acknowledgment Appreciation is expressed to the staff of the premature nursery at North Carolina Memorial Hospital, especially Ernest N. Kraybill, M.D., and Martha G. Russell, R.N., and to the parents of N.M. for their cooperation and support of this project.

References

1. Michaelis, R, Parmalee, AH, Stern, E, et al: Activity states in premature and term infants. Psychobiol 6:209–215, 1973.

2. Saint-Anne Dargassies, S: The Development of the Nervous System in the Foetus. Monograph available from the author, centre neonatal de l'Association Claude Bernard, 123 Boulevard de Port-Royal, 75014 Paris, France. Switzerland, Nestle.

3. Saint-Anne Dargassies, S: Neurological Maturation of the Premature Infant of 28 to 41 Weeks Gestational Age. In Human Development, edited by Falkner, F. Philadelphia. W.B. Saunders Company, 1966.

4. Apgar, V: The newborn (Apgar) scoring system. Pediatr Clin North Am 13:645, 1966.

5. Meadow, R: Phototherapy and hyperbilirubinemia. Dev Med Child Neurol 12:802–804, 1970.

6. Prechtl, H and Beintema, DJ: The Neurological Examination of the Full Term Newborn Infant. Little Club Clinics in Developmental Medicine, no 12. London, National Spastics Society, 1964.

7. André-Thomas, Chesni Y and Saint-Anne Dargassies, S: The Neurological Examination of the Infant. Little Club Clinics in Developmental Medicine, no 1. London, National Spastics Society, 1960.

8. Kraybill, EN: Personal communication, 1973.

9. Hutt, SJ, Lenard, HG, and Prechtl, HFR: Psychophysiological Studies in Newborn Infants. In Advances in Child Development and Behavior Vol 4, edited by Lipsitt LP and Reese, HW. New York, Academic Press, 1969, pp 128–172.

10. Beintema, DJ: A Neurological Study of Newborn Infants. Little Club Clinics in Developmental Medicine, no 28. London, National Spastics Society, 1968.

11. Milani-Comparetti, G and Gidoni, EA: Routine developmental examination in normal and retarded children. Dev. Med Child Neurol 9:631–638, 1967.

12. Escardó, F and de Coriat, LF: Development of postural and tonic patterns in the newborn infant. Pediatr Clin North Am 7:511–525, 1960

13. Yang, DC: Neurologic status of newborn infants on first and third day of life. Neurology 12:72–77, 1962.

14. Illingworth, RS: The Development of the Infant and Young Child: Normal and Abnormal. 5th ed. Baltimore, The Williams & Wilkins Company, 1972.

15. Piaget, J: The Origins of Intelligence in Children. New York, International Universities Press, 1952.

16. Brazelton, TB: Neonatal Behavioral Assessment Scale. Little Club Clinics in Developmental Medicine, no 50. Philadelphia, JB Lippincott Company, 1973.

17. Burpee, B: Hand-mouth Behaviors of Premature and Full Term Infants. Unpublished research, University of North Carolina at Chapel Hill, Chapel Hill, NC, 1974.

18. Moore, KL: The Developing Human: Clinically Oriented Embryology. Philadelphia, W.B. Saunders Company, 1973.

19. Rosenblith, JF: Manual for Behavioral Examination of the Neonate as Modified by Judy F. Rosenblith (unpublished) from Graham, FK: Behavioral differences between normal and traumatized newborns: 1. The test procedures. Psychol Monogr 70:6–15 (no 427), 1956. Manual available from author: Institute for Research in the Health Sciences, Brown University, Providence, RI.

20. Arcangel, CD, Johnston, R, and Bishop, B: The Achilles tendon reflex and the H-response during and after tendon vibration. Phys Ther 51:889–902, 1971.

21. Johnston, RM, Bishop, B, and Coffey, GH: Mechanical vibration of skeletal muscles. Phys Ther 50:499–505, 1970.

22. Bishop, B: Vibratory stimulation: Part I. Neurophysiology of motor responses evoked by vibratory stimulation. Phys Ther 54:1273–1282, 1874.

23. Bishop, B: Vibratory stimulation: Part II. Vibratory stimulation as an evaluation tool. Phys Ther 55:28–34, 1975.

Low-Load Prolonged Stretch vs. High-Load Brief Stretch in Treating Knee Contractures

KATHYE E. LIGHT, SHARON NUZIK,
WALTER PERSONIUS, and
AUBYN BARSTROM

Key Words • Contracture • Knee • Physical therapy

*This study was designed to compare the results of a tradi-
tional method of stretching knee flexion contractures by
high-load brief stretch (HLBS) with the results of an experimental method of prolonged knee extension by skin traction, low-load prolonged stretch (LLPS). End range of passive knee extension was measured by standard goniometry.
Subjects were 11 nonambulatory residents of a nursing
home who had demonstrated gradually progressive bilateral knee contractures. Each subject served as his or her
own control with one lower limb receiving LLPS and the
other limb receiving HLBS and passive range of motion
(PROM). Sequential medical trials were used as the clinical
research design. Whether comparing the LLPS limb PROM
measurements pretreatment and posttreatment (p ≤ .05) or
the HLBS to the LLPS limb PROM recordings posttreatment*

Ms. Light is Assistant Professor, Physical Therapy Program, University of Texas Health Science
Center at San Antonio, 7703 Floyd Curl Drive, San Antonio, TX 78284 (USA).

Ms. Nuzik is Research Physical Therapist, Medical College of Virginia Hospitals, Virginia
Commonwealth University, Richmond, VA 23298.

Mr. Personius is Assistant Professor, Department of Physical Therapy, School of Allied Health
Professions, Medical College of Virginia, Virginia Commonwealth University.

Ms. Barstrom is a graduate student in the Department of Physical Therapy, School of Allied
Health Professions, Medical College of Virginia, Virginia Commonwealth University.

The results of this study were presented in poster format at the Annual Conference of the
American Physical Therapy Association, Anaheim, CA, June 19–23, 1982, and at the 1982
State Meeting of the Virginia Chapter of the American Physical Therapy Association,
Williamsburg, VA, where Ms. Nuzik was awarded Best Clinical Research Paper.

273

(p ≤ .05), the results demonstrated a preference for LLPS in the treatment of knee contractures in the immobile nursing home resident.

1 Many elderly individuals demonstrate limited movement abilities; a frequent consequence is the development of knee contractures. Despite the efforts of an active physical therapy maintenance program at a county nursing home, including daily range of motion (ROM) and passive stretching techniques, these chronic knee contractures continued to be a problem. This study was designed to compare a more traditional method of stretching knee contractures, high-load brief stretch (HLBS), with an experimental method of prolonged knee extension, low-load prolonged satretch (LLPS).

Literature Review

2 Experimental and clinical data suggest that the tissue changes, which may cause restricted joint motion in the bedridden elderly, are physiological[1-3] or morphological[4-9] and involve intra-articular,[5] periarticular[4,6,9] and extra-articular structures.[7,8]

3 Neuromuscular dysfunction appears to be a common cause of extra-articular physiological joint restriction. This physiological restriction of muscle length may be a consequence of spinal segment and supraspinal inputs on the gamma loop gain set mechanism.[10-12] The result is an alteration of extrafusal muscle fiber resting length. Therapeutic exercise techniques have been hypothesized to affect this mechanism directly. The therapeutic techniques of contract-relax[2] and proprioceptive neuromuscular facilitation (PNF),[3] as well as the application of fluorimethane spray and stretch,[1] have all been shown to assist a rapid improvement of restricted joint-range excursion.

4 Gross anatomical, histological, and mechanical data implicate abnormal intra-articular, periarticualr, and extra-articular connective tissue structures as the cause of limited passive ROM (PROM). These structures include intra-articular adhesions,[5] periarticular jopint capsule stiffness,[4,6,9] and shortened extra-articular skeletal muscle.[7,8] After four weeks of immobilization in a shortened position, cat soleus muscle demonstrated a 40 percent decrease in the number of sarcomeres in series[7] and, therefore, a decrease in length of the parallel elastic component.[8] The decrease in cat soleus muscle length resulted in a shift of its passive length-tension curve to the left and a concomitant decrease in ankle ROM. After four weeks release from immobilization (and nor-

mal activity by the cats in their cages during the interim), muscle extensibility and sarcomere number were restored to normal.[7] In another study, joints of monkeys immobilized in shortened positions exhibited decreased ROM, decreased joint capsule length, and loss of extensibility.[6] Reduction of joint ROM and strength of the medial posterior capsule was reported by Lavigne and Watkins to be appreciable at 16 days and marked after 32 days of immobilization.[6]

5   The mechanism for immobilization-induced capsular restriction of ROM is not well understood and may be multifactorial. Histological studies of immobilized tissue have demonstrated capsular fibrofatty infiltrate,[6] decreased matrix water and glycosaminoglycans, increased major collagen cross-links,[4] and increased total amount of collagen.[9]

6   Warren et al used rat-tail tendons as an experimental model for clinical stretching techniques.[13] The rat-tail tendonms were used to compare two elongation methods similar to those used in this study. Application of low-load, long-duration tension at elevated temperatures, followed by cooling with the load maintained, produced significantly greater residual elongation with less tearing damage to the tissue than high-load, short-duration tension at lower temperatures. The present study included two of the four elements tested by Warren et al: low-load and long-duration tension.

7   Existing literature supports LLPS as the preferred method of lengthening immobilized, shortened tissues in animal models. Because the very common clinical practice of stretching contractures with manual high loads for periods of a minute or less was contradictory to findings in the literature, this study sought to compare the PROM effects between the clinical treatments of briefly applied manual high loads versus prolonged low loads by skin traction. We hypothesized that if chronic knee flexion contractures of at least 30 degrees in nonambulatory geriatric nursing home subjects are treated with LLPS instead of HLBS, then the passive knee extension ROM will increase significantly.

Method

SUBJECTS

8   Criteria for admission to this study were 1) the presence of bilateral knee flexion contractures of at least three-months duration and at least 30 degrees short of full passive extension and 2) the inability to walk or pivot transfer without maximal assistance. Eleven geriatric subjects who were nonambulatory and who had demonstrated gradually progressive bilateral chronic knee-flexion contractures ranging

from 30 degrees to 132 degrees short of full passive end-range extension participated in this study. Subjects served as his or her own control with one lower extremity receiving the LLPS and the other receiving a traditional combination of both HLBS and PROM. The choice of treatment for each limb was randomly determined. Each treatment was performed twice daily, five days a week for four weeks.

PROCEDURES

9 The lower extremity not chosen to receive LLPS was treated with a traditional regimen of 10 repetitions of passive lower extremity flexion, adduction, and external rotation using PNF diagonals that were followed by the HLBS. The HLBS procedure was considered to be a routine, forced, passive, manual-stretching technique. A maximum manual force was used that did not cause injury. The muscles on stretch were palpably very tight. With the LLPS, this was not the case. The patient's limb was moved manually at a force and velocity that allowed the soft tissue structures to accommodate to the change in ROM without resulting in excessive resistance, pain on the part of the patient, or the possibility of injury. Once the end range was achieved, this position was manually maintained for one minute. The force was then reduced for 15 seconds. The sequence of HLBS followed by a 15-second rest was repeated three times each treatment session. The total time required for the HLBS and PROM was approximately 15 minutes of patient-practitioner time.

10 Transmission of LLPS to the limb was accomplished by applying a modified Buck's skin traction technique with the patient in bed. A foam strip measuring 60 in by 3 in by 1 in* was applied to the subject's lower extremity in a stirrup-like fashion. The central portion of the foam strip was placed at the subject's heel; its length extended alongside the medial and lateral aspects of the limb. Taped to the center of the foam and positioned at the subject's heel was a 3-in by 3-in by 0.75-in padded wooden block. A screw eye extended outward from the center of the block and served as an attachment for the pulley rope. The foam strip and block were secured to the limb by two or three 6-in ace bandages. The rope was threaded through a single pulley and a weight was attached to the end. Plastic milk cartons filled with sand were used as weights. The length of each LLPS treatment was one hour; the patient-practitioner setup time required only two to five minutes. Each week the traction weight was increased as follows: week

---

*One inch = 2.54 cm.

one, 2.27 kg (5 lb); week two, 3.18 kg (7 lb); week three, 4.08 kg (9 lb); and week four, 5.44 kg (12 lb).

11 In addition to the two methods of stretching described, each subject received a standard upper extremity and trunk program of guided passive movement once daily. This program included 10 repetitions of pelvis-on-trunk rotation and upper extremity PNF diagonals bilaterally.

12 Standard manual goniometric measurements of the limbs were taken before treatment began and after four weeks of treatment. With the subject in the supine position, a physical therapist moved one limb to its end range of knee extension while also progressing toward maximal hip extension. This end position was maintained for one minute. The knee-extension range was then measured by a second physical therapist. The goniometer arms were aligned parallel to the long axis of the femur and the tibia with the axis at midknee joint. These two tasks were performed by the same individuals throughout the experiment.

DATA ANALYSIS

13 Sequential medical trials (SMT) were chosen to be the method of experimental design and statistical analysis.[14,15] This sequential design was considered ideal because 1) subjects could be admitted to the study as they became available, 2) comparisons could be made within the same subject, 3) no statistical computations were necessary, and 4) the experiment could be terminated as soon as statistical significance was achieved (ie, a predetermined number of subjects was not required).

14 The SMT plan was designed by Bross.[14] Significance levels were preestablished at the $p \leq .05$ level. The outcome measure, passive knee-extension end range, was assessed in two separate test situations. Each test had its own criterion for improvement: Test 1, difference between pretreatment and posttreatment PROM recordings of the LLPS leg must be $\geq 15°$; Test 2, difference in PROM posttreatment change between LLPS and HLBS limbs must $\geq 10°$.

Results

15 A total of 11 subjects participated in this study before a $p \leq .05$ significance level was attained with SMT. The SMT grids for Test 1 (Fig. 1) and Test 2 (Fig. 2) demonstrate how quickly and directly the

TEST 1: Increase in PROM of LLPS limb > 15°

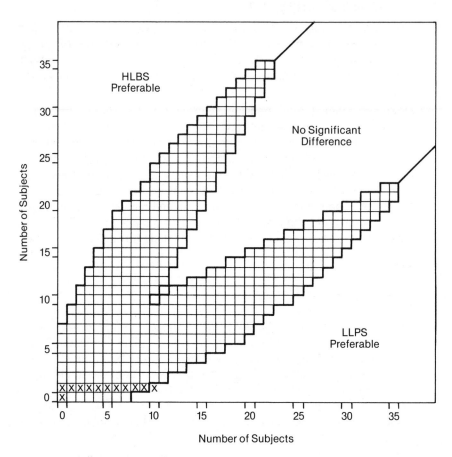

FIGURE 1   Sequential medical trials grid with a significance level of $P \leq 0.5$ comparing pretreatment and posttreatment LLPS for Test 1 criterion. Statistical significance is established when the demarcation lines are passed to the lower right or upper left of the grid.

LLPS was found to be the superior treatment. In Test 1, when comparing pretreatment and posttreatment knee extension of the LLPS limb, 10 of the 11 subjects demonstrated greater than a 15-degree increase in PROM. When comparing the HLBS with the LLPS limb in Test 2, a 10-degree PROM difference in favor of LLPS was demonstrated in the same 10 subjects. Whether comparing the LLPS limb measurements pretreatment and posttreatment (Fig. 1) or the increase in limb measurement of the LLPS versus HLBS limbs posttreatment (Fig. 2), the results demonstrated a preference (greater increase in PROM) for

TEST 2: PROM increase of LLPS limb at least
10° > PROM increase of HLBS limb

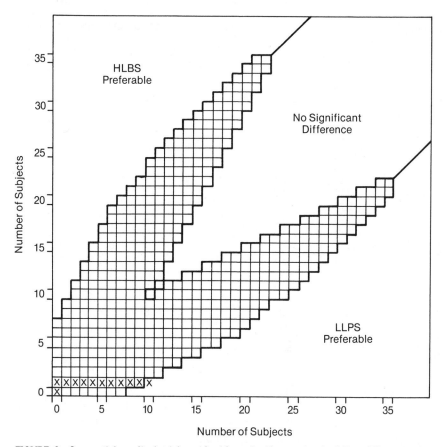

FIGURE 2   Sequential medical trials grid with a significance level of $P \leq 0.5$ comparing posttreatment results of LLPS with HLBS for Test 2 criterion.

LLPS in treatment of knee contractures of the immobile nursing home resident. The Table offers a synopsis of raw data from this study.

Discussion

16   A simple, noninvasive, nonstressful treatment is always desirable, especially in an elderly group. In this sample, patients did not appear to experience pain while receiving LLPS treatment. Trained physical

TABLE **PASSIVE RANGE OF MOTION CHANGES OF EACH SUBJECT**

Subject No.	Rx	PROM (° from 180°)		Change between Pre Rx and Post Rx	Post Rx Difference between LLPS and HLBS
		Pre Rx	Post Rx		
1	LLPS	− 50	− 46	4	
	HLBS	− 75	− 57	18	−14
2	LLPS	−132	−102	30	
	HLBS	−113	− 99	14	16
3	LLPS	− 95	− 80	15	
	HLBS	−102	− 97	5	10
4	LLPS	− 99	− 70	29	
	HLBS	− 80	− 67	13	16
5	LLPS	− 45	− 27	18	
	HLBS	− 48	− 40	8	10
6	LLPS	− 82	− 64	18	
	HLBS	− 70	− 67	3	12
7	LLPS	− 92	− 57	35	
	HLBS	− 60	− 56	4	31
8	LLPS	− 69	− 50	19	
	HLBS	− 68	− 74	− 6	25
9	LLPS	− 75	− 58	17	
	HLBS	− 60	− 70	−10	27
10	LLPS	− 53	− 20	33	
	HLBS	− 54	− 36	18	12
11	LLPS	−112	− 80	32	
	HLBS	−105	−108	3	29

therapy aides were instructed to implement the exercise program and apply the traction apparatus. Inconvenience to the nursing staff was minimal, and the LLPS device did not impede primary care needs of the patients, such as bathing and elimination.

17 Most of the subjects were characterized by a history of progressive mental confusion, reduction of mobility, and subsequent physical dependence. The use of traction as a treatment for knee contractures in this patient group was initiated long after the early physiological and possible morphological effects of immobility had developed. The goals of this treatment approach were to 1) reduce contractures to aid in ease of nursing care and 2) increase active movement abilities, including standing transfers.

18 Changes in activities of daily living (ADL) were not objectively measured in this study. None of these subjects, however, became ambulatory, and all continued to require maximal assistance in transferring. Considering the severity and duration of the contractures, as well as the general mental and physical debilitation of these subjects, the reduction in contractures was probably inadequate to affect functional level. With another group, ADL changes might have been used as a criterion for improvement. Further investigations could consider the effects of LLPS for early treatment of contractures in mentally alert hospitalized patients.

19 Individuals with severe joint restrictions, subjects 2 and 11 in the Table, demonstrate greater improvement with the LLPS treatment than those subjects whose initial restrictions were less dramatic. The number of subjects and study procedures cannot confirm this observation, but it does raise the question of whether contractures of different degrees of severity respond better to different stretching procedures. Other possible explanations may lie in the morphological and physiological changes specific to a given disease process. Patients in this study had a variety of diagnoses, as do most geriatric nursing home residents.

20 We presumed that the effects obtained in this study were the direct result of connective tissue lengthening. Alterations in neurophysiological input, and consequently, the gamma loop, may also have been a factor. Neurological changes occur rapidly and accommodate quickly, and, therefore, were not measured or focused on in this study.[12] The results of this study are in accordance with those of Warren et al who used a rat-tail tendon model to study the effects of load on tissue elongation.[13] Low-load, long-duration tension produced greater elongation of tissues than high-load, short-duration tension. Temperature, a variable not considered in this experiment with humans, was found by Warren et al to enhance tissue elongation in rats.[13]

21 Sapega et al have published a treatment protocol designed to increase ROM in the postreconstructed and immobilized knee.[16] Their protocol was based on principles evolved from the results of in vitro, connective-tissue studies in animals, including the study of Warren et al, and involved the use of heat in addition to low-load, long-duration tension. Their recommended treatment sequence is 1) heating of the shortened tissues, 2) applying the load while maintaining the elevated tissue temperature, 3) maintaining both the load and heat throughout the treatment period, 4) cooling the tissue below the normal body temperature before the load is removed, and 5) removing the load. No experimental data were presented. Sapega et al did not incorporate a traction component into their stretching technique.[16] We believed joint mechanics to be an important consideration. We attempted to apply the load in line with the tibia, so as to distract the knee, and reduce compressive forces that may be created by lengthening of imbalanced shortened tissues. The results of this study may partially reflect the difference in treatment times between the two groups. A future study is planned to compare results of light-load versus heavy-load, skin-traction progression with equal treatment time for groups.

Conclusion

22 Chronic knee flexion contractures are a familiar clinical problem to most physical therapists. This study was performed to compare the results of two methods of treatment (LLPS vs HLBS) in increasing the passive knee extension ROM of knee flexion contractures in a group of elderly, nonambulatory, nursing-home patients. The SMT design allowed the obvious preference for LLPS to be attained at the $p \leq .05$ significance level after only 11 subjects were assessed. The LLPS was found to be the more effective, acceptable, nonstressful treatment to the patient over a four-week period.

References

1. Halkovich, LR, Personius, WJ, Clamann, HP, et al: Effect of fluorimethane spray on passive hip flexion. Phys Ther 61:185–189, 1981.
2. Medeiros, JM, Smidt, GL, Burmeister, LF, et al: Influence of isometric exercise and passive stretch on hip joint motion. Phys Ther 57:518–523, 1977.
3. Tanigawa, MC: Comparison of the hold-relax procedure and passive mobilization on increasing muscle length. Phys Ther 52:725–735, 1972.
4. Akeson, W, Amiel, D, and Woo, S: Immobility effects on synovial joints: The pathomechanics of joint contracture. Biorheology 17:95–110, 1980.
5. Enneking, WF and Horowitz, M: The intra-articular effects of immobilization on the human knee. J Bone Joint Surg [Am] 57:973–985, 1972.
6. Lavigne, AB and Watkins, RP: Preliminary results on immobilization-induced stiffness of monkey knee joints and posterior capsules. In Perspectives in Biomedical Engineerings: Proceedings of a Symposium. Biological Engineering Society University of Strathclyde, Glascow, Scotland, Baltimore, MD, University Park Press, 1972, pp 177–179.
7. Tabary, JC, Tabary, C, and Tardieu, C: Physiological and structural changes in the cat's soleus muscle due to immobilization at different lengths by plaster casts. J Physiol 224:231–244, 1972.
8. Tardieu, C, Tabary, JC, Tabary, C, et al: Adaptation of connective tissue length to immobilization in the lengthened and shortened positions in cat soleus muscle. J Physiol 78:214–220, 1982.
9. Peacock, E: Comparison of collagenous tissue surrounding normal and immobilized joints. Surgical Forum 14:440–441, 1963.
10. Granit, R and Burke, RE: The control of movement and posture. Brain Res 53:1–28, 1973.
11. Kots, YM: The Organization of Voluntary Movement: Neurophysiological Mechanisms, New York, NY, Plenum Publishing Corp, 1977, pp 5–25.
12. Matthews, PBC: Mammalian Muscle Receptors and Their Central Actions. Baltimore, MD, Williams & Wilkins, 1972, pp 143–192, 481–606.

13. Warren, CG, Lehman, JF, and Koblanski, JN: Heat and stretch procedures: An evaluation using rat tail tendon. Arch Phys Med Rehabil 57:122–126, 1976.
14. Bross, I: Sequential medical plans. Biometrics 8:189–205, 1952.
15. Gonnella, C: Designs for clinical research. Phys Ther 53:1276–1283, 1973.
16. Sapega, AA, Quedenfeld, TC, Moyer, RA, et al: Biophysical factors in range-of-motion exercise. Physician and Sports Medicine 9:57–65, 1981.

The Effectiveness of Spinal Mobilisation in the Treatment of Low Back Pain: A Single Case Study

ALASDAIR J. M. BEATTIE

An ABAB single case study was conducted to assess the effectiveness of Maitland spinal mobilisation techniques in the treatment of lumbar back pain. Left-side lumbar flexion was taken as the dependent variable. It was predicted that implementation of treatment would result in an increase in left-side lumbar flexion not seen when treatment was withdrawn. This prediction is supported by the data collected. It was concluded that Maitland spinal mobilisation techniques were effective in the short-term treatment of low back pain, although it was suggested that further studies should re-examine subjects at set periods following termination of treatment to assess long-term effects.

Introduction

1 Low back pain is among the most common rheumatological complaints and is responsible for a substantial proportion of total morbidity and loss of work through illness. Frymoyer (1983, quoted in Pedretti, 1985) estimated that 217 million working days are lost annually in the USA due to back pain. However, objective data evaluating the treatment of low back pain through physiotherapeutic procedures are few. Of the many treatment modalities available to the clinician, the mobilisation technique as described by Maitland (1986) was selected for effectiveness assessment in this case.

2 Maitland (1977) defines mobilisation as 'passive movements performed in such a way (particularly in relation to speed of the movements) that at all times they are within the control of the patient so that he

A. J. M. Beattie, Department of Physiotherapy, North Middlesex Hospital, Sterling Way, London N18 1QX, UK
Accepted for publication October 1990

can prevent the movement if he so chooses'. In his application of graded passive movement, Maitland uses a set sequence determined by the site of pain and the behaviour of the joint to the testing movement. These considerations are secondary to the information gained from the examination.

3   Maitland (1977) described the three main roles of mobilisation as follows:

   (1) The restoring of structures within a joint to their normal positions or pain-free positions so as to allow a full range of painless movement.
   (2) Stretching a stiff painless joint to restore range.
   (3) The relieving of pain.

4   Grieve (1986) also postulated that repetitive rhythmical movement would:
   - Affect the hydrostatics of the disc and the vertebral bodies;
   - Activate the type I and II mechanoreceptors in the capsule of the facet joint influencing the spinal gaiting mechanisms; and
   - Assist in the pumping effect on the venous plexus of the vertebral segment.

5   Historically, however, the whole subject of manual treatment has always been contentious, with much factional and inter-professional rivalry.

6   In relation to common vertebral syndromes, physiotherapy has undergone very considerable changes. In the critical evaluation of treatment results, Grieve (1986) quotes his work and that of other clinicians (Cyriax, 1975; Maitland, 1977; Kaltenborn, 1970) as showing the inadequacy of the universal application of, for example, thermal techniques, back extension exercises, lumbar flexion exercises, and a new systematic treatment approach has been developed. This approach has remained non-doctrinal, based on careful analysis establishing dysfunction of the vertebral segment with consequential changes in the neuro-musculoskeletal structures. Appropriate physiotherapy techniques such as manual mobilisation are then supposedly used to normalise the function.

7   Sims-Williams and colleagues conducted studies in 1978 and 1979 that took the form of controlled double-blind trials of mobilisation and manipulation for low back pain compared with placebo physiotherapy. The clinicians concluded in 1978 that a course of mobilisation and manipulation may hasten improvement of nonspecific lumbar pain symptoms. However, in 1979, following the same procedure, they concluded that no definite advantage could be associated with mobilisation and manipulation compared with placebo.

8   Glover et al (1974) compared manipulation with short-wave diathermy

in factory workers complaining of low back pain. Immediately after manipulation, many subjects obtained pain relief, though there was little difference between the two groups a few days post-treatment. Bergquist and Larsson (1977), however, concluded from their studies that spinal mobilisation was more beneficial than placebo physiotherapy in the treatment of low back pain.

9   This single case study tried to assess the effectiveness of spinal mobilisation in the treatment of low back problems in a single subject. It was predicted that the implementation of treatment would result in an increase in left-side lumbar flexion, not seen when treatment was withdrawn.

Method

SUBJECT

10 A.L. was an unemployed 20-year-old female who complained of low back pain of 2 months' duration and was identified from the waiting list of a physiotherapy out-patient department. The patient complained of episodic back pain for 1 year, the present exacerbation having no recallable precipitating injury or factor. Though the pain level had reached a static state, the patient complained of pain on the left lumbar area, left buttock and thigh when bending or twisting to the left. The patient had been out of work for 18 months, leading a fairly sedentary life-style, notably watching television in a soft armchair for 2–3 hours per day. She was able to carry out all activities of daily life, though was unable to sit for longer than 30 minutes.

11 None of the exclusion criteria used in this study for Maitland manipulations were relevant to the present case (see Appendix). The relevant findings from preliminary examinations are summarised below.

(1) *Pain.* The patient presented with pain in the left lumbar area, occasionally radiating to the left buttock.

(2) *Posture.* The patient's spine was laterally shifted to the right with a decreased lumbar lordosis. The patient stood with very little weight-bearing through her left leg.

(3) *Active measurements.* A.L.'s range of motion was restricted in the following movements:
- Left-side flexion (three-quarters range of movement, pain end of range);
- Left rotation (half range of movement, pain end of range); and
- Flexion (half range of movement, pain end of range).

(4) Left straight leg raising was limited to 50 degrees.

(5) Palpation according to the Maitland method of examination repro-
duced pain with posterior anterior central vertebral pressure
(PACVP) at the L_4/L_5 level and left unilateral pressure at the L_4/L_5 lumbar level in the outer range.

12   A.L.'s consent was obtained prior to the study taking place.

PROCEDURE

13   An ABAB design single case study was used, in which:
   - A1 = baseline phase;
   - B1 = primary intervention phase;
   - A2 = withdrawal of treatment phase; and
   - B2 = reintroduction of treatment phase.

14   The parameter measured was left-side lumbar flexion, this being one
of the limited ranges of motion. Pain was not selected because objective measurement is difficult. Left-side lumbar flexion was recorded
as follows:
   (1) The patient stood erect, hands by her side.
   (2) The patient then slid her left hand down along the lateral aspect
   of her left leg as far as possible.
   (3) The final position of the tip of the middle finger was then marked
   with a pen and the patient was allowed to straighten once more.
   (4) The perpendicular distance from this mark to the floor was then
   recorded.

15   Right-side lumbar flexion was also recorded in the same manner. Both
the patient and a relative were instructed in this measurement technique. During the initial baseline phase, the patient received no contact
with the physiotherapist for 5 days. The patient collected the baseline
measurements (A1 phase) with the aid of a relative. The data were
collected twice a day at 10.00 and 14.00 h for 5 days for a total of 15
measures.

16   On day 7, the patient attended the out-patient department. Prior to
treatment, both left- and right-side lumbar flexion were recorded. The
patient received treatment in the form of Maitland mobilisation on
days 7, 9, 12, 14 and 18 of the study and the data were recorded. On
each occasion, three mobilisations were performed and three measurements taken, and any subjective change in symptoms noted.

17   Throughout the study, grade and duration of mobilisation were adapted,
guided by the therapist's clinical knowledge as signs and symptoms
altered. Initially, the patient was treated with grade II Maitland right
lumbar rotation techniques as the underlying problem appeared to be
pain. After two therapy sessions, the grade of mobilisation was sub-

sequently increased to grade III, as the patient's pain had resolved sufficiently to enable treatment to increase the range of lumbar side flexion.

18 During the A2 phase—days 18–28—treatment was withdrawn. Treatment and measurement resumed on days 28, 30, 32 and 35, when the patient was discharged (the B2 phase).

Results

19 Data were collected on both left- and right-side flexion using the procedure described above for the duration of the study. Over this time period, the value (50 cm) observed for right-side flexion did not vary; for this reason, only the data for left-side flexion will be considered in the discussion below.

20 During the baseline period (A1), data were collected twice a day (10.00 and 14.00 h) on 5 consecutive days (see Table 1). A mean value of 62 cm was observed for left-side flexion during phase A1.

21 During the first treatment phase (B1), the data were again collected twice per day, once before treatment and once after treatment for 5 consecutive therapy sessions (see Table 2). The mean value for left-side flexion during phase B1 was 56.8 cm. The data demonstrate a relatively regular pattern (improvement followed by some deterioration, etc.), and this must be taken to reflect the fact that while performance improved as a result of treatment, this improvement was not maintained to the same level by the time measurement was taken on the subsequent day (see Fig. 1).

22 During the second baseline phase (A2), the data were again collected on a twice-daily basis at the same time intervals given above (see Table 3). The mean value for left-side flexion during phase A2 was 53.2 cm.

TABLE 1 **LEFT-SIDE LUMBAR FLEXION (cm): BASELINE PHASE (A1)**

	Recorded Measurement (cm)	
Day	**10.00 h**	**14.00 h**
1	62.0	62.0
2	61.0	62.0
3	64.0	63.0
4	62.0	62.0
5	61.0	62.0

TABLE 2   **LEFT-SIDE LUMBAR
FLEXION (cm): PRIMARY
INTERVENTION PHASE (B1)**

	Recorded Measurement (cm)	
Day	Prior to Treatment	Following Mobilisation
7	62.0	60.0
9	62.0	57.0
11	58.0	54.0
14	56.0	53.0
18	54.0	52.0

23 During the final treatment phase (B2), the data were collected both before and after treatment on 4 consecutive days. The mean value for left-side flexion during this period was found to be 51 cm. Performance during phase B2 did not show the same variability as performance during phase B1. It should be noted that for five of the eight observations, the degree of left-side flexion equalled the degree of right-side flexion (see Fig. 1).

24 Autocorrelation coefficients were computed for each phase of the study to determine whether the data were serially dependent. No significant autocorrelations were found. Autocorrelations of 0.27, 0.51, 0.4 and 0.5 were found for A1, B1, A2 and B2 respectively (Bartlett's test figures for these conditions being 0.63, 0.63, 0.82 and 0.71 respectively).

25 Because there was no serial dependency, a one-factor ANOVA was performed. A highly significant F value was obtained [$F(3,30) = 42.25$, $P<0.0001$]. A *post-hoc* comparison of the different conditions using the Student–Newman–Keuls test revealed that all the conditions were significantly different from each other at the 0.05 level apart from A2 and B2. The failure to find significance here probably reflects the small number of observations in A2.

26 An assessment of linearity revealed marked differences between the different phases. For A1 and A2, the slopes of side flexion against

TABLE 3   **LEFT-SIDE LUMBAR
FLEXION (cm): WITHDRAWAL
PHASE (A2)**

	Recorded Measurement (cm)	
Day	10.00 h	14.00 h
21	52.0	52.0
23	54.0	54.0
25	54.0	53.0

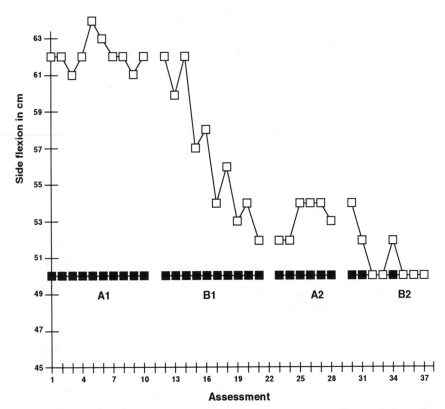

FIGURE 1   Changes in left-side flexion with respect to time and physiotherapeutic intervention. ■, right-side flexion; □, left-side flexion.

assessment were close to 0 or positive (− 0.02 for A1 and 0.30 for A2).
This indicates that performance during these phases was either static
(in the case of A1) or deteriorating (in the case of A2). For B1 and B2,
the slopes of side flexion against assessment were both larger and
negative (− 1.12 for B1 and − 0.52 for B2). This suggests an improvement in side flexion during these two phases. The percentage of variance that could be accounted for by linearity was 0.4, 86, 38 and 72%
for A1, B1, A2 and B2 respectively.

Discussion

27   The results from the study show that at the two phases where physiotherapeutic intervention occurred, left-side lumbar flexion markedly
increased in its range of movement. From Fig. 1 it can be seen that

patient improvement was attained more rapidly at the initial treatment stage compared with the reintroduction stage. At the baseline stage, the condition was static.

28 It could be argued that the patient's condition recovered spontaneously over the study period. This is unlikely in this case, however, as the latest episode had developed into a chronic, static problem and would be unlikely to resolve in such a short time period. If the back condition was demonstrating spontaneous recovery, this would become apparent during the baseline phase of the study. As range of movement did not improve over this period, we can assume this is not the case.

29 The 'placebo effect'—referring to any effect of intervention which cannot be attributed to the specific action of treatment given—could also be cited as a possible confounding variable. In some cases, simply a visit to the hospital and a consultation with a health care professional is sufficient to cause a remission of signs and symptoms. If a placebo effect was occurring in this study, we would have expected to see a significant improvement in the patient's condition over the baseline period, after the initial consultation. There was no such improvement and therefore this effect had been controlled, as far as was possible.

30 The patient was questioned at each treatment session as to whether her daily pattern of life with respect to her back had altered since the previous consultation. She claimed neither to have changed her daily pattern of life or her position of rest throughout the day.

31 A.L. was always treated at the same time of day to ensure that her back would be in the same approximate condition with regards to daily pattern of pain at each consultation. The surrounding environment was also kept constant throughout the study period. Sabshin and Ramot (1956) found through their studies that a varying hospital environment can affect treatment results. It appears, therefore, that the study was well controlled and that the treatment results were due to physiotherapeutic intervention.

32 The implications of these findings first suggest that the role of mobilisation described by Maitland (1977) stands up—a full range of painless movement was achieved through the techniques employed. The results would seem to support the views of Bergquist and Larsson (1977), that intervention produces more beneficial treatment results than placebo physiotherapy or non-intervention.

33 Sims-Williams et al (1979) postulated that the benefits of mobilisation were probably restricted to patients likely to recover spontaneously and that patients that had required specialist referral were not likely to benefit. During the intervention phase, A.L. did not seem to recover spontaneously, but had reached a long-term static level, which appears

contrary to Sims-Williams et al (1979). Furthermore, A.L. had been referred to physiotherapy by a specialist, a consultant rheumatologist.

34   Further studies should follow-up patients at set intervals post-discharge to determine whether or not mobilisations have a long-term effect.

Conclusion

Considering this evidence, the null hypothesis can be rejected. The findings of this study suggest consistency with the prediction that implementation of treatment results in an increase in left-side lumbar flexion not seen when treatment is omitted.

References

Bergquist-Ullman M, Larsson U 1977 Acute low back pain in industry. Acta Orthopaedica Scandinavica 170 (Suppl):1–117

Cyriax J 1975 Textbook of orthopaedic medicine, Vol. 1, 6th edn. Ballière Tindall, London

Glover JR, Morris JG, Khosla T 1974 Back pain: A randomised clinical trial of rotational manipulation of the trunk. British Journal of Industrial Medicine 31:59–64

Grieve GP 1986 Modern manual therapy of the vertebral column. Churchill Livingstone, Edinburgh

Kaltenborn EM 1970 Mobilisation of the spinal column. New Zealand University Press, Wellington

Maitland GD 1977 Peripheral manipulation, 2nd edn. Butterworths, London

Maitland GD 1986 Vertebral manipulation, 5th edn. Butterworths, London

Pedretti LW 1985 Occupational therapy: Practice skills for physical dysfunction, 2nd edn. CV Mosby, St Louis

Sabshin M, Ramot J 1956 Pharmacotherapeutic evaluation and the psychiatric setting. Archives of Neurology and Psychiatry 75:362–370

Sims-Williams H, Jayson MIV, Young SMS, Baddeley H, Collins E 1978 Controlled trial of mobilisation and manipulation for patients with low back pain in general practice. British Medical Journal xi:1338–1340

Sims-Williams H, Jayson MIV, Young SMS, Baddeley H, Collins E 1979 Controlled trial of mobilisation and manipulation for low back pain: Hospital patients. British Medical Journal xi:1318–1320

Appendix: Exclusion Criteria for Maitland Manipulations

1   Pregnancy.

2   Disorders of the spinal cord or cauda equina.

3   Spinal disease.

4 Inflammatory or other specific disorders of the spine, e.g. ankylosing spondylitis, Paget's disease, vertebral collapse.

5 Marked obesity.

6 Previous back surgery.

7 Previous spinal physiotherapy.

8 Disability income or pending litigation.

9 Long-term steroid prescription.

10 Long-term anti-coagulant prescription.

11 Recent marked weight loss.

Exercise Response in Children with and without Juvenile Rheumatoid Arthritis: A Case-Comparison Study

MANUELA JASSO GIANNINI and
ELIZABETH J PROTAS

Key Words • Bicycle ergometer • Child • Exercise • Juvenile arthritis • Oxygen consumption

The primary purpose of the study was to compare the response to bicycle ergometer exercise in children with and without juvenile rheumatoid arthritis (JRA). Heart rate, exercise duration, highest work load completed, and peak oxygen consumption (peak $\dot{V}O_2$) were compared. A secondary purpose of the study was to determine the relationship between peak $\dot{V}O_2$ and articular disease severity. Thirty children with JRA and 30 controls matched for age, sex, and body surface area (BSA) were the subjects. Peak $\dot{V}O_2$ was determined by an open-circuit computerized gas analysis system. Peak $\dot{V}O_2$, highest work load completed, exercise duration, and peak heart rate were significantly lower among the children with JRA than their respective controls.

M Jasso Giannini, PhD, PT, was a doctoral student, School of Physical Therapy, Texas Woman's Univeristy, 1130 MD Anderson Blvd, Houston, TX 77030-2897, when this study was completed in partial fulfillment of her degree requirements. Address all correspondence to Ms Jasso Giannini at 3513 Telford St, Cincinnati, OH 45220 (USA).

EJ Protas, PhD, PT, is Professor and Assistant Dean, School of Physical Therapy, Texas Woman's University.

This work was supported by a grant from the Arthritis Health Professions Association, National Office of the Arthritis Foundation.

This study was approved by the institutional review boards of Texas Woman's University, Baylor College of Medicine, Texas Children's Hospital, and Kelsey-Seybold Clinic, Houston, TX.

This article was submitted May 16, 1991, and was accepted January 16, 1992.

294

Submaximal heart rate was significantly higher for the children with JRA. There was no difference in resting heart rate between the two groups. There was no relationship between peak $\dot{V}o_2$ and articular disease severity among the children with JRA. The results suggest that aerobic conditioning programs may be indicated soon after diagnosis for patients with JRA, regardless of the severity of their articular disease. One subject with JRA and 2 control subjects reported light-headedness and dizziness, and 1 subject with JRA complained of increased knee swelling. We recommend that physical therapists monitor patients for signs of exercise intolerance and joint symptoms during exercise training sessions. [Jasso Giannini M, Protas EJ. Exercise response in children with and without juvenile rheumatoid arthritis: a case-comparison study. Phys Ther 1992;72:365–372.]

1 Juvenile rheumatoid arthritis (JRA) is the most common of the pediatric rheumatic diseases, with an annual incidence of approximately 1.4 cases per 10,000 children and a prevalence of 0.5 to 1 case per 1,000 in the United States.[1-3] Chronic pain, synovitis, deformity, and growth disturbances are common manifestations of the disease.[4,5] It has been documented in the literature that children with a chronic illness are unable to tolerate as much exercise as their "healthy" peers.[6,7] Bar-Or[6,7] hypothesizes that this lower tolerance is a result of hypoactivity, which leads to deconditioning, and specific pathophysiologic factors that limit one or more exercise-related functions.

2 We have previously shown that peak oxygen consumption ($\dot{V}o_2$) is significantly lower in children with JRA than in children without JRA.[8] Physical therapists prescribe exercise programs for children with JRA routinely. These exercise programs are aimed at improving range of motion (ROM), muscle strength, and cardiovascular endurance. There is, however, little quantitative information on cardiovascular response to exercise for this group of children. Characterization of exercise response in this pediatric population and comparison with a control group are essential for identification of functional exercise deficits in children with JRA. Heart rate, exercise duration, and work load are clinical variables that can then be monitored easily to provide the clinician with useful information about the patient's functional exercise tolerance.

3 The primary purpose of this investigation was to characterize the exercise response of a group of patients with JRA and compare this

exercise response with that of a group of healthy controls matched for age, sex, and body surface area (BSA). The variables examined were (1) heart rate (resting, submaximal, and peak), (2) peak $\dot{V}O_2$, (3) highest work load completed, and (4) exercise duration. We hypothesized that heart rate would be of greater magnitude in the children with JRA and that they would not be able to exercise as long as their matched controls. Additionally, we expected that our earlier findings of lower aerobic capacity and lower work load completed[8] would be confirmed in a separate and larger sample of subjects. A secondary purpose of this study was to determine the relationship between peak $\dot{V}O_2$, the "gold standard" for measuring aerobic conditioning, and two commonly used measures of articular disease severity. We hypothesized that a strong, inverse correlation exists between peak $\dot{V}O_2$ and articular disease severity. That is, a patient with more severe joint disease will be more hypoactive and thus will become deconditioned to a greater extent than a patient with less severe joint disease. Although our previous research[8] did not support this hypothesis, we believed that the small sample size warranted further testing of our hypothesis.

Method

4   Our data were obtained as part of a larger study that compared exercise response and muscle performance in children with JRA and in matched controls. All data for an individual subject were collected during a single day.

SUBJECTS

5   The subjects were 30 patients with JRA and 30 controls with no history of an acute or chronic illness matched by age, sex, and BSA. All patients were within 1 year of age of their respective controls (mean difference = 0.29 year); all subjects were between 7 and 17 years of age. Additionally, all patients had a BSA within 0.4 m² of their respective controls (mean difference = 0.04 m²). The patient population was recruited from the Pediatric Rheumatology Center, Texas Children's Hospital (Houston, Tex), and all patients fulfilled the 1977 revised American Rheumatism Association criteria for a diagnosis of JRA.[9]

6   Patients who, in the opinion of the examining physician, required a change in their current medical therapy were excluded from the study. Additional exclusion criteria were (1) insufficient lower-extremity ROM to pedal a bicycle, (2) insufficient mouth-opening capability (for the mouthpiece) attributable to temporomandibular joint involvement, (3)

bilateral knee pain on resisted extension (for purposes of muscle performance testing, and (4) lower-extremity surgery in the previous 6 months. Subjects with contraindications to or special precautions for exercise, as established by the Ad Hoc Committee on Exercise Testing in the Pediatric Age Group,[10] were also excluded. Consecutive patients (and their parents) who were scheduled to be seen by the pediatric rheumatologist and who met the criteria for diagnosis, age, and stable medical status (ie, required no change in their current medical therapy) were informed about the study and asked to participate. The controls were recruited through professional colleagues from The Texas Medical Center (Houston, Tex).

7 No attempt was made to control the antirheumatic drug therapy of the patients. Many of the patients were taking a combination of nonsteroidal anti-inflammatory drugs and disease-modifying antirheumatic drugs. Twenty-three patients were taking a variety of nonsteroidal anti-inflammatory agents, 8 were taking oral gold, 3 were taking injectable gold, 2 were taking low-dose prednisone, 3 were taking low-dose methotrexate, and 1 was taking hydroxychloroquine. Three patients were not receiving medication at the time of testing. Written informed consent was obtained from the children and their parents. Verbal assent was also obtained from the children.

ASSESSMENT OF ARTICULAR DISEASE ACTIVITY

8 A joint evaluation was performed by the same physical therapist (MJG) for all patients. Two measures of articular disease severity commonly used by clinicians and researchers were derived from the joint evaluation: (1) the number of joints with active arthritis and (2) the articular disease severity score. The joint evaluation and the articular disease severity grading were performed according to the standardized methodology used by the Pediatric Rheumatology Collaborative Study Group.[11] Four clinical indexes of articular inflammation were assessed: swelling, pain on passive motion (POM), tenderness to palpation, and passive limitation of motion (LOM). A joint with active arthritis is defined as a joint with swelling or, if no swelling is present, a joint with passive LOM accompanied by either heat, pain, or tenderness. Severity of joint involvement is graded on a four-point scale (ie, 0–3) for swelling, POM, and tenderness to palpation. Swelling is graded as follows: 0 = no swelling, 1 = mild swelling (definite swelling, but with no loss of bony contour), 2 = moderate swelling (loss of distinctiveness of bony contour), and 3 = marked swelling (bulging synovial proliferation with cystic characteristics or effusion). Pain on motion and tenderness to palpation are graded as follows: 0 = no POM or tenderness, 1 = mild POM or tenderness (patient complains of pain or tenderness), 2 = moderate POM or tenderness (patient withdraws or changes facial expression upon joint motion or palpation), and 3 = severe POM or tenderness (patient responds markedly to joint motion or palpation). Passive LOM was graded on the following scale: 0 = full ROM, 1 = 1% to 25% LOM, 2 = 26% to 50% LOM, 3 = 51% to 75% LOM, and 4 = 76% to 100% LOM (fibrous or bony ankylosis). The articular disease severity score is calculated by summing all the scores.

INSTRUMENTATION

9 An open-circuit computerized gas analysis system[*] was used to measure $\dot{V}O_2$. The system consists of a 10-L spirometer that measures gas volume, an oxygen analyzer that measures oxygen concentration, and a carbon dioxide analyzer that measures carbon dioxide concentration. The air-collection equipment consisted of a two-way respiratory valve that collects the expired air, a rubber mouthpiece, a noseclip, and a flexible connecting hose to the gas analyzers (Fig. 1). Before testing a subject, the spirometer and gas analyzers were calibrated with known air volumes and gas concentrations according to the manufacturer's specifications. A Monark bicycle ergometer[†] was used to measure work load. The ergometer was calibrated prior to the beginning of the study and checked weekly throughout the study. Heart rate was monitored with the Narco Physiograph CMP-4A[‡] using a CM5 chest lead configuration.

BICYCLE ERGOMETER PROTOCOL

10 We chose cycling as an exercise in order to avoid weight-bearing stress to arthritic joints. A continuous graded bicycle ergometer exercise protocol was used, modified from the continuous graded exercise test used by James et al.[12] The exercise protocol involved increasing the work load by 25-W increments every 2 minutes while pedaling at a constant rate of 60 rpm. The work loads were increased until voluntary exhaustion or until the child was no longer able to pedal at a constant rate. The starting work load was determined by the BSA of the child.

[*]Sensormedics Manufacturing Co, 1630 S State College Blvd, Anaheim, CA 92806.
[†]Monark Model 5134530, Quinton Instruments Co, 3051 44th Ave W, Seattle, WA 98199.
[‡]Narco Biosystems, PO Box 12511, Houston, TX 77061.

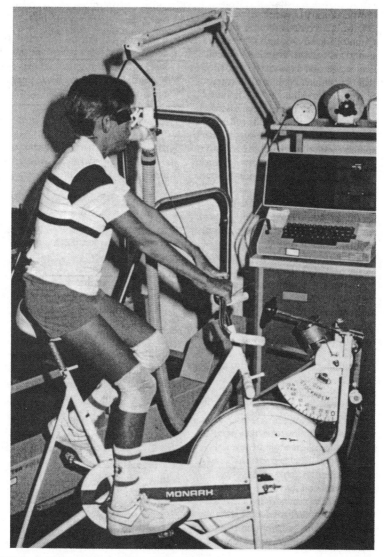

FIGURE 1   Subject undergoing bicycle ergometer test.

The BSA was calculated from the Du Bois nomogram, using height and weight according to the following formula:

$$\text{Surface area} = \text{weight}^{0.425} \times \text{height}^{0.725} \times 71.84$$

11 Children with a BSA of less than 1.2 m² started at 25 W; those with a BSA greater than 1.2 m² started at 50 W. Each subject was given a chance to establish the pedaling rate with verbal cues from the investigator before beginning the exercise test. The investigator monitored pedaling rate with a stopwatch and verbally cued each subject periodically during the test. The seat of the bicycle was adjusted so that the subject's knee was in 15 degrees of flexion when the pedal was in the down position. The children were encouraged verbally to continue throughout the exercise procedure. During the first 2 minutes after stopping exercise, the subjects continued to pedal slowly at 20 rpm to prevent blood pooling. Heart rate was recorded with subjects in the seated position at 1-minute intervals at rest, during exercise, and during recovery for 10 minutes. Oxygen consumption was recorded every 20 seconds during exercise and recovery. Blood pressure was measured manually with a mercury sphygmomanometer[*] to monitor clinical response to exercise.

12 Peak $\dot{V}O_2$ was defined as the highest rate of $\dot{V}O_2$ achieved in any 20-second period. The highest work load completed was the highest rate of work that was reached and maintained for the 2-minute duration of each stage of exercise. Peak heart rate was determined for the final minute of exercise of the highest work load. Submaximal heart rate was recorded at the end of the second stage of exercise.

RELIABILITY TESTING

13 The test-retest reliability for the open-circuit method of determining maximal oxygen consumption ($\dot{V}O_2$max) had yielded a Pearson product-moment correlation coefficient (r) of .95 with a standard error of $0.84 \text{ mL·kg}^{-1}\text{·min}^{-1}$.[13] When the computerized gas analysis system used in our study is compared with the $\dot{V}O_2$max values of a referee system (Applied Electrochemistry oxygen analyzer,[†] Beckman LB-2 carbon dioxide analyzer,[‡] and Parkinson-Cowan CD4 gasometer[||]), a Pearson correlation coefficient of .989 and a standard error of $1.1 \text{ mL·kg}^{-1}\text{·min}^{-1}$ result, demonstrating concurrent validity.[14] This finding demonstrates that the gas analysis system used in our study yields reliable and valid measurements during maximum exercise of nondisabled adults.

14 The reliability of peak $\dot{V}O_2$ measurements in the JRA population using the computerized gas analysis system was determined in a separate group of patients performing the exercise protocol described earlier. Peak $\dot{V}O_2$ was recorded during three test trials within a 3-week period in 10 children with JRA. The mean age for this group was 10.9 years

---

[*]Baumamometer Standley Model, WA Baum Co, Copiaque, NY 11726.

[†]Applied Electrochemistry, 735 N Pastoria Ave, Sunnyvale, CA 94086.

[‡]Beckman Instruments Inc, 2500 Harbor Blvd, Fullerton, CA 92634.

[||]Sensormedics Manufacturing Co, State College Blvd, Anaheim, CA 92806.

TABLE 1 **MEANS,**[a] **STANDARD DEVIATIONS, AND COEFFICIENTS OF VARIATION FOR PEAK OXYGEN CONSUMPTION**[b] **IN PATIENTS WITH JUVENILE RHEUMATOID ARTHRITIS (N = 10)**

Patient No.	$\overline{X}$	SD	CV[c]
1	52.0	2.3	4.5
2	30.4	8.7	28.5
3	39.2	11.9	30.5
4	24.8	1.3	5.2
5	37.3	2.6	6.9
6	33.5	2.6	7.7
7	30.1	0.4	1.3
8	24.8	5.8	23.2
9	37.4	4.8	12.8
10	32.8	2.6	7.9

[a]Mean of three trials.
[b]Measured in mL $O_2 \cdot kg^{-1} \cdot min^{-1}$.
[c]Coefficient of variation expressed as a percentage.

(SD = 2.4, range = 8.3–14.8). The mean disease duration was 5.5 years (SD = 3.7, range = 1.4–11.4), and the mean age at disease onset was 5.6 years (SD = 2.5, range = 1.1–8.9). The mean number of active joints was 13 (SD = 12, range = 0–35), and the mean articular disease severity score was 35 (SD = 33, range = 2–95). The means, standard deviations, and coefficients of variation of the three test trials were calculated for each subject to determine the within-subject variability and are presented in Table 1. The coefficient of variation for the group was 12.8%, and the standard error for the group was 3.4. Rothstein[15] notes that the coefficient of variation can be used to estimate the percentage of variation that can be expected in a measurement solely because of measurement error when no intersubject variability is expected and is a useful way to analyze the reliability of instrument-based measurements.

15 The reliability of $\dot{V}O_2$ measurements in nondisabled children has been investigated using the bicycle ergometer; the mean coefficients of variation between tests ranged from 2% to 5.3%.[16,17] Cumming et al[16] reported a mean coefficient of variation of 4.5% (range = 2%–9%) for children exercising to exhaustion on 12 different occasions (over a 6-day period) on the bicycle ergometer. Subjects exercised 6 minutes at a submaximal work load, immediately followed by a maximal work load. Boileau et al[17] reported a group mean coefficient of variation of 5.3% for the bicycle ergometer when two tests were administered within a 2-week period. Subjects were 21 boys with a mean age of 12.8 years. The bicycle test began at an initial load of 1.5 kilopond-meters, and the resistance thereafter was increased by 0.5 kilopond-meter every 3 minutes until voluntary exhaustion or until the subject could not maintain a pedaling rate of 60 rpm.

16 The intrasubject variability of children with chronic disease can be higher than that of children without chronic disease.[18] Measurements obtained from seven of our subjects had a mean coefficient of variation of 6.6%, which is within the range of children without chronic disease. Three subjects had variations on the order of 23% to 30% between trials. We believe that this finding may reflect variations in their articular disease during the 3-week testing period. Our data did not show any trend for trial. We chose to limit our measures to a single testing day for any one subject in order to limit intrasubject variability.

17 The reliability of our measurements of maximal heart rate was established in a previous study of 15 adults aged 20 to 30 years.[19] These subjects underwent maximal exercise tests once a week for a 3-week period. Heart rates were monitored continuously during the tests. Peak heart rates were calculated for the final minute of the last work load completed. The means and standard deviations of peak heart rates for each testing session were calculated. A one-way analysis of variance (ANOVA) for repeated measures on heart rate was used to compare the means, and an intraclass correlation coefficient ($ICC[1,1]$) was performed to determine the strength of the relationship between the three grand means of heart rate.[19] The means and standard deviations for the three test sessions were 193 ± 7.2, 194 ± 9.9, and 194 ± 9.9. There were no significant differences between the means ($F = 0.10$, $df = 2$). Using an upper limit of $+1.00$ and a lower limit of -0.50, the ICC was $-.43$, indicating a very strong correlation of peak heart rates for the three test sessions. Our method for measuring heart rate yields reliable measurements.

DATA ANALYSIS

18 Differences in peak $\dot{V}O_2$, exercise duration, and heart rate (resting, peak, and submaximal) between the patients and their respective controls were tested for statistical significance using a Student's paired t test for one-tailed comparison. The distribution of paired differences was tested for normality by the Anderson-Darling test prior to conducting statistical procedures that require a Gaussian distribution (as performed by the PC!INFO Retriever Data Systems version 3.0 computer program*). The Wilcoxon matched-pairs signed-rank test was

---

*PC!INFO Retriever Data Systems, 1102 33rd Ave S, Seattle, WA 98144.

TABLE 2   **COMPARISON OF MATCHING VARIABLES BETWEEN PATIENTS WITH JUVENILE RHEUMATOID ARTHRITIS (JRA) AND THEIR MATCHED CONTROLS**

Variable	JRA Group (n = 30)	Control Group (n = 30)	t[a]
Age (y)			
$\overline{X}$	11.4	11.1	0.3[b]
SD	2.7	2.8	
Range	7.2–17.3	7–17.4	
BSA[c] (m²)			
$\overline{X}$	1.23	1.27	0.3[b]
SD	0.26	0.29	
Range	0.83–1.74	0.78–1.72	

[a]One-tailed t test.
[b]Not significant.
[c]Body surface area.

used to test for paired differences in the highest work load completed. The alpha, or Type I error, level was set at .05.

19 Pearson's product-moment correlation (r) was used to determine the relationship between peak $\dot{V}O_2$ and the number of joints with active arthritis. Spearman rank-order correlation was used to describe the relationship between peak $\dot{V}O_2$ and the severity score.

Results

20 There were no significant differences in mean age of BSA between the two groups (Tab. 2). The clinical characteristics of the patients with JRA are shown in Table 3. Three distinct types of JRA are recognized: systemic JRA, which is characterized by intermittent fever (>39.4°C), rheumatoid rash, and arthritis; polyarticular JRA, in which five or more joints are affected with arthritis without systemic manifestations; and

TABLE 3   **CLINICAL CHARACTERISTICS AMONG PATIENTS WITH JUVENILE RHEUMATOID ARTHRITIS (n = 30)**

	Disease Duration (y)	Age at Disease Onset (y)	Number of Joints with Active Arthritis	Articular Disease Severity Score
$\overline{X}$	5.3	6.1	16	48
SD	3.3	4.4	19	56
Range	0.3–13.2	0.9–15.6	0–60	0–181

TABLE 4   **FREQUENCY OF JOINTS IN PATIENTS WITH ACTIVE JUVENILE RHEUMATOID ARTHRITIS (n = 30)**

Joint	Percentage of Patients
Temporomandibular joint	6.7
Shoulder	3.3
Elbow	23.3
Wrist	60.0
Fingers	56.6
Hip	13.3
Knee	66.7
Ankle	50.0
Toes	53.3
Cervical spine	6.7
Sacroiliac joint	3.3

pauciarticular JRA, in which arthritis alone is present in four or fewer joints.[4,9] Seventeen children had polyarticular JRA, 11 children had pauciarticular JRA, and 2 children had systemic JRA with polyarticular manifestations. The distribution of the joints with active arthritis is shown in Table 4.

21 Comparisons of heart rates between the two groups are shown in Table 5. Peak heart rate attained by the patients was significantly lower than that achieved by the controls. In the patient group, peak heart rate averaged 185 bpm (SD = 16, range = 170–210) versus 195 bpm (SD = 10, range = 132–208) for the controls. The patients exercised at a significantly higher percentage of their maximal heart rate than did the controls during submaximal exercise. Submaximal heart rate in the patients averaged 176 bpm (SD = 17, range = 132–199) and 163 bpm (SD = 16, range = 135–195) in the controls. There was no difference in the resting heart rate between the two groups.

TABLE 5   **COMPARISON OF HEART RATE[a] (HR) BETWEEN PATIENTS WITH JUVENILE RHEUMATOID ARTHRITIS (JRA) AND THEIR MATCHED CONTROLS**

Variable	JRA Group (n = 30)		Control Group (n = 30)		t^b
	X̄	SD	X̄	SD	
Resting HR	85	14	84	12	1.51
Peak HR	185	16	195	10	−2.645[c]
Submaximal HR	176	17	163	16	3.528[c]

[a]Measured in beats per minute.
[b]Paired one-tailed t test, df = 29.
[c]$p < .05$.

TABLE 6 **COMPARISON OF PEAK OXYGEN CONSUMPTION ($\dot{V}o_2$)[a] AND EXERCISE DURATION[b] BETWEEN PATIENTS WITH JUVENILE RHEUMATOID ARTHRITIS (JRA) AND THEIR MATCHED CONTROLS**

Variable	JRA Group (n = 30)		Control Group (n = 30)		t[c]
	X̄	SD	X̄	SD	
Peak $\dot{V}o_2$	32.0	8.8	36.9	6.5	−3.573[d]
Exercise duration	5.4	1.6	7.1	1.4	−4.957[d]

[a]Measured in mL $O_2 \cdot kg^{-1} \cdot min^{-1}$.
[b]Measured in minutes.
[c]Paired, one-tailed t test, $df = 29$.
[d]$P < .05$

22 The patients achieved significantly lower peak $\dot{V}o_2$ than their respective controls (Tab. 6). The patients failed to exercise as long as their respective controls. The control group exercised for an average of 7.1 minutes (SD = 1.4, range = 4.8–10), as compared with 5.4 minutes (SD = 1.6, range = 2.3–9.3) for the patients.

23 There was no significant correlation between peak $\dot{V}o_2$ measurements and (1) the number of joints with active arthritis ($r = -.33$) and (2) the articular disease severity score ($r - .29$) among the children with JRA.

24 The controls were usually able to complete higher work loads compared with the children with JRA. Three patients completed higher work loads than did their respective controls, 4 patients completed the same work loads as their respective controls, and 23 patients completed lower work loads than did their respective controls (Fig. 2).

Discussion

25 The literature on cardiovascular response to exercise in both healthy and sick children is limited. A majority of the reported studies were conducted outside the United States, and the subjects were often athletic or their level of physical activity was often greater than that of most American children. Variation in equipment, data-collection methods, and exercise protocols as well as regional and sample differences made comparison of published normative values with values obtained from our patient sample difficult. Thus, a control group was essential in our study. The control group was not a random sample and thus may not be representative of the general population for socioeconomic

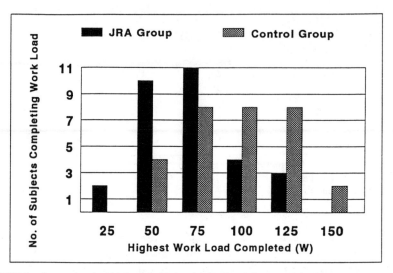

FIGURE 2   Comparison of highest work load completed (in watts) between patients with juvenile rheumatoid arthritis (JRA) and their matched controls.

status. Matching, however, was performed on the basis of age, gender, and BSA, the variables known to exert the greatest influence on exercise performance in children.[20–24]

26   Because of the small sample size, individual exercise variables were not compared statistically with regard to gender, age, and BSA. The mean peak heart rate for the control group, however, was consistent with heart rates previously reported by other investigators using a bicycle ergometer protocol.[12,25] The lower peak heart rate achieved in the JRA group, in combination with a lower work load achieved and shorter duration of exercise, may suggest deconditioning. Because the patient group exercised at a significantly higher percentage of their peak heart rate than did the control group while performing submaximal work, they appear to be at a lower level of conditioning. Initiation of conditioning programs for children with JRA soon after their diagnosis may prevent the cycle of hypoactivity and deconditioning often experienced by individuals with a chronic illness.[7]

27   We reported, in our earlier study,[8] mean peak $\dot{V}O_2$ values of 33 and 47 mL $O_2 \cdot kg^{-1} \cdot min^{-1}$ for children with and without JRA, respectively. It is unclear why our two control groups achieved different mean peak $\dot{V}O_2$ levels. Both samples were recruited from the same geographical area, and identical protocols and equipment were used by the same observers. A possible explanation for the difference in peak $\dot{V}O_2$ achieved by the two control groups is sampling. It is noteworthy, however, that

the conclusions of both studies were similar—the patients with JRA had significantly lower peak $\dot{V}O_2$ levels than did their matched controls.

28 The values for peak $\dot{V}O_2$ obtained for both groups in this study are lower than those reported in the literature for healthy children. In a recent study of aerobic and anaerobic characteristics of North American children, Washington et al[20] found mean $\dot{V}O_2$ values of 41 to 47 $mL\cdot kg^{-1}\cdot min^{-1}$ in healthy children aged 7 to 12 years. Maximum heart rates reported by Washington et al were 191 to 196 bpm, similar to the control group heart rates in our study. Possible reasons for the differences in $\dot{V}O_2$ values obtained in these two studies include the use of different bicycle ergometer protocols, gas analysis equipment, and sample characteristics.

29 We agree with Bar-Or's[6,7] hypothesis that the lower aerobic capacity often seen in children with chronic illnesses is due to both hypoactivity and specific pathophysiological factors. Bar-Or postulates that deficient oxygen extraction from the exercising muscle or low blood flow to the exercising muscle results in a high mixed venous oxygen content and subsequently a lower aerobic capacity. This is thought to occur in conditions such as arthritis, spina bifida, and poliomyelitis, in which the skeletal muscles are atrophied.[7] No data are available for children with these conditions to confirm this hypothesis. Further research involving the assessment of metabolic variables is needed.

30 We did not evaluate the difference in submaximal work efficiency between the two groups; however, comparison of $\dot{V}O_2$ values obtained during submaximal exercise was possible in 18 pairs of subjects. In 10 pairs of subjects, the $\dot{V}O_2$ values were higher for the children with JRA than for the control subjects, indicating that efficiency was lower for the subjects with JRA. In 2 pairs of subjects, submaximal $\dot{V}O_2$ values were essentially the same. In the remaining 6 pairs of subjects, the $\dot{V}O_2$ values obtained during submaximal exercise were higher for the controls than for the children with JRA. Further study is needed during submaximal work to determine whether a difference in exercise efficiency exists between the two groups.

31 Low muscle force production and endurance may contribute to the low aerobic capacity observed in children with JRA.[6] Additionally, clinical observations suggest that children with JRA may have poor mechanical efficiency attributable to joint deformity, resulting in a high metabolic cost in performing submaximal activities. We hypothesize that the child with arthritis will have to work at a higher percentage of her or his aerobic capacity than a child without arthritis during functional activities.

32 The use of the joint evaluation for reliable measurement of articular

disease severity is supported by the literature, provided the same clinician performs the evaluation on all subjects.[11,26–28] Although the validity of the joint evaluation has not been demonstrated conclusively by scientific study, this tool is used by researchers and clinicians alike to measure and monitor articular disease severity.[11,26–28]

33 Articular disease severity does not appear to be useful for predicting peak $\dot{V}O_2$. Similar to our previous study,[8] no significant correlation was found between peak $\dot{V}O_2$ and measures of articular disease severity. Because of the small sample size, we did not examine the relationship between lower-extremity joint involvement and peak $\dot{V}O_2$. Results of this study indicate that deconditioning occurs in the patient with JRA regardless of the severity of the articular disease. Thus, intervention should occur soon after diagnosis to prevent the cycle of hypoactivity and deconditioning.

34 During recovery, two control subjects and one subject with JRA complained of dizziness, nausea, and light-headedness. The subjects were assisted to the supine position, and their systolic blood pressure values were found to be between 80 and 90 mm Hg. The symptoms occurred during recovery while the subjects were performing slow cycling. Blood pressure, heart rate, and signs and symptoms were monitored for 20 minutes, and all three subjects recovered within a 5- to 10-minute period. One subject with JRA reported increased knee swelling, which resolved within 24 hours. The exercise protocol involved exercising to voluntary exhaustion; thus, all subjects were monitored closely for exercise intolerance. Although exercise training sessions may be of lesser intensity than an exercise test to voluntary exhaustion, the clinical implications are that patients with JRA should be monitored closely for signs and symptoms of exercise intolerance and joint symptoms.

Conclusions

35 This study documented differences in exercise responses between children with and without JRA. Peak $\dot{V}O_2$, highest work load completed, exercise duration, and peak heart rate were significantly lower in the children with JRA than in their matched controls. Submaximal heart rates were also higher for the children with JRA. These findings suggest a lower aerobic capacity in children with JRA. The decreased aerobic capacity was unrelated to the severity of the articular disease. This is in contrast to the commonly held belief that a patient with more severe articular disease will be more hypoactive and will become more deconditioned than a patient with less severe joint disease. Results of this study indicate that deconditioning occurs in children with JRA regardless of the severity of the articular disease: The clinical implications are that aerobic conditioning programs may be indicated for children with JRA in order to improve their exercise capacity. Intervention should occur soon after diagnosis to prevent the cycle of hypoactivity and deconditioning that commonly occurs in individuals with a chronic illness.

Acknowledgments

We thank the Pediatric Rheumatology Center at Texas Children's Hospital, Houston, Tex, for their assistance in subject recruitment. Appreciation is extended to Edward H Giannini, DrPH, for his assistance with data analysis. We also thank Patricia Taylor, PT; Kimberly Dorsey, PT; Miriam Garson, PT; and Carolyn Hendrix, PT, for their contributions to this project.

References

1. Towner SR, Michet CJ Jr, O'Fallon WM, et al. The epidemiology of juvenile arthritis in Rochester, Minnesota 1960–1979. *Arthritis Rheum.* 1983;26:1208–1213.
2. Gewanter HL, Roghmann KJ, Baum J. The prevalence of juvenile arthritis. *Arthritis Rheum.* 1983;26:599–603.
3. Petty RE. Epidemiology and genetics of the rheumatic diseases of childhood. In: Cassidy JT, ed. *Textbook of Pediatric Rheumatology.* New York, NY: John Wiley & Sons Inc; 1982.
4. Brewer EJ, Giannini EH, Person DA. *Juvenile Rheumatoid Arthritis.* 2nd ed. Philadelphia, Pa: WB Saunders Co; 1982.
5. Cassidy JT. Juvenile rheumatoid arthritis. In: Cassidy JT, ed. *Textbook of Pediatric Rheumatology.* New York, NY: John Wiley & Sons Inc; 1982.
6. Bar-Or O. Pathophysiological factors which limit the exercise capacity of the sick child. *Med Sci Sports Exerc.* 1986;18:276–282.
7. Bar-Or O. *Pediatric Sports Medicine for the Practitioner: From Physiologic Principles to Clinical Applications.* New York, NY,: Springer-Verlag New York Inc; 1983.
8. Giannini MJ, Protas EJ. Aerobic capacity in juvenile rheumatoid arthritis patients and healthy children. *Arthritis Care and Research.* 1991;4:131–135.
9. Brewer EJ, Bass J, Baum J, et al. Current proposed revision of JRA criteria. *Arthritis Rheum.* 1977;20:195–199.
10. Ad Hoc Committee on Exercise Testing. Standards for exercise testing in the pediatric age group. *Circulation.* 1982;66:1377A–1397A.
11. Brewer EJ, Giannini EH. Methodology and studies of children with juvenile rheumatoid arthritis. *J Rheumatol.* 1982;9:107–113.
12. James FW, Kaplan S, Glueck CJ, et al. Responses of normal children and young adults to controlled bicycle exercise. *Circulation.* 1980;61:902–912.
13. Taylor HL, Buskirk E, Henschel A. Maximal oxygen intake as an objective measure of cardio-respiratory performance. *J Appl Physiol.* 1955;8:73–80.
14. Bradley PW, Jackson AS, Hartung GH. *An Evaluation of an Automated System for Mea-*

surement of Cardiorespiratory Function During Exercise. Anaheim, Calif: Sensormedics Manufacturing Co; 1984.

15. Rothstein JM. Measurement and clinical practice: theory and application. In: Rothstein JM, ed. *Measurement in Physical Therapy.* New York, NY: Churchill Livingstone Inc; 1985:40.

16. Cumming GR, Goodwin A, Baggley G, et al. Repeated measurements of aerobic capacity during a week of intensive training at a youth track camp. *Can J Physiol Pharmacol.* 1967;45:805–811.

17. Boileau RA, Bonen A, Heyward VH, Massey BH. Maximal aerobic capcity on the treadmill and bicycle ergometer of boys 11–14 years of age. *J Sports Med.* 1977;17:153–162.

18. Nickerson BJ, Lemen RJ, Gerdes CB, et al. Within-subject variability and percent change for significance of spirometry in normal subjects and in patients with cystic fibrosis. *Am Rev Respir Dis.* 1980;12:859.

19. Shrout PE, Fleiss JL. Intraclass correlations: uses in assessing rater reliability. *Psychol Bull.* 1979;86:420–426.

20. Washington RL, van Gundy JC, Cohen C, et al. Normal aerobic and anaerobic exercise data for North American school-age children. *J Pediatr.* 1988;112:223–233.

21. Bouchard C, Malina RM, Hollmann W, et al. Submaximal working capacity, heart size and body size in boys 8–18 years. *Eur J Appl Physiol.* 1977;36:115–126.

22. Sunnegardh J, Bratteby L-E. Maximal oxygen uptake, anthropometry and physical activity in a randomly selected sample of 8 and 13 year old children in Sweden. *Eur J Appl Physiol.* 1987;56:266–272.

23. Nagle FJ, Hagberg J, Kamei S. Maximal O_2 uptake of boys and girls—ages 14–17. *Eur J Appl Physiol.* 1977;36:75–80.

24. Matsui H, Miyashita M, Miura M, et al. Maximal oxygen uptake and its relation to body weight of Japanese adolescents. *Med Sci Sports Exerc.* 1972;4:29–32.

25. Pels AE, Gilliam TB, Freedson PS, et al. Heart rate response to bicycle ergometer exercise in children ages 6–7 years. *Med Sci Sports Exerc.* 1981;13:299–302.

26. Eberl DR, Fasching V, Rahlfs V, et al. Repeatability and objectivity of various measurements in rheumatoid arthritis: a comparative study. *Arthritis Rheum.* 1976;19:1278–1286.

27. Ritchie DM, Boyle JA, McInnes JM, et al. Clinical studies with an articular index for the assessment of joint tenderness in patients with rheumatoid arthritis. *Q J Med.* 1968;23:393–406.

28. Lansbury J. Report of a three-year study on the systemic and articular indexes in rheumatoid arthritis: theoretic and clinical considerations. *Arthritis Rheum.* 1958;1:505–522.

Self-Esteem of Persons with Cerebral Palsy: from Adolescence to Adulthood

JOYCE E. MAGILL-EVANS and GAYLE RESTALL

Key Words • Cerebral palsy • Self-concept • Social adjustment

A longitudinal study of self-esteem in 22 adolescents with cerebral palsy is reported. The subjects were matched with nondisabled adolescents by age, sex, IQ, and school. Seven years later, 39 of the 44 subjects (mean age = 22.8 years) completed the Tennessee Self-Concept Scale (Roid & Fitts, 1988), the Social Support Inventory (McCubbin, Patterson, Rossman, & Cooke, 1982), and a demographic question-naire with some open-ended questions. As adolescents, the girls with cerebral palsy scored significantly lower than the other groups on physical, social, and personal self-esteem; however, as adults, these subjects were no longer signifi-cantly different from other groups. Male subjects with cere-bral palsy had self-esteem scores similar to those of the nondisabled groups in both adolescence and adulthood. Demographic information is summarized. The factors that the subjects identified as leading to changes in self-esteem were relationships and experiences. The low self-esteem scores indicate that psychosocial occupational therapy intervention with adolescent girls with cerebral palsy and with some adults with cerebral palsy would be appropriate.

1   Occupational therapists who provide intervention to persons with

---

Joyce E. Magill-Evans, PhD, OT(C), is Assistant Professor, Department of Occupational Ther-apy, Faculty of Rehabilitation, University of Alberta, Edmonton, Alberta, Canada T6G 2G2.

Gayle Restall, OT(C), is Assistant Director of Occupational Therapy, Health Sciences Centre, Winnipeg, Manitoba, Canada.

This article was accepted for publication March 28, 1991.

cerebral palsy often heed Carrasco's (1989) injunction to look beyond posture and tone and provide holistic treatment. Mayberry (1990) believed that most pediatric therapists include goals related to self-esteem in their treatment. Consideration of self-esteem in persons with cerebral palsy is necessary; studies of nondisabled persons' attitudes toward persons with disabilities have shown that cerebral palsy is one of the least favorably viewed physical disabilities (Abroms & Kodera, 1979; Strohmer, Grand, & Purcell, 1984; Tringo, 1970). If one tends to shift toward the values held in one's environment as a result of interactions with others (Barris, Kielhofner, Levine, & Neville, 1985; Heiss, 1981), then persons with cerebral palsy can be expected to have lower self-esteem than those who are viewed more positively or who do not have disabilities. Because self-esteem is associated with effective functioning (Gurney, 1988) and personal satisfaction (Coopersmith, 1967), an understanding of this aspect of the client is appropriate in planning occupational therapy intervention. Therefore, it is important to determine whether the self-esteem of persons with cerebral palsy is indeed lower than that of their nondisabled peers as well as whether the level of self-esteem varies in periods of vulnerability to societal views (e.g., adolescence) or is consistent throughout the life span.

2   In this study, we measured the self-esteem of persons with cerebral palsy who had participated in a study of adolescent self-esteem 7 years previously (Magill & Hurlbut, 1986). We used Mayberry's (1990) definition of self-esteem, namely, how one feels about oneself. The purpose of the present study was to determine how self-esteem scores changed from adolescence to adulthood, how the changes compared to those of nondisabled peers, and the relationship of demographic variables (i.e., years of education, employment status, weekly contacts with friends) and social support to self-esteem. This study continues the work of identifying a population for occupational therapy intervention (e.g., adolescent girls with cerebral palsy, adolescent boys with cerebral palsy, women with cerebral palsy, men with cerebral palsy), thus ensuring that intervention is directed appropriately.

Literature Review

3   The terms *self-concept* and *self-image* are used as reported by the authors referenced. The authors measured how the subjects felt about themselves, which, for the purposes of the present study, we have defined as *self-esteem*. This study addresses a void in the literature: There are no longitudinal studies of self-esteem in persons with cere-

bral palsy and few cross-sectional studies comparing persons with cerebral palsy with nondisabled persons. A study of 15 children with cerebral palsy between the ages of 4 and 8 years revealed that the children with cerebral palsy tended to have lower self-concepts than did those in the control group (Teplin, Howard, & O'Connor, 1981). Scores for girls and boys were not analyzed separately. In contrast, a study of 30 children with cerebral palsy between ages 9 and 13 years reported self-esteem scores that were similar to those of the control group (Ostring & Nieminen, 1982).

4 Resnick and Hutton (1987) examined the relationship of self-image and demographic variables in 60 adolescents with cerebral palsy using open-ended interviews. They found no relationship between self-image and severity of disability and a significant positive relationship between self-image and having both friends who were disabled and friends who were nondisabled. No comparisons to nondisabled adolescents were made. Magill and Hurlbut (1986) examined the self-esteem of 22 adolescents with cerebral palsy, ages 13 to 18 years, and found no significant differences as compared with nondisabled peers on overall self-esteem, as measured by the Tennessee Self-Concept Scale (Roid & Fitts, 1988). However, the 11 girls with cerebral palsy scored significantly lower on social self-esteem than did the boys with cerebral palsy and the nondisabled boys and girls. Differences between boys and girls with cerebral palsy did not follow the pattern of higher social self-esteem for girls that has been found in studies of nondisabled adolescents (Dusek & Flaherty, 1981; Osborne & LeGette, 1982). The girls with cerebral palsy also scored significantly lower than the boys with cerebral palsy and the nondisabled girls on physical self-esteem, but did not differ from the nondisabled boys. Adolescent girls tend to have lower physical self-esteem than boys (Rosenberg, 1986), and the girls and boys with cerebral palsy followed this pattern. However, the physical self-esteem of the girls with cerebral palsy was lower than their same-sexed nondisabled peers, whereas the boys with cerebral palsy were similar to their nondisabled peers. It is important to determine if differences in self-esteem persist into adulthood.

5 Longitudinal studies of nondisabled adolescents have reported more positive self-esteem with age (Cairns, McWhirter, Duffy, & Barry, 1990; McCarthy & Hoge, 1982; O'Malley & Bachman, 1983; Savin-Williams & Demo, 1984). However, the rank ordering of self-esteem scores tends to remain fairly stable from adolescence to adulthood (O'Malley & Bachman, 1983; Tashakkori, Thompson, Wade, & Valente, 1990). Thus, nondisabled adolescents appear to experience a relatively stable growth in self-esteem (Savin-Williams & Demo, 1984). It is important to determine if this same growth occurs in those with cerebral palsy and if

adolescents with low self-esteem continue to have low self-esteem as adults.

6   When investigating self-esteem in adulthood, one must consider other variables. Social support has been identified as having a positive effect on adolescent self-esteem (e.g., Hoelter & Harper, 1987) and adult psychological functioning (Kaplan, Robbins, & Martin, 1983; Schultz & Saklofske, 1983). Employment and marital situation are also important, although the effects on self-esteem appear to vary with the person's sex (Stein, Newcomb, & Bentler, 1990).

Study Purpose

7   In this paper, we have addressed the following questions:
   (1) Will women with cerebral palsy continue to have lower social and physical self-esteem scores than men with cerebral palsy and nondisabled men and women, as measured by the Tennessee Self-Concept Scale?
   (2) Will self-esteem scores remain stable over 7 years?
   (3) Is there a difference between persons with and without cerebral palsy in educational achievement, employment status, number of weekly contacts with friends (as measured by a demographic questionnaire), and satisfaction with social support (as measured by the Social Support Inventory [McCubbin, Patterson, Rossman, & Cooke, 1982])? Is there a relationship between self-esteem scores and these variables?

Method

SUBJECTS

8   The subjects were contacted through their parents and telephone directories. Thirty-nine of the 44 adults who had participated in the adolescent study were located and agreed to participate. Of those who did not participate, one nondisabled man declined to participate, one man with cerebral palsy agreed to participate but did not return the materials, and one man with cerebral palsy had committed suicide while in high school. Two subjects could not be located.

9   In the adolescent study, 22 subjects with cerebral palsy who were in integrated classrooms were matched by age, sex, school, and IQ with 22 nondisabled adolescents. For the present study, 9 female and 8 male pairs were represented (see Table 1 for the ages and IQ scores

TABLE 1 **AGE AND IQ SCORES OF SAMPLE**

	Females		Males	
Variable	Cerebral Palsy ($n = 10$)	Non-disabled ($n = 10$)	Cerebral Palsy ($n = 9$)	Non-disabled ($n = 10$)
Age				
M	22.8	23.2	22.7	22.6
SD	1.8	1.4	1.6	1.7
IQ[a]				
M	100.4	102.2	96.7	102.4
SD	9.5	12.8	8.4	12.0

[a]Intelligence quotient as measured in adolescent study.

of the sample). No significant differences were found between the groups on age [$F(3,35) = 0.20, p = .90$; Cochran's C, $p = .87$] or IQ [$F(3,35) = 0.56, p = .65$; Cochran's C, $p = .67$] despite the loss of some matched pairs.

10 The severity of disability for the men and women with cerebral palsy was similar. Eight persons (4 men, 4 women) had mild, 7 persons (3 men, 4 women) had moderate, and 4 persons (2 men, 2 women) had severe disabilities (definitions are provided in Magill & Hurlbut, 1986). Equal numbers of men and women had conditions diagnosed as hemiplegia ($n = 4$), spastic diplegia ($n = 8$), and spastic quadriplegia ($n = 4$). One man and 2 women had conditions diagnosed as athetoid quadriplegia.

MATERIALS

11 The Tennessee Self-Concept Scale, an ordinal Likert-type index with 100 items, measures aspects of self-concept (identity, behavior) and self-esteem. The scores related to self-esteem were used in both this study and the adolescent study. The Tennessee Self-Concept Scale is suitable for persons aged 12 to 68 years and allows for a comparison of scores across developmental stages. Scores on all subscales were calculated, but only physical (health, appearance, sexuality), social (general relationships), personal (personality apart from body and roles), family, and overall self-esteem scores were considered.

12 Information about years of education, employment status (i.e., employed, student, or unemployed), living arrangements (i.e., alone, with spouse, with parents, or in an institution), and number of weekly contacts with friends was collected with a forced-choice questionnaire. The questionnaire included open-ended questions on perceptions of change in self-esteem and reasons for change.

13   Social support was measured with the Social Support Inventory, which
     has three response categories—no, yes, and yes a lot. The following
     four scores from this self-report pen-and-paper measure were used in
     the analysis: total score, support from friends, support from relatives,
     and feelings of being valued and respected (similar to self-esteem).

PROCEDURE

14   Each subject who consented to participate received $15 upon com-
     pletion of the questionnaires. For subjects in the vicinity, a research
     assistant delivered the questionnaires at a mutually agreed-on time
     and made sure that all of the subjects were able to complete them (2
     persons required physical assistance). For subjects residing out of
     town, questionnaires were mailed along with instructions about the
     order in which they were to be completed.

15   The data were analyzed with the SPSSx program (SPSS, 1986). A one-
     way analysis of variance (ANOVA) was used to measure group differ-
     ences for age and IQ. Two repeated-measures multivariate analyses
     of variance (MANOVAs) were done with the independent variables of
     sex, disability, and time. The dependent measures in one of these
     MANOVAs were the physical, social, personal, and family self-esteem
     scores and, in the other MANOVA, total self-esteem. A MANOVA was
     done with the independent variable of disability and dependent var-
     iables of social support scores, years of education, and number of
     contacts with friends. Pearson correlations were used to measure the
     relationship of total self-esteem in adolescence with total self-esteem
     in adulthood; adolescent and adult physical, social, personal, and fam-
     ily self-esteem; and total self-esteem and education, number of friends,
     and social support scores. Chi-square analyses were used to examine
     employment.

Results

OVERALL SELF-ESTEEM: GROUP DIFFERENCES AND
CHANGE OVER TIME

16   As expected, overall self-esteem scores increased significantly from
     adolescence to adulthood $[F(1,35) = 14.02, p = .001]$. No main effects
     for disability or sex and no significant interactions were found. As in
     the prior adolescent study, no significant differences between the groups
     were found on overall self-esteem. Women with cerebral palsy con-
     tinued to have the lowest mean scores (see Table 2).

TABLE 2   **ADOLESCENTS'[a] (N = 44) AND ADULTS' (N = 39)
MEAN SCORES ON THE TENNESSEE SELF-CONCEPT SCALE[b]**

	Female		Male	
Category	Cerebral Palsy	Non-disabled	Cerebral Palsy	Non-disabled
Overall				
Adult	342.0	362.3	354.4	352.5
Adolescent	319.5	335.9	346.8	341.4
Physical				
Adult	65.8	71.9	70.2	70.0
Adolescent	60.8	67.4	69.9	70.7
Personal				
Adult	67.8	70.5	70.2	68.7
Adolescent	61.7	65.5	69.7	71.0
Social				
Adult	67.9	73.7	71.9	70.8
Adolescent	62.6	69.7	67.8	66.1
Family				
Adult	69.2	72.6	73.8	71.4
Adolescent	68.2	65.7	70.8	69.3

[a]Adolescents' mean scores are based on those persons who were included in both the adult and adolescent studies.
[b](Roid & Fitts, 1988).

17   Overall self-esteem scores were expected to increase but remained relatively stable from adolescence to adulthood. The correlation between adolescent and adult overall self-esteem was significant ($r = .49; p = .001$). Overall self-esteem scores were rank ordered and divided into thirds. Seven girls with cerebral palsy were in the lower third of the adolescent sample and none were in the middle third. By early adulthood, women with cerebral palsy were more evenly distributed throughout the sample. There were more nondisabled men and men with cerebral palsy in the lower third of the adult sample than there were in the adolescent sample.

18   A comparison of individual scores over time revealed that 18 subjects remained in the same third of the sample distribution and 17 moved to an adjacent third. Four persons, three of whom had cerebral palsy, had substantial changes, moving from the upper to the lower third or vice versa. One woman with mild cerebral palsy had an increase of 78 points, thereby moving from one standard deviation below the normative mean to one standard deviation above the mean. She attributed the change to more self-reliance and an enjoyable part-time job. A moderately disabled woman with a much lower score reported an increase in self-esteem, although in conversation she mentioned embarrassing moments related to attendance at a university. The man with cerebral palsy whose score dropped substantially had recently lost his job.

TENNESSEE SELF-CONCEPT SCALE SUBSCALES: GROUP DIFFERENCES AND CHANGE OVER TIME

19 The women with cerebral palsy no longer differed significantly from the other groups in social and physical self-esteem although they continued to have the lowest mean scores (see Table 2). Planned post hoc multiple comparisons with the Student-Newman-Keuls test revealed that the physical and personal self-esteem scores of the women with cerebral palsy had increased significantly ($p < .05$) more than did those of the other groups. Although the social self-esteem of these women had improved, the improvement was not significantly more than that of the other groups. The women with cerebral palsy had a greater range of social self-esteem scores ($SD = 12.1$; Cochran's C = $.65, p = .001$) than did the other adult groups ($SD = 4.6, 4.3, 6.2$).

20 Pearson correlation coefficients measuring the relationship of adolescent and adult subscale scores were all significant (physical = $.35, p = .02$; personal = $.34, p = .02$; family = $.37, p = .01$; social = $.35, p = .02$).

DEMOGRAPHIC AND SOCIAL SUPPORT VARIABLES

21 No significant differences were found between the cerebral palsy and nondisabled groups on years of education, weekly contacts with friends, or satisfaction with social support (see Table 3). Total self-esteem was

TABLE 3 **DEMOGRAPHICS AND SOCIAL SUPPORTS**
(N = 39)

	Women		Men	
Variable	Cerebral Palsy	Non-disabled	Cerebral Palsy	Non-disabled
Employment				
Student	8	4	2	1
Working	2	5	4	8
Unemployed	0	1	3	1
Years of Education (*SD*)	13.5 (2.2)	14.2 (2.0)	13.4 (1.6)	13.6 (1.6)
No. of Weekly Contacts				
With friends (*SD*)	4.5 (3.2)	4.8 (2.7)	5.8 (3.8)	5.2 (2.5)
With family (*SD*)	6.2 (4.2)	6.7 (5.1)	4.0 (2.6)	3.4 (2.7)
Married/Partner	0	6	1	5

significantly correlated with total social support ($r = .62, p < .01$) and feelings of being valued by persons in the social network ($r = .59, p < .01$) for the group with cerebral palsy. Correlations of self-esteem with other social support variables, education, and contacts with friends were not significant (range = .16 to .46). There were no significant correlations for the nondisabled group (range = .07 to .36).

22 The chi-square analysis of employed persons versus students in the cerebral palsy and nondisabled groups was significant [$\chi^2(1, n = 34) = 4.04, p < .05$]. As shown in Table 3, more of the group with cerebral palsy, particularly the women, were students. The numbers of unemployed persons in each group were not compared due to the small numbers. The unemployed men with cerebral palsy included 2 mildly disabled men who had been unemployed for a few months and 1 severely disabled man who had never worked.

23 The groups also differed significantly as to whether they had a spouse or partner [$\chi^2(1, N = 39) = 11.2, p < .001$]. As shown in Table 3, only 1 person with cerebral palsy—a man—was married, whereas 11 subjects from the nondisabled group had a spouse or partner. Twelve persons with cerebral palsy (7 women, 5 men) were living at home, compared with 7 nondisabled subjects (3 women, 4 men). One man with cerebral palsy was living in an institution.

SUBJECTIVE REPORTS

24 None of the subjects reported a decrease in self-esteem since adolescence. Four persons (1 woman with cerebral palsy, 3 men with cerebral palsy) believed that their self-esteem had not changed since adolescence. A woman with cerebral palsy who was severely disabled had the lowest overall score and her self-esteem had decreased. The scores of the men had remained in a similar range. The factors that the subjects associated with an increase in self-esteem are summarized in Table 4. The nondisabled adults identified family and friends as having had positive effects on their self-esteem more often than did the subjects with cerebral palsy. Nondisabled men tended to identify general life experiences and maturation as the primary causes of changes, whereas the other groups gave a variety of responses.

Discussion

25 It is encouraging to see that adolescents with cerebral palsy show expected increases in self-esteem as they move into early adulthood. For many of these persons, their self-esteem does not differ signifi-

TABLE 4   SUBJECTS' EXPLANATIONS FOR CHANGES IN
THEIR SELF-ESTEEM

	Women		Men	
Explanation	Cerebral Palsy ($n = 8$)	Non-disabled ($n = 10$)	Cerebral Palsy ($n = 6$)	Non-disabled ($n = 9$)
People	4	8	3	5
Experiences				
General	1	3	1	5
Education	3	2	2	1
Work	4	2	1	1
Leisure[a]	2	0	1	0
Move	1	1	0	0
Personal Growth				
More independence	1	2	0	0
Maturation	3	3	2	5

[a]Two of these subjects were involved in competitions for persons with disabilities. One had
won international gold medals.

cantly from that of their peers despite their having a negatively perceived disability. The increase self-esteem, which was seen particularly
in women with cerebral palsy, might be due to the subjects' increased
ability to defend their self-esteem from negative perceptions in their
environment. One must consider this defensiveness when measuring
self-esteem and interpreting the results (Mayberry, 1990). The Tennessee Self-Concept Scale includes a self-criticism scale that measures
willingness to acknowledge minor faults. An ANOVA and subsequent
Student-Newman-Keuls tests revealed that the women with cerebral
palsy were actually more self-critical than were nondisabled women
and men with cerebral palsy [$F(3,35) = 4.68, p = .01$]. All scores were
within the normal ranges; the increases in self-esteem cannot be attributed simply to defensiveness.

26   The increase in self-esteem may be related to a greater choice of
environments within which to interact once high school has been
completed. As one tends to assimilate the views of others into one's
self-esteem (Heiss, 1981), the independence of adulthood may allow
one to reduce exposure to negative situations and choose environments with values and interests similar to one's own (Barris et al.,
1985). As adults, 3 persons with cerebral palsy in the present study
chose to be involved with fitness programs for persons with disabilities. This environment allows them to interact with persons with
similar interests and to experience positive interactions. Twelve of the
19 persons with cerebral palsy were still living at home, thus it does

not appear to be necessary to change living environments in order to experience an increase in self-esteem.

27 Considering the increases in self-esteem with age, one might argue that intervention is not required. However, the relative stability of the self-esteem scores, as evidenced by the significant correlations between adult and adolescent scores in this study and others (e.g., Keltikangas-Jarvinen, 1990), indicates that problems in adolescence do not all disappear over time. Indeed, some of the adolescents with low self-esteem relative to their cohort and the normative sample continue to have low self-esteem in adulthood. It is these persons who must be identified and included in intervention programs. One woman with severe disabilities had percentile scores that ranged from 1 to 5, placing her below 95% to 99% of the normal population. Another woman with mild disabilities scored below the normative range on social self-esteem. The lower self-esteem of some of the adolescent girls continued into adulthood, whereas some of the boys with cerebral palsy faced decreases in self-esteem in early adulthood.

28 Occupational therapy programs should include an assessment of self-esteem when they involve persons with cerebral palsy, in light of such persons' long-term physical and social difficulties (Thomas, Bax, & Smyth, 1989) and the negative perceptions of cerebral palsy. Adolescence may be a period of greater vulnerability due to the emphasis on appearance and physical abilities (Thomas et al., 1989). Intervention should be provided to ameliorate the difficulties that many adolescent girls with cerebral palsy experience, especially in the areas of physical and social self-esteem. Persons with very low self-esteem and severe disabilities are of particular concern. As suggested previously (Magill & Hurlbut, 1986), girls with cerebral palsy need help in redefining attractiveness in themselves and others and to develop the social skills they need for healthy relationships. Several adolescent subjects with cerebral palsy, most of whom had been mainstreamed for all of their education, mentioned that they did not know anybody else with cerebral palsy and wanted to get together with others to talk about their difficulties. An informal group led by a young adult with cerebral palsy may be a helpful part of therapeutic programming during adolescence. Therapists working in school systems may have opportunities to address the self-esteem needs of mainstreamed adolescents and ensure that they have opportunities to choose positive environments within which to interact.

29 Consideration of self-esteem must continue into adulthood: 4 subjects with cerebral palsy had scores below the normative range in some or all areas. Although the differences between groups in the present study were found to be no longer statistically significant, the female subjects

with cerebral palsy continued to have the lowest scores. Differences between groups in physical self-esteem may be considered realistic, but lower social self-esteem in persons with cerebral palsy should be addressed, particularly in light of the lower rate of the reporting of a spouse or partner among the subjects with cerebral palsy, as compared with the nondisabled persons in this and other studies (e.g., Thomas et al., 1989). The significant positive relationship between social support and self-esteem for adults with cerebral palsy indicates that therapists should consider the client's social network in assessment and treatment. Clients may need help in developing substitute social networks to provide the support that would normally come from the traditional sources of a spouse, a partner, or co-workers. Clients with cerebral palsy may benefit from positive interactions with disabled and nondisabled friends and participation in meaningful productive activity.

Conclusion

30   In this study, we addressed a void in the rehabilitation literature by looking at the self-esteem of persons with cerebral palsy from adolescence to adulthood, as measured by the Tennessee Self-Concept Scale. The results indicate that self-esteem increases as persons move out of adolescence. Whether persons with cerebral palsy continue to score similarly to their nondisabled peers on self-esteem measures in later adulthood and whether they find someone with whom to share their lives and find fulfillment in meaningful, productive work remains to be seen. Other longitudinal studies that follow persons with cerebral palsy from early childhood into adolescence might identify strategic periods for intervention. Replication of our study with a larger sample and different self-esteem measures would enhance our understanding of the development of self-esteem over time for persons with physical disabilities such as cerebral palsy.

Acknowledgments

We are grateful to each of the study participants. Special thanks to Jim Vargo for editorial suggestions.

This project was made possible by a grant from the Small Faculties Endowment Fund, University of Alberta, Edmonton, Alberta, Canada.

References

Abroms, KI & Kodera, TL (1979). Acceptance hierarchy of handicaps: Validation of Kirk's statement, "Special education often begins where medicine stops." *Journal of Learning Disabilities, 12,* 24–29.

Barris, R, Kielhofner, G, Levine, RE & Neville, AM (1985). Occupation as interaction with the environment. In G Kielhofner (ed), *A Model of Human Occupation: Theory and application* (pp. 43–62). Baltimore: Williams & Wilkins.

Cairns, E, McWhirter, L, Duffy, U, & Barry, R (1990). The stability of self-concept in late adolescence: Gender and situational effects. *Personality and Individual Differences, 11,* 937–944.

Carrasco, R (1989). Children with cerebral palsy. In P Pratt & A Allen (eds), *Occupational therapy for children* (2nd ed., pp. 396–421). St. Louis: Mosby.

Coopersmith, S (1967). *The antecedents of self-esteem.* San Francisco: Freeman.

Dusek, JB & Flaherty, JF (1981). The development of the self-concept during the adolescent years. *Monograph of the Society for Research in Child Development, 46*(4).

Gurney, PW (1988). *Self-esteem in children with special educational needs.* London: Routledge.

Heiss, J (1981). *The social psychology of interaction.* Englewood Cliffs, NJ: Prentice-Hall.

Hoelter, J & Harper, L (1987). Structural and interpersonal family influences on adolescent self-conception. *Journal of Marriage and Family, 49,* 129–139.

Kaplan, HB, Robbins C, & Martin, SS (1983). Antecedents of psychological distress in young adults: Self-rejection, deprivation of social support, and life events. *Journal of Health and Social Behavior, 24,* 230–244.

Keltikangas-Jarvinen, L (1990). The stability of self-concept during adolescence and early adulthood: A six-year follow-up study. *Journal of General Psychology, 117,* 361–368.

Magill, J & Hurlbut, N (1986). The self-esteem of adolescents with cerebral palsy. *American Journal of Occupational Therapy, 40,* 402–407.

Mayberry, W (1990). Self-esteem in children: Considerations for measurement and intervention. *American Journal of Occupational Therapy, 44,* 729–734.

McCarthy, JD & Hoge, DR (1982). Analysis of age effects in longitudinal studies of adolescent self-esteem. *Developmental Psychology, 18,* 372–379.

McCubbin, HI, Patterson, JM, Rossman, MM, & Cooke, B (1982). Social Support Inventory. In D Olson, H McCubbin, H Barnes, A Larson, M Muxon, & M Wilson (eds), *Family inventories: Inventories used in a national survey of families across the family life cycle.* St. Paul: University of Minnesota.

O'Malley, PM & Bachman, JG (1983). Self-esteem: Change and stability between ages 13 and 23. *Developmental Psychology, 19,* 257–268.

Osborne, WL & LeGette, HR (1982). Sex, race, grade level, and social class differences in self-concept. *Measurement and Evaluation in Guidance, 14,* 195–201.

Ostring, H & Nieminen, S (1982). Concept of self and the attitude of school age CP children towards their handicap. *International Journal of Rehabilitation Research, 5,* 235–237.

Resnick, M & Hutton, L (1987). Resiliency among physically disabled adolescents. *Psychiatric Annals, 17,* 796–800.

Roid, GH & Fitts WH (1988). *Tennessee Self-Concept Scale: Revised manual.* Los Angeles: Western Psychological Services.

Rosenberg, M (1986). Self-concept from middle childhood through adolescence. In J Suls & AG Greenwald (eds), *Psychological perspectives of the self* (Vol. 3, pp 107–136). Hillsdale, NJ: Erlbaum.

Savin-Williams, RC & Demo, DH (1984). Developmental change and stability in adolescent self-concept. *Developmental Psychology, 20,* 1100–1110.

Schultz, BJ & Saklofske, DH (1983). Relationship between social support and selected measures of psychological well-being. *Psychological Reports, 53,* 847–850.

SPSS, Inc. (1986). *SPSSx.* Chicago: Author.

Stein, JA, Newcomb, MD, & Bentler, PM (1990). The relative influence of vocational behavior and family involvement on self-esteem: Longitudinal analyses of young adult women and men. *Journal of Vocational Behavior, 36,* 320–338.

Strohmer, DC, Grand, SA, & Purcell, MJ (1984). Attitudes toward persons with a disability: An examination of demographic factors, social context, and specific disability. *Rehabilitation Psychology, 29,* 131–145.

Tashakkori, A, Thompson, V, Wade, J, & Valente, E (1990). Structure and stability of self-esteem in late teens. *Personality and Individual Differences, 11,* 885–893.

Teplin, SW, Howard, JA, & O'Connor, M (1981). Self-concept of young children with cerebral palsy. *Developmental Medicine and Child Neurology, 23,* 730–738.

Thomas, AP, Bax, M, & Smyth, DP (1989). *The health and social needs of young adults with physical disabilities.* Cambridge, MA: Blackwell Scientific.

Tringo, JL (1970). The hierarchy of preference toward disability groups. *Journal of Special Education, 4,* 295–306.

Volumetric Comparison of Seated and Standing Test Postures

ERICA B. STERN

Key Words • Assessment process • Occupational therapy • Edema • Hand evaluation

Published protocols for the volumetric assessment of upper-extremity edema differ regarding patients' posture. The present study was designed to determine the effect of posture on test-retest reliability and mean volume. Thirty women were tested in both seated and standing postures. For the dominant hand, test-retest reliabilities for the seated posture were identical to those for the standing posture. Test-retest reliability was slightly stronger for the nondominant hand in sitting than for the same hand in standing. Both postures afforded clinically acceptable test-retest reliabilities. The mean volumes in sitting were significantly lower than those in standing (p < .0001), thus suggesting that volumetric measures should be considered discontinuous if the patient's test posture is altered. Mean volumes of the dominant hand averaged 9.3 ml more than those of the nondominant hand. It is suggested that this discrepancy be considered in the establishment of goals for edema control and in the determination of the need for continued edema treatment.

1 Upper extremity edema is a common problem in the rehabilitation of persons with burns (Malick & Carr, 1982), cerebrovascular accident,

Erica B. Stern, PhD, OTR, is Assistant Professor, Program in Occupational Therapy, University of Minnesota, 271 Children's Rehabilitation Center, Box 388 UMHC, 426 Church Street, SE, Minneapolis, Minnesota 55455. At the time of this study, she was Associate Professor, Occupational Therapy Education Department, University of Kansas Medical Center, Kansas City, Kansas.

This article was accepted for publication April 18, 1991.

325

gouty arthritis (Smyth, Velayos, & Amoroso, 1963), rheumatoid arthritis (McKnight & Schomburg, 1982), mastectomy (Engler & Sweat, 1962), generalized lymphedema (Bunchman & Lewis, 1974), and soft-tissue trauma associated with sprains (Cote, Prentice, Hooker, & Shields, 1988) and surgery (Barclay, 1959; Hunter & Mackin, 1990; Nicholas, 1977). Edema is most commonly attributed to an inadequate or compromised pumping mechanism acting on the venous and lymphatic system (Vasudevan & Melvin, 1979). Edema reduces the functional abilities of the hand by predisposing the metacarpophalangeal joints toward extension, thus contributing to collateral ligament shortening (Nicholas, 1977; Strickland, 1987).

2 Although high-technology options exist for the evaluation of upper extremity edema (Goltner, Gass, Haas, & Schneider, 1988), occupational therapists most commonly measure edema using the less expensive and more accessible options of either circumferential or volumetric assessment. In *circumferential assessment,* edema is evaluated through the measurement of the circumference of hand segments. Greenhill (1979) noted poor test-retest reliability in the circumferential measurement of the edematous hand and wrist. She attributed much of the variability in this assessment to inconsistent placement and tension of the measuring tape. In cases in which edema is localized in the fingers, Kasch (1990) suggested that a jeweler's ring sizer could be used, thus reducing the error associated with tape tension. In *volumetric assessment,* edema is evaluated through the measurement of the water displace when a limb is immersed. Several authors have promoted volumetric assessment over circumferential evaluation, especially when edema involves the hand and wrist in addition to the digits (Bear-Lehman & Abreu, 1989; Greenhill, 1979; Swedborg, 1977). Even those who consider volumetric assessment to be overly complicated and time consuming concede that the tool is "an accurate way of following the progression of the disease [lymphedema] and the outcome of any therapy" (Bunchman & Lewis, 1974, p. 64).

3 Commercially available volumeters were first manufactured in 1977 (J. Creelman, personal communication, July 1, 1990). They have since become a ubiquitous clinical tool as well as a frequently used measure among researchers. Although Eccles (1956) is credited with developing the earliest clinical volumeter, the commercial volumeter is based on Brand and Cohen's (nee Ramsammy) prototype (Creelman, 1989; Hunter & Mackin, 1990). The commercial hand-forearm volumeter consists of a plastic tank ($3\frac{1}{2}$ in. by 5 in. $\times$ 11 in.) with a dowel centered in the lower third of the container to control the depth of hand immersion (Creelman, 1989). A spout at the top of the container allows the displaced water to drain and to collect in the 500-ml graduated cylinder

that accompanies the volumeter in the commercial set. The cylinder is marked by 5-ml graduations.

4 Several sources of variability have been noted in volumetry, and a protocol of administration has been developed to reduce the effect of these variables during volumetric assessment. The variables cited most frequently are orientation of the hand in the device, speed of immersion, verticality of the forearm axis, aeration of the water, forearm stillness during the assessment, pressure against the dowel, placement of the volumeter in the test environment, and placement of the graduated cylinder during reading (Fess & Moran, 1981; Hunter & Mackin, 1990; Smyth et al., 1963; Waylett-Rendall & Seibly, 1991). Interestingly, despite detailed descriptions of volumetric procedure, authors usually do not report whether the subject was seated or standing while the test was conducted (McKnight & Schomburg, 1982; Schultz-Johnson, 1988; Smyth et al., 1963; Waylett-Rendall & Seibly, 1991). Indeed, the most authoritative voices disagree on the correct patient posture for testing. For example, the American Society of Hand Therapists specified the seated position for the assessment, noting that "the patient, with dressings and jewelry removed from the extremity, should then be seated comfortably next to the volumeter and instructed to slowly immerse the hand and forearm until a firm pressure from the stop rod is perceived in the third web space" (Fess & Moran, 1981, p. 8). Likewise, Hunter and Mackin recommended that the evaluation be performed while seated, with the use of a chair that "easily allows the lowering of one third of the forearm into the plastic hand volumeter" (p. 190), and that the volumetric tank be positioned on a stable stand. They even specified that the patient be "instructed to sit with the back well against the chair and the feet flat on the floor" (p. 190).

5 Conversely, the manufacturer of the volumeter specifies that the standing posture be used (Creelman, 1989). The photographs in Eccles's (1956) article attest to his preference for the standing posture as well.

6 Volumetric assessment is used by occupational therapists and physical therapists throughout the United States and internationally. It was my belief, therefore, that clinical practice might benefit from a clarification of the effects that test posture could have on the assessment. The present study was conducted to determine whether test posture would significantly affect either test-retest reliability or volumetric results.

Method

SUBJECTS

7 Thirty right-hand-dominant women ranging from 18 to 25 years of age volunteered for and participated in the study. The subjects reported

themselves to be in good health and without any known injury or disease affecting either upper extremity.

INSTRUMENT

8   In keeping with the literature's recommendation, a commercially available plastic hand-sized volumetric tank was used for the present study (Fess & Philips, 1987; Hunter & Mackin, 1990; Schultz-Johnson, 1988). The accuracy of this assessment tool is reported as $\pm 1\%$ (Creelman, 1989; J. Creelman, personal communication, July 1, 1990; Hunter & Mackin, 1990; Schultz-Johnson, 1988). Because the volume of an average hand has been reported as 500 ml, this accuracy is sometimes reported as being ± 5 ml in the adult hand (Creelman, 1989; Creelman, personal communication, July 1, 1990; Hunter & Mackin, 1990; Schultz-Johnson, 1988). Waylett-Rendall and Seibly's (1991) research suggested that up to 10 ml of difference may be expected when normal hands are repeatedly measured by the same examiner.

PROCEDURE

9   In addition to a commercial hand volumeter set (i.e., volumeter tank, graduated cylinder, and filling pitcher), testing in the seated posture required two identical standard armless chairs with firm backs and seats and a stable wooden support to raise the volumeter from the floor. Testing in the standing posture required a stable, level table 32-in. high and a commercial hand volumeter set. A single volumeter and graduated cylinder were used during the study.

10 The table and floor surfaces of the assessment area were marked with tape to ensure consistent placement of the subjects, volumeter, chairs, and wooden support. When testing subjects in the seated position, I placed the volumeter on a wooden support between two chairs. The subjects alternated between the chairs, thus permitting standard volumetric assessment of both the dominant and nondominant hands without necessitating movement of the volumeter.

11 Three data gatherers were trained and tested until they reached 100% agreement on both administration procedure and measurement for volumetric assessment. In situations where the water line fell between the 5 ml markings, the readings were recorded to the lower number.

12 Each subject had a single test session in which three measurements were taken in the seated and standing positions for both the dominant and nondominant hands. For each assessment, the volumeter was filled with room-temperature tap water from a still source until the water

overflowed from the spout. The subjects (a) removed all jewelry, (b) were oriented to the assessment procedure, (c) slowly immersed the hand (thumb toward spout) without contacting the sides of the device, (d) continued immersion until the dowel rod rested firmly in the web space between the middle and ring fingers, (e) maintained the hand immobile in this position until the flow of water had been collected and the measuring cylinder removed, and (e) withdrew the hand. Each subject's arm, along with the graduated cylinder, was thoroughly dried between measurements.

13 When measures were being performed in the seated test position, the subject sat with her back against the chair and her feet flat on the floor. In the standing position, each subject stood within a square marked by tape that had been placed on the floor.

14 The order of testing was individually assigned for each subject with the use of a modified Latin square to control for both test order and relative position within order (Keppel, 1982).

Results

RELIABILITY

15 Test-retest reliability for each test condition was established with the use of a Pearson correlation coefficient, which was performed on the first two of the three measurements. The test-retest correlations in sitting for the nondominant hand ($r = .99$), sitting for the dominant hand ($r = .99$), standing for the nondominant hand ($r = .91$), and standing for the dominant hand ($r = .99$) were all significant at the $p < .0001$ level. These high correlations indicate an extremely strong test-retest reliability regardless of test posture or hand being tested.

COMPARISON OF MEAN VOLUME

16 A 2×2 (Posture $\times$ Hand) analysis of variance (ANOVA) with repeated measures was performed with the mean value from the three measurements in each condition. This ANOVA was performed with the Biomedical Data Processing Statistical Software Package, Program 2V (Dixon, 1983). Each of the two main effects (posture and hand) significantly influenced the volumetric results (see Table 1). The posture effect showed a significant difference in hand volumes when the subjects were measured while seated versus while standing ($p < .0001$), with the mean seated volume averaging 5.3 ml less than the mean standing volume (see Table 2). The second main effect demonstrated

TABLE 1 **VOLUME ANALYSIS OF VARIANCE WITH TWO**
LEVELS OF REPEATED MEASURES ($N = 30$)

Source	SS	df	MS	F	p
Posture	842.70	1	842.70	46.52	.0001
Error	525.30	29	18.11		
Hand	2650.80	1	2650.80	14.71	.0006
Error	5224.20	29	180.14		
Posture × Hand	4.80	1	4.80	0.58	.4517
Error	239.20	29	8.25		

that the dominant and nondominant hands produced significantly different volumetric readings ($p = .0006$) (See Table 1), with the nondominant hand averaging 9.4 ml less than the dominant hand (see Table 2).

17 The interaction effect of posture and hand was not significant ($p = .45$) (see Table 1). Therefore, the volumes of the dominant and nondominant hands were not significantly different when taken in the seated or standing postures.

Discussion

18 On the basis of the Pearson correlation coefficients, the test-retest reliability of volumetry appears equally acceptable in both the seated and standing postures. Both postures offer highly reliable test-retest assessment of hand volume. Even the nondominant hand in standing, which received the lowest test-retest value ($r = .91$), was well within the range of reliability acceptable for clinical assessments. Clinicians who frequently have to defend their test procedures in court, however, may wish to ensure the highest level of test-retest reliability by consistently performing the test in the seated posture.

19 The stability of the seated posture may contribute to its greater test-retest reliability by permitting the patient consistent control of dowel

TABLE 2 **VOLUMES FOR THREE MEASUREMENTS OF**
DOMINANT AND NONDOMINANT HANDS IN THE SEATED
AND STANDING POSTURES ($N = 30$)

	M (SD)		
Posture	Dominant	Nondominant	Combined
Seated	370.60 (40.62)	360.80 (38.65)	365.70 (39.62)
Standing	375.50 (41.58)	366.50 (39.41)	371.00 (40.42)
Combined	373.05 (40.83)	363.65 (38.80)	—

pressure against the web space. Possibly, when subjects are tested in the standing posture, they press more firmly against the dowel, thereby using it as a supporting surface during the minor balance shifts that accompany less-controlled upper extremity movements in standing. This may explain why a slightly reduced reliability is seen when the nondominant hand is tested in a standing posture but not when the dominant hand is assessed in the same posture.

20 Therapists who conduct volumetric tests using a standing posture may be unwittingly encouraging their patients to press more forcefully against the web stop or to move more during immersion as a result of the less-stable standing posture. Because test posture has a statistically significant effect on volumetric assessment, with volume consistently higher when standing than when sitting, therapists should note the client's assessment posture on the record forms and view only those measurements taken in the same posture as continuous measures of the edema trend. In cases in which a patient's status requires a change in test posture, the therapist should acknowledge that the postural change is likely to influence the volume reading and that the measurements should not be considered continuous.

21 The results of this study support van Velze, Kluever, van der Merwe, and Mennen's (1991) finding that a significant difference exists in the volumes of dominant and nondominant hands. The expected difference between dominant and nondominant hands has important ramifications when one considers that therapists often compare volumes of affected and unaffected arms to monitor progress in addition to "comparing the injured extremity to itself over time" (Schultz-Johnson, 1988, p. 26). The realistic establishment of goals for edema treatment and timing for discontinuation of treatment may be assisted by the recognition that the nondominant hand of women averages 10 ml smaller than the dominant when measured with a commercially available instrument.

Study Limitations

22 This study was conducted on a small and homogeneous group of subjects. All of the subjects were right handed, female, and college aged. Other populations' results could differ significantly. For example, van Velze et al. (1991) noted a smaller volume difference between dominant and nondominant hands of left-handed men as compared with right-handed men.

Conclusion

23 The greatest reliability in testing is afforded when volumetric assessment is performed in the seated posture. Additionally, measurements taken in the standing posture are consistently and significantly larger than those seen when the subject is seated. As a result, therapists may wish to conform to the American Society of Hand Therapists' guidelines (Fess & Moran, 1981) (including the seated posture) when performing a volumetric assessment. If for some reason the subject cannot be tested in the seated posture, the therapist should record that the assessment was performed in a standing posture and continue future volumetric measurement in that posture. If the test posture is changed because the patient's status alters, the therapist should record the change in posture and consider only those measurements taken in the same posture as reflective of a trend of volume change.

Acknowledgments

I thank Greg Goertzen, OTR, Erin Henry, OTR, and Michelle Knoblich, OTR, for gathering data; Krista Coleman, MS, PT, and Cheryl Meyers, MA, OTR, for editorial assistance; and the University of Kansas Medical Center's Department of Biometry for statistical assistance.

I gratefully acknowledge the University of Kansas School of Allied Health Research Fund for its supporting grant.

This paper is based on a poster session presented in April 1989 at the 69th Annual Conference of the American Occupational Therapy Association in Baltimore, Maryland.

References

Barclay, TL (1959). Edema following operation for Dupuytren's contracture. *Plastic and Reconstructive Surgery, 23,* 348–360.

Bear-Lehman, J & Abreu, BC (1989). Evaluating the hand: Issues in reliability and validity. *Physical Therapy, 69,* 1025–1033.

Bunchman, HH & Lewis, SR (1974). The treatment of lymphedema. *Plastic and Reconstructive Surgery, 54,* 64–69.

Cote, DJ, Prentice, WE, Hooker, DN, & Shields, EW (1988). Comparison of three treatment procedures for minimizing ankle sprain swelling. *Physical Therapy, 68,* 1072–1076.

Creelman, J (1989, April). *Hand volumeter: Directions for use* [Instructions included with hand volumeter set]. Idyllwild, CA: Volumeters Unlimited.

Dixon, WJ (1983). *Biomedical data processing statistical software.* Berkeley, CA: University of California Press.

Eccles, MV (1956). Hand volumetrics. *British Journal of Physical Medicine, 19,* 5–8.

Engler, HS & Sweat, RD (1962). Volumetric arm measurements: Technique and results. *American Surgeon, 28,* 465–468.

Fess, EE & Moran, CA (1981). *Clinical assessment recommendations.* Garner, NC: American Society of Hand Therapists.

Fess, EE & Philips, CA (1987). *Hand splinting principles and methods.* St. Louis: Mosby.

Goltner, E, Gass, P, Haas, JP, & Schneider, P (1988). The importance of volumetry, lymphscintigraphy and computer tomography in the diagnosis of brachial edema after mastectomy. *Lymphology, 21,* 134–143.

Greenhill, A (1979). Clinical note: The hand. *Physiotherapy Canada, 31,* 34–35.

Hunter, JM & Mackin, EJ (1990). Management of edema. In JM Hunter, LH Schneider, EJ Mackin, & AD Calahan (eds), *Rehabilitation of the hand: Surgery and therapy* (3rd ed., pp. 187–194). St Louis: Mosby.

Kasch, MC (1990). Acute hand injuries. In LW Pedretti & B Zoltan (eds), *Occupational therapy practice skills for physical dysfunction* (3rd ed., pp. 477–506). St. Louis: Mosby.

Keppel, G (1982). *Design and analysis: A researcher's handbook* (2nd ed). Englewood Cliffs, NJ: Prentice-Hall.

Malick, MH & Carr, JA (1982). *Manual on management of the burn patient.* Pittsburgh: Harmarville Rehabilitation Center.

McKnight, PT & Schomburg, FL (1982). Air pressure splint effects on hand symptoms of patients with rheumatoid arthritis. *Archives of Physical Medicine and Rehabilitation, 63,* 560–563.

Nicholas, JS (1977). The swollen hand. *Physiotherapy, 63,* 285–286.

Schultz-Johnson, K (1988). *Volumetrics: A literature review.* Santa Monica, CA: Upper Extremity Technology.

Smyth, CJ, Velayos, EE, & Amoroso, C (1963). A method for measuring swelling of hands and feet. *Acta Rheumatologica Scandinavia, 9,* 306–322.

Strickland, JW (1987). Anatomy and kinesiology of the hand. In EE Fess & CA Philips (eds), *Hand splinting principles and methods* (pp 3–41). St Louis: Mosby.

Swedborg, I (1977). Voluminometric estimation of the degree of lymphedema and its therapy by pneumatic compression. *Scandinavian Journal of Rehabilitation Medicine, 9,* 131–135.

van Velze, CA, Kluever, I, van der Merwe, CA, & Mennen, U (1991). The difference in volume of dominant and nondominant hands. *Journal of Hand Therapy, 1,* 6–9.

Vasudevan, SV & Melvin, JL (1979). Upper extremity edema control: Rationale of the techniques. *American Journal of Occupational Therapy, 33,* 520–523.

Waylett-Rendall, J & Seibly, D (1991). A study of the accuracy of a commercially available volumeter. *Journal of Hand Surgery, 4,* 10–13.

Statistical and Writing References

Statistical References

These are *roughly* in order of difficulty, from easy to hard.

Stahl, SM and Hennes, JD: Reading and Understanding Applied Statistics: A Self-Learning Approach. CV Mosby, St. Louis, 1980.
This book is out of print, but worth searching out of the library because of its clarity of presentation.

Shott, S: Statistics for Health Professionals. WB Saunders, Philadelphia, 1990.
Each chapter provides the reader with problems to solve in order to test understanding.

Wang, M, Airhihenbuwa, CO, and Okolo, EN: Data analysis and selection of statistical methods. In Okolo, EN (ed): Health Research Design and Methodology. CRC Press, Ann Arbor, 1990.

Schefler, WC: Statistics for Health Professionals. Addison-Wesley, Reading, MA, 1984.

Sellers, GR: Elementary Statistics. WB Saunders, Philadelphia, 1977.

Kuebler, RR and Smith, H: Statistics: A Beginning. John Wiley & Sons, New York, 1976.

Spence, JT, Cotton, JW, Underwood, BJ, and Duncan, CP: Elementary Statistics, ed 4. Prentice-Hall, Englewood Cliffs, NJ, 1983.

Siegel, S: Nonparametric Statistics for the Behavioral Sciences. McGraw-Hill, New York, 1956.

Daniel, WW: Applied Nonparametric Statistics. Houghton Mifflin, Boston, 1978.

Daniel, WW: Biostatistics: A Foundation for Analysis in the Health Sciences, ed 3. John Wiley & Sons, New York, 1983.

Dotson, CO, and Kirkendall, DR: Statistics for Physical Education, Health and Recreation. Harper & Row, New York, 1974.
Out of print, but good.

Duncan, RC, Knapp, RG, and Miller, MC: Introductory Statistics for the Health Sciences, ed 2. John Wiley & Sons, New York, 1983.

Conover, WJ: Practical Nonparametric Statistics, ed 2. John Wiley & Sons, New York, 1980.

Trochim, WMK: Advances in Quasi-Experimental Design and Analysis. Jossey-Bass, San Francisco, 1986.

Kilpatrick, SJ: Statistical Principles in Health Care Information, ed 2. University Park Press, Baltimore, 1977.

Foreman, EK: Survey Sampling Principles. Marcel Dekker, New York, 1991.

Tabachnick, BG and Fidell, LS: Using Multivariate Statistics. Harper & Row, New York, 1983.

Robinson, PW: Fundamentals of Experimental Psychology, ed 2. Prentice-Hall, Englewood Cliffs, NJ, 1981.

John, JA and Quenouille, MH: Experiments: Design and Analysis, ed 2. Macmillan, New York, 1977.

Regier, MH, Mohapata, RN, and Mohapata, SN: Biomedical Statistics and Computing. John Wiley & Sons, New York, 1982.

Kerlinger, FN: Foundations of Behavioral Research. Holt, Rinehart & Winston, New York, 1967.

Remington, RD, and Schosk, MA: Statistics with Applications to the Biological and Health Sciences, ed 2. Prentice-Hall, Englewood Cliffs, NJ, 1985.

Weinberg, GM and Schumaker, JA: Statistics: An Intuitive Approach, ed 3. Brooks-Cole, Belmont, CA, 1974.

Kirk, RE: Experimental Design: Procedures for the Behavioral Sciences, ed 2. Brooks-Cole, Belmont, CA, 1982.

Keppel, G: Design and Analysis: A Researcher's Handbook, ed 2. Prentice-Hall, Englewood Cliffs, NJ, 1982.

Winer, BJ: Statisitcal Principles in Experimental Design, ed 2. McGraw-Hill, New York, 1971.

Rosner, B: Fundamentals of Biostatistics, ed 2. Duxbury Press, Boston, 1986.

Writing

American Physical Therapy Association: Style Manual. Author, Alexandria, VA, latest edition.

Barzun, J: The Modern Researcher, ed 3. Harcourt, Brace, Jovanovich, New York, 1977.

Barzun, J: Simple and Direct: A Rhetoric for Writers. Harper & Row, New York, 1975.

University of Chicago Press: A Manual of Style. Author, Chicago, latest edition.

Campbell, WG and Ballou, SV: Form and Style. Houghton Mifflin, Boston, latest edition.

Day, RA: Scientific English: A Guide for Scientists and other Professionals. Oryx Press, Pheonix, AZ, 1992.

DeBakey, L: Competent medical exposition: The need and the attainment. Bull Am Col Surg 52(2):85, 1967.

Fink, J: Writing for the Allied Health Professional. Prentice-Hall, Englewood Cliffs, NJ, 1990.

Harbert, EN and Digaetani, JL: Writing for Action: A Guide for the Health Care Professional. Dow-Jones-Irwin, Homewood, IL, 1984.

Huth, EJ: How to Write and Publish Papers in the Medical Sciences, ed 2. Williams & Wilkins, Baltimore, 1990.

Meador, R: Guidelines for Preparing Proposals. Lewis, Chelsea, MI, 1991.

Ogden, TE: Research Proposals: A Guide to Success. Raven Press, New York, 1991.

Robinson, AM, and Notter, LE: Clinical Writing for Health Professionals. Prentice-Hall, Englewood Cliffs, NJ, 1982.

Sheen, AP: Breathing Life into Medical Writing: A Handbook. CV Mosby, St. Louis, 1981.

Stein, MD and Smith, JL: Instructions for Authors: Biomedical Journals. Academic Press, New York, 1986.

Turabian, KL: A Manual for Writers. University of Chicago Press, Chicago, latest edition.

Zeiger, M: Essentials of Writing Biomedical Research Papers. McGraw-Hill, New York, 1991.

Zinsser, W: On Writing Well. Harper & Row, New York, 1980.

*Glossary**

Alternate Hypothesis   An intelligent guess as to the nature of the answer to the basic question; it predicts the outcome of the study.

Applied Research   Concerned with the solution of immediate problems without necessarily being concerned for the basic reason as to why the solution works. Also called *action research.*

Assumptions   Facts taken for granted and thus not demonstrated.

Basic Research   Interest in the acquisition of knowledge for its own sake without any concern for the utility of that knowledge.

Bivariate or Multivariate Analysis   The act of relating two (or more) variables to each other mathematically as well as logically.

Cluster Sampling   Sampling using predefined groups of individuals, for example, classrooms.

Cohort   A defined sample followed over a period of time.

Concept   Describes some regularity or relationship within a group of facts and is designated by some sign or symbol, usually verbal.

Concurrent Validity   Refers to the relationship between test scores (or other measures) and either criterion states or measurements whose validity is known.

Confounding Variables   Variables that will confound or confuse the interpretation of the data if not controlled.

Constant Comparative Analysis   A qualitative research technique in which the researcher simultaneously codes and analyzes data in order to develop concepts.

Construct Validity   The extent to which a tool measures what it claims to measure, defines what we wish to measure, and tests behavior in theory.

Content Validity   Regulates the sampling of a construct and raises the question, Does this measure truly sample the behavior that I want to study?

Control   All aspects of the research project *except* the one being studied. This is often referred to as the control of confounding variables.

---

*For a more detailed discussion of these terms, please see the appropriate section of the text and references cited there, as applicable.

Correlation Coefficient   A mathematical measure of the extent to which two or more paired phenomena or events tend to occur together.

Correlation Matrix   A table of all possible correlations among given data sets.

Correlational Research   Answers the generic question, To what extent do two (or more) characteristics tend to occur together by association?

Criterion   The dependent variable.

Criterion Measure   That which quantifies the criterion.

Cross-sectional Study   Collecting data on several cohorts at the same time for a relatively short period of time.

Data   Measurements or records of facts made under specific conditions.

Data Set   A group (2 or more) of recorded observations made on a defined sample of subjects.

Deductive Logic   Application of a general rule to particular instances.

Dependent Variable (DV)   The result or measured outcome of the action of the independent variable. Also called the *criterion.*

Descriptive Research   Answers the generic question, What are the existing characteristics of the real world relative to the specific question?

Developmental Research   Describes a sequence of events over a long period of time.

Dichotomy   Having two mutually exclusive classes.

Double-Blind Study   A study in which neither patient nor researcher knows who gets the treatment and who gets the placebo.

Double Sampling   The retesting of individuals who respond in a certain way on the first sample.

Ethnographic Descriptive Research   Research that tries to render a true-to-life picture of what people say and how they act; people's words and actions are left to speak for themselves.

Experimental Controls   Those mechanisms that regulate or guide every aspect of the experimental situation such that changes in the observed measurement can be attributed only to the uncontrolled or independent variables in the study.

External Validity   Generalization from the sample to the population.

Face Validity   The appearance of a test or measure: does it look like it will test what it is supposed to test?

Facts   Records of events.

Factorial Designs   Research designs in which there are a number of independent variables, and each variable may have two or more levels.

Grounded Theory Research   Qualitative research as a process of building theory that is inductively derived from the study of the phenomenon it represents.

Historical Research   Descriptive research that focuses on past rather than present events.

Hypothetical Construct A verbal symbol for something that cannot be seen. Examples are intelligence and motivation.

Hypothetico-Deductive Research Places an emphasis on quantitative deductions based on data gathered in response to a specific hypothesis.

Hypothesis A possible relationship between concepts; an assumption not proved by experiment or observation. It is assumed for the sake of testing or to facilitate investigation of a class of phenomena—a conclusion drawn before all the facts are established and tentatively accepted as a basis for further investigation.

Independent Variable (IV) The experimental variable being studied. It is often manipulated by the researcher to see what effect that manipulation will have on the dependent variable.

Inductive Logic Logic that draws a general rule from particular instances.

Intensive Case Study Repeated measures on the same individual with deliberate attempts to define the parameters measured in operational terms and to quantify observation at a level that is intellectually defensible.

Internal Validity The relationship between the independent and the dependent variables. A study is internally valid when the differences that are measured in the dependent variable are accounted for by differences in the independent variables.

Interrater Reliability Consistency of measurement between two or more raters.

Interval Scale A form of metric measurement in which both unit of measurement and absolute zero are arbitrary.

Intrarater Reliability Consistency of measurement recorded by one rater.

Logic The science that deals with the criteria for valid inferences. Logic instructs us in the methodology for making inferences based on reason.

Longitudinal Studies Data collected on a cohort for an extended period of time.

Level of Significance The chance of being wrong in accepting or rejecting an hypothesis. The significance level is best regarded as a measure of the conflict between the evidence and the null hypothesis.

Life History Another approach to qualitative research.

Matching Method of sampling in which the researcher imposes his or her own criteria and attempts to force the groups into equivalency along dimensions or characteristics that the researcher believes to be important.

Measurement The process of quantifying people, objects, events, or their characteristics.

Meta-Analysis A step beyond an interpretative review of literature. The reviewer establishes criteria for evaluating the quality or the validity of the studies reviewed.

Metric Scale of Measurement Data that are distributed into independent, mutually exclusive, and exhaustive categories. There is a qualitative relationship (rank order) between categories, and the distance between any two numbers on the scale are of known and equal size, so they may be properly treated with arithmetical procedures. The quantification of data.

Mixed Factorial Design A design in which one factor is not randomized and the other is.

Model A representation of complex phenomena in a simpler way.

Nominal Descriptive Research Studies of one or a few samples, often in form of case studies.

Nominal Scale of Measurement The weakest level of measurement in which the data are placed into broad categories that are mutually exclusive, independent, and exhaustive. It classifies data.

Nonparametric Statistics Statistics that require few assumptions about the data; used with nominal and ordinal data.

Nonprobability Samples Samples taken from a population for which there is no frame, for example, osteoarthritic patients.

Nonrelational Propositions Propositions that state the existence of a relationship, its direction, shape, strength, or symmetry.

Normative Descriptive Research Research that defines the average or typical characteristics of a given sample that may be inferred to the population.

Null Hypothesis Prediction that there will be no statistically significant difference between two or more sets of data. The only form of the question to which a statistical test can be applied.

Operational Definition Phenomena that are concrete, observable, and measurable at some level.

Ordinal Scale of Measurement Data that are not only distributed into independent, mutually exclusive and exhaustive categories, but also into a qualitative relationship between categories; a ranking scale.

Parameter An estimation of the value of some variable in a population.

Parametric Statistics Statistics that require several specific conditions in the data, including a metric scale of measurement.

Population The members of a clearly defined set or class of people, objects, or events that are the focus of an investigation; all the actual data that could potentially be collected on a well-described variable.

Post-Hoc Test Test performed to see where in the data the greatest difference lies. Examples: the Newman-Keuls, Tukey or Scheffe tests.

Postulate States demonstrated relationships between the concepts defined. Also called the *principle, proposition, or generalization.*

Predictive Research Research wherein the generic question is generally one of comparison: Is treatment A different from treatment B?

Predictive Validity Future-oriented statement made on the basis of a measure made today. Predictive validity is also criterion-related; it is related to outside objective criteria or direct measures of performance.

Principle   Expression of a correct relationship between two or more concepts. Also called a rule, a generalization, or, sometimes, a law.

Probability   The long-run proportion of times some event of interest will occur. The science of probability is concerned with allowing you to know how large a risk you are taking in making a deduction from data.

Probability Sampling   Sampling that allows every member of the population to have an equal opportunity to be in the sample.

Qualitative Research   A form of descriptive research that studies people, individually or collectively, in their social and cultural context. Qualitative research has been called holistic-inductive because it is interested in rich verbal descriptions of people and phenomena based on direct observation.

Quasi-Experimental Design   A design in which some of the essential controls are missing but which still has some resemblance to, and possesses some of the attributes of, true experimental design.

Quota Sampling   Wherein the researcher specifies that the sample of convenience will contain certain quotas or proportions.

Random Error   Sampling error due to chance.

Randomization   The process of assigning to groups so that each individual object or event has an equal chance of being assigned to each group.

Ranking Scale   See *ordinal scale.*

Ratio Scale   A form of metric measurement in which only the unit of measurement is arbitrary. There is an absolute zero.

Regression   The establishment of a mathematical relationship between two or more variables that best describes the total group.

Relational Postulates   Concurrent or sequential relationships, deterministic or probabilistic relationships, sufficient or contingent relationships.

Relational Propositions   Propositions that state the existence of a relationship, its direction, shape, strength, symmetry.

Reliability   Stability, repeatability, dependability.

Reliability of Parallel Forms   Obtaining the same results from two versions of the same test.

Replicability   Other people can repeat the experiment using the same controls and measurements and come out with the same results that the first researcher obtained.

Research   Goal-directed process of looking for a specific answer to a specific question in an organized, objective, reliable way; the discovery and validation of the concepts and principles on which practice is based.

Research Design   Those concepts and techniques that make research organized, objective, and reliable.

Research Hypothesis   See *alternate hypothesis.*

Retrospective Descriptive Research   A data set gathered from already existing records or data.

Review of Literature   The process whereby experts in a given field have read, understood, integrated, and summarized for the busy reader a significant body of literature.

Sample   All the observations of a variable actually measured, or all those subjects selected from a population for study. Usually a sample is a subset of a population, but occasionally sample and population are identical.

Sample of Convenience   Sampling from limited but available resources.

Sampling Error   The error of measurements on different individuals, i.e., group data. Sampling errors may be of two kinds: random and systematic.

Sequential Clinical Trials Design   A research design for two data sets in which the statistical test is incorporated into a graph on which decisions about pairs of data are recorded.

Single-Blind Study   A study in which the patients do not know whether they are getting treatment or placebo.

Single-Subject Designs   Predictive research designs intended to study one (or a very few) individuals.

Standard Deviation   The square root of the variance of a data set.

Standard Error of Estimate   A statistic describing the extent of error in predicting a score on one variable or characteristic based on the score from another variable or characteristic. Also called the *standard error of prediction.*

Standardized Measure   A measure in which the procedure has been described in detail in a protocol, allowing others to follow the same protocol.

Statistic   A numerical statement about observations actually made on a sample.

Stratified Random Sampling   Sampling from predefined subclasses.

Survey Research   Research that exposes the sample to a predetermined set of questions, the answers to which can be quantified with descriptive statistics.

Systematic Error   Sampling error caused by bias, either conscious or unconscious.

Systematic Sampling   Sampling by using a table of random numbers in a systematic way.

Taxonomy   Classification of any set of related phenomena.

Tests of Homogeneity   Tests that demonstrate that two or more groups are equal on some variable.

Theory   A set of interrelated principles (in this context often called postulates or propositions) that are based on solid evidence. A theory
organizes what is known about the subject of the theory and it acts
as a stimulus to research; its purpose is to explain, predict, and control
behavior.

Type 1 Error   The chance of rejecting a null hypothesis and saying that
indeed there is a difference when in fact there is not. In other words,
we run the risk of backing a loser. The risk of committing a type 1
error is symbolized by the Greek letter alpha (α).

Type 2 Error   The chance of not rejecting a null hypothesis and saying
that there is no difference when in fact there is. We run the risk of
missing a winner. The risk of a type 2 error is symbolized by the Greek
letter beta (β).

Univariate Analysis   Examinination of one variable at a time.

Validity   Appropriateness, truthfulness, authenticity, effectiveness.

Variable   An observable and measurable characteristic or event that can
assume a range of values on some dimension.

Variance   A measure of variability, of real differences in a characteristic
in a sample or population.

Summary of Statistical Concepts[*]

Autocorrelation   The possibility that two data points on a graph may not be independent of each other. Also called *serial dependency.*

Central Tendency   A measure of the average or most representative score in a distribution.

Chi-square   A nonparametric predictive statistical test of the similarity between two sets of data measured at the nominal level.

$$\chi^2 = \frac{(O - E)^2}{E}$$

Cochran Q Test   A nonparametric predictive statistical test of the similarity between three sets of data measured at the nominal level.

Coefficient of Determination   The square of the correlation coefficient; also expressed as r^2.

Correlation Coefficient   A mathematical measure of the extent to which two or more paired phenomena or events tend to occur together.

"An index of the degree of association between two variables or the extent to which the order of individuals on one variable is similar to the order of individuals on a second variable."

"The ratio of the amount of information that two variables measure jointly, compared with the average amount of information measured individually by each of the two variables."

"The correlation coefficient provides a quantitative description of how well the regression line fits the actual data."

Correlation Matrix   A table of all possible correlations among given data sets.

Cronbach's Coefficient Alpha   A correlation coefficient for dichotomous or discrete data.

F Test (ANOVA)   A parametric predictive statistical test of the similarity between three or more sets of data measured at the metric level.

Friedman Test   A nonparametric predictive statistical test of the similarity between three sets of data measured at the ordinal level.

---

[*]For more detailed discussion of these concepts, please see text and the references cited there, as applicable.

Intraclass Correlation (ICC)   A measure of agreement (not just association) for metric data.

$$ICC = \frac{BMS - WMS}{BMS + (k-1)WMS}$$

Kappa   A correlation coefficient for two or more nominal classifications. Its basic formula is

$$\kappa = \frac{p_o - p_c}{1 - p_c}$$

where p_o = proportion of observed agreements and p_c = proportion of agreements expected due to chance.

Kendall's Coefficient of Concordance   A correlation coefficient for three or more sets of ranked (ordinal) data; also expressed as w.

Kendall's Tau   A correlation coefficient for small samples of ordinal data.

Kruskal-Wallis Test   A nonparametric predictive statistical test of the similarity between three sets of data measured at the ordinal level.

McNemar Test   A nonparametric predictive statistical test of the similarity between two sets of data measured at the nominal level.

Mann-Whitney U Test   A nonparametric predictive statistical test of the similarity between two sets of data measured at the ordinal level.

Mean   An arithmetic measure of central tendency for metric data; the set of scores is summed and divided by n.

Median   A statistic of central tendency of a set of ordinal data. It is the middle of the range of recorded measurements, listed in order.

Median Test   A nonparametric predictive statistical test of the similarity between two sets of data measured at the ordinal level.

Mode   A measure of central tendency for nominal data; the score(s) that appear(s) most often.

n The number of observations in the sample.

N The number of observations possible in the population.

Parameter   An estimate, based on a sample, of the value of some variable in a population.

Pearson Product Moment Correlation   A correlation coefficient that is appropriate for metric variables that are continuous. The *conceptual model* for the Pearson Product Moment Correlation coefficient is

$$r_{xy} = \frac{(x - \bar{x})(y - \bar{y})}{ns_x s_y}$$

Another more useful formula is

$$r_{xy} = \frac{n\Sigma xy - \Sigma x \Sigma y}{[n\Sigma x^2 - (\Sigma x)^2][n\Sigma y^2 - (\Sigma y)^2]}$$

Phi Coefficient   A correlation coefficient for ordinal data.

Power of a Statistical Test   The probability of reaching a correct decision and rejecting the null when it should be rejected, symbolized as $1 - \beta$. Correctly accepting the null is symbolized as $1 - \alpha$.

Probability   Chance of occurrence. The most basic formula for probability is

$$\frac{\text{Number of observations of an event}}{\text{Number of observations}}$$

Range   The extremes of a data set.

Regression   A mathematical relationship between two or more variables that best describes the total group. Metric data are required. The general formula for a (straight) regression line is

$$y = a + bx$$

where a is the point where the line intercepts the y axis, and b is the slope of the line.

Sign Test   A nonparametric predictive statistical test of the similarity between two sets of data measured at the ordinal level.

Spearman Rank Order Correlation   A correlation coefficient that is appropriate for two variables measured at the ordinal level.

$$\rho = \frac{1 - 6\Sigma d^2}{n(n^2 - 1)}$$

Standard Deviation   A measure of variability in a data set; it is the square root of the variance.

Statistic   A numerical statement computed from actual observations made on a sample.

t-test   A parametric predictive statistical test between two means.

$$t = \frac{x_1 - x_2}{\sqrt{\dfrac{n_1 s^2_1 + n_2 s^2_2}{n_1 + n_2 - 2}} \sqrt{\dfrac{n_1 + n_2}{n_1 n_2}}}$$

Variance   A numerical measure of the variability in real differences of a characteristic in a sample or population. The formula for variance is

$$\frac{(x - \bar{x})^2}{n - 1}$$

Wilcoxon Signed-Rank Test   A nonparametric predictive statistical test of the similarity between two sets of data measured at the ordinal level.

Yule's q   A correlation coefficient for two nominal scale measures.

Index

A "t" following a page number indicates a table; an "f" indicates a figure.